# Current Topics in Pathology
# 93

Springer-Verlag Berlin Heidelberg GmbH

A. Desmoulière · B. Tuchweber (Eds.)

# Tissue Repair and Fibrosis

## The Role of the Myofibroblast

Contributors

P.D. Arora, F.A. Auger, M. Aumailley, C.B. Ballas, G. Bellon,
S.I. Benn, F. Berthod, C. Betsholtz, H. Boström, G. Castilloux,
J.J. Cho, J.F. Cordier, A.M.A. Costa, J.M. Davidson, A. Desmoulière,
D. Dogic, B. Eckes, M. El Nahas, S. Eming, H. Emonard, S. Faouzi,
J.M. Foidart, G. Gabbiani, B. Ganss, D. Garrel, J. Gauldie, L. Germain,
M. Gharaee-Kermani, P. Gillery, M. Golgauer, A.I. Gotlieb, F. Goulet,
D. Goumenos, F. Grinnell, J. Guirouilh, E.G. Hahn, M. Hellström,
W. Hornebeck, J.D. Jia, M. Kalén, L. Karlsson, F. Kebers, T.Y.J. Lee,
A. Lew, Z. Li, P. Lindahl, R.B. Low, L. Luo, F.X. Maquart, E. Maquoi,
B. Marr, C.A.G. McCulloch, M. Mericskay, J.C. Monboisse,
F. Monier, A. Monvoisin, V. Moulin, E.C. Muchaneta-Kubara, N. Narani,
V. Neaud, A. Noel, M. O'Connor-McCourt, D. Paulin, B. Pennington,
S.H. Phan, J. Rosenbaum, D. Schuppan, W. Schürch, P.J. Sime,
A. Siméon, N. Tamimi, G.M. Tremblay, B. Tuchweber, Y. Wegrowski,
J.S. Whitsitt, Z. Xing, I.M. Yousef, H.Y. Zhang, K. Zhang

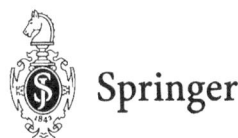

Springer

Dr. ALEXIS DESMOULIÈRE
GREF
Université Victor Segalen Bordeaux 2
146, Rue Léo-Saignat
33076 Bordeaux Cedex, France

Professor BEATRIZ TUCHWEBER
Départment de Nutrition
Université de Montréal
Pavillon Liliane-de-Stewart
C. P. 6128, Succursale Centre-Ville
Montréal, Québec H3C 3J7
Canada

With 53 Figures and 18 Tables

ISBN 978-3-540-65244-1

CIP data applied for
Die Deutsche Bibliothek – CIP-Einheitsaufnahme

**Tissue repair and fibrosis** : the role of the myofibroblast / ed.: Alexis
Desmoulière ; Beatriz Tuchweber. – Berlin ; Heidelberg ; New York ; Barcelona ;
Hongkong ; London ; Mailand ; Paris ; Singapur ; Tokio : Springer, 1999
(Current topics in pathology ; Vol. 93)
ISBN 978-3-540-65244-1     ISBN 978-3-642-58456-5 (eBook)

DOI 10.1007/978-3-642-58456-5

Production: PRO EDIT GmbH, Heidelberg
Cover design: Design & Production GmbH, Heidelberg
Typesetting: Fotosatz-Service Köhler GmbH, Würzburg
Computer to film: Konrad Triltsch, Druck- und Verlagsanstalt GmbH, Würzburg

SPIN  10689872        81/3135 – 5 4 3 2 1 0 – Printed on acid-free paper

# Contributors

P. D. ARORA

MRC Group in Periodontal Physiology,
Faculty of Dentistry, Room 4384,
Medical Sciences Building,
University of Toronto,
8 Taddle Creek Road,
Toronto, Ontario,
M5G 1G6, Canada

F. A. AUGER

Laboratoire d'Organogénèse
Expérimentale/LOEX,
Hôpital du Saint-Sacrement, 1050,
Chemin Sainte-Foy,
Québec,
G1S 4L8, Canada

M. AUMAILLEY

Institut für Biochemie II,
Joseph-Stelzmann-Str. 52,
50931 Köln, Germany

C. B. BALLAS

Department of Pathology, C-3321 MCN,
Vanderbilt University School of Medicine,
Nashville, TN 37232–2561, USA

G. BELLON

Laboratory of Biochemistry – UPRESA,
CNRS 6021, Faculty of Medicine,
IFR 53-Biomolécules, 51 Rue Cognacq-Jay,
51095 Reims Cedex, France

S. I. BENN

Department of Pathology, C-3321 MCN,
Vanderbilt University School of Medicine,
Nashville, TN 37232–2561, USA

F. BERTHOD

Laboratoire d'Organogénèse
Expérimentale/LOEX,
Hôpital du Saint-Sacrement, 1050,
Chemin Sainte-Foy,
Québec, G1S 4L8, Canada

C. Betsholtz

Department of Medical Biochemistry,
University of Göteborg,
Medicinaregatan 9A, Box 440,
405 30 Göteborg, Sweden

H. Boström

Department of Medical Biochemistry,
University of Göteborg,
Medicinaregatan 9A, Box 440,
405 30 Göteborg, Sweden

G. Castilloux

Laboratoire de Recherche des Grands
Brûlés/LOEX and Département
de Chirurgie, Université Laval,
Hôpital du Saint-Sacrement,
1050 Chemin Sainte-Foy,
Québec, G1S 4L8, Canada

J. J. Cho

Department of Gastroenterology
and Hepatology,
Klinikum Benjamin Franklin,
Free University of Berlin,
Berlin, Germany

J. F. Cordier

Department of Respiratory Medicine,
Hôpital Louis Pradel,
69394 Lyon Cedex 03, France

A. M. A. Costa

Departamento de Histologia
e Embriologia, Universidade do Estado
do Rio de Janeiro, Rio de Janeiro, Brazil

J. M. Davidson

Department of Pathology, C-3321A MCN,
Vanderbilt University School of Medicine,
Nashville, TN 37232–2561, USA

A. Desmoulière

GREF, Université Victor Segalen
Bordeaux 2, 146, Rue Léo-Saignat,
33076 Bordeaux Cedex, France

D. Dogic

Institut de Biologie et Chimie des
Protéines, CNRS-UPR 412,
7 Passage du Vercors, 69367 Lyon, France

B. Eckes

Department of Dermatology,
Medical Faculty, Köln, Germany

M. El Nahas

Sheffield Kidney Institute,
Northern General Hospital,
Herries Road,
Sheffield S5 7AU,
United Kingdom

S. EMING            Department of Pathology, C-3321 MCN,
                    Vanderbilt University School of Medicine,
                    Nashville, TN 37232–2561, USA

H. EMONARD          Laboratory of Biochemistry – UPRESA,
                    CNRS 6021, Faculty of Medicine,
                    IFR 53-Biomolécules, 51 Rue Cognacq-Jay,
                    F-51095 Reims Cedex, France

S. FAOUZI           Groupe de Recherches pour l'Etude
                    du Foie, Université Victor Segalen
                    Bordeaux 2, 33076 Bordeaux, France

J. M. FOIDART       Laboratory of Tumor and Developmental
                    Biology, University of Liège,
                    Sart-Tilman 4000 Liège, Belgium

G. GABBIANI         Department of Pathology,
                    University of Geneva-CMU,
                    1 Rue Michel-Servet, 1211 Geneva 4,
                    Switzerland

B. GANSS            MRC Group In Periodontal Physiology,
                    Faculty of Dentistry, Room 4384,
                    Medical Sciences Building, University
                    of Toronto, 8 Taddle Creek Road,
                    Toronto, Ontario, M5G 1G6, Canada

D. GARREL           Centre des Grands Brûlés,
                    Hôtel-Dieu de Montréal, Montréal, Canada

J. GAULDIE          Department of Pathology 2N16,
                    McMaster University,
                    1200 Main Street West,
                    Hamilton, Ontario, L8N 3Z5, Canada

L. GERMAIN          Laboratoire de Recherche des Grands
                    Brûlés/LOEX and Département
                    de Chirurgie, Université Laval,
                    Hôpital du Saint-Sacrement,
                    1050 Chemin Sainte-Foy,
                    Québec, G1S 4L8, Canada

M. GHARAEE-KERMANI  Department of Pathology, University
                    of Michigan Medical School,
                    Ann Arbor, MI 48109–0602, USA

P. GILLERY          Laboratory of Biochemistry – UPRESA,
                    CNRS 6021, Faculty of Medicine,
                    IFR 53-Biomolécules, 51 Rue Cognacq-Jay,
                    51095 Reims Cedex, France

M. Glogauer                MRC Group in Periodontal Physiology,
                           Faculty of Dentistry, Room 4384,
                           Medical Sciences Building,
                           University of Toronto,
                           8 Taddle Creek Road,
                           Toronto, Ontario, M5G 1G6, Canada

A. I. Gotlieb               Department of Laboratory Medicine
                           and Pathobiology, The Toronto Hospital
                           Research Institute, 200 Elizabeth Street,
                           CCRW 1-857, Toronto, Ontario,
                           M5G 2C4, Canada

F. Goulet                  Laboratoire d'Organogénèse
                           Expérimentale/LOEX,
                           Hôpital du Saint-Sacrement, 1050,
                           Chemin Sainte-Foy,
                           Québec, G1S 4L8, Canada

D. Goumenos                Sheffield Kidney Institute,
                           Northern General Hospital,
                           Herries Road, Sheffield S5 7AU,
                           United Kingdom

F. Grinnell                Department of Cell Biology and
                           Neuroscience, University of Texas
                           Southwestern Medical Center,
                           Dallas, TX 75235–9039, USA

J. Guirouilh               Groupe de Recherches pour l'Etude
                           du Foie, Université Victor Segalen,
                           Bordeaux 2, France

E. G. Hahn                 Department of Medicine I,
                           University of Erlangen-Nürnberg,
                           Krankenhausstr. 12D, 91054 Erlangen,
                           Germany

M. Hellström               Department of Medical Biochemistry,
                           University of Göteborg,
                           Medicinaregatan 9A, Box 440,
                           405 30 Göteborg, Sweden

W. Hornebeck               Laboratory of Biochemistry – UPRESA,
                           CNRS 6021, Faculty of Medicine,
                           IFR 53-Biomolécules,
                           51 Rue Cognacq-Jay,
                           51095 Reims Cedex, France

J. D. JIA                        Department of Gastroenterology
                                 and Hepatology
                                 Klinikum Benjamin Franklin,
                                 Free University of Berlin,
                                 Berlin, Germany

M. KALÉN                         Department of Medical Biochemistry,
                                 University of Göteborg,
                                 Medicinaregatan 9A, Box 440,
                                 405 30 Göteborg, Sweden

L. KARLSSON                      Department of Medical Biochemistry,
                                 University of Göteborg,
                                 Medicinaregatan 9A, Box 440,
                                 405 30 Göteborg, Sweden

F. KEBERS                        Laboratory of Tumor and Developmental
                                 Biology, University of Liège,
                                 Sart-Tilman, 4000 Liège, Belgium

T. Y. J. LEE                     Department of Laboratory Medicine and
                                 Pathobiology, The Toronto Hospital
                                 Research Institute, 200 Elizabeth Street,
                                 CCRW 1–857, Toronto, Ontario,
                                 M5G 2C4, Canada

A. LEW                           MRC Group in Periodontal Physiology,
                                 Faculty of Dentistry, Room 4384,
                                 Medical Sciences Building,
                                 University of Toronto,
                                 8 Taddle Creek Road, Toronto,
                                 Ontario, M5G 1G6, Canada

Z. LI                            Biologie Moléculaire de la Différenciation,
                                 Institut Pasteur – Université Paris 7,
                                 Case 7136, 2 Place Jussieu,
                                 75251 Paris Cedex 05, France

P. LINDAHL                       Department of Medical Biochemistry,
                                 University of Göteborg,
                                 Medicinaregatan 9A, Box 440,
                                 405 30 Göteborg, Sweden

R. B. LOW                        Department of Molecular Physiology
                                 and Biophysics, Given E-217,
                                 University of Vermont,
                                 Burlington, VT 05405, USA

L. Luo                          MRC Group in Periodontal Physiology,
                                Faculty of Dentistry, Room 4384,
                                Medical Sciences Building, University of
                                Toronto, 8 Taddle Creek Road, Toronto,
                                Ontario, M5G 1G6, Canada

F. X. Maquart                   Laboratory of Biochemistry – UPRESA,
                                CNRS 6021, Faculty of Medicine,
                                IFR 53-Biomolécules, 51 Rue Cognacq-Jay,
                                51095 Reims Cedex, France

E. Maquoi                       Laboratory of Tumor and Developmental
                                Biology, University of Liège,
                                Sart-Tilman, 4000 Liège, Belgium

B. Marr                         Department of Pathology,
                                McMaster University,
                                1200 Main Street West,
                                Hamilton, Ontario, L8N 3Z5, Canada

C. A. G. McCulloch              MRC Group In Periodontal Physiology,
                                Faculty of Dentistry, Room 4384,
                                Medical Sciences Building,
                                University of Toronto,
                                8 Taddle Creek Road, Toronto, Ontario,
                                M5G 1G6, Canada

M. Mericskay                    Biologie Moléculaire de la Différenciation,
                                Institut Pasteur – Université Paris 7,
                                Case 7136, 2 Place Jussieu,
                                75251 Paris Cedex 05, France

J. C. Monboisse                 Laboratory of Biochemistry – UPRESA,
                                CNRS 6021, Faculty of Medicine,
                                IFR 53-Biomolécules, 51 Rue Cognacq-Jay,
                                51095 Reims Cedex, France

F. Monier                       Laboratory of Biochemistry – UPRESA,
                                CNRS 6021, Faculty of Medicine,
                                IFR 53-Biomolécules, 51 Rue Cognacq-Jay,
                                51095 Reims Cedex, France

A. Monvoisin                    Groupe de Recherches pour l'Etude
                                du Foie, Université Victor Segalen
                                Bordeaux 2, 33076 Bordeaux, France

V. Moulin                       Laboratoire de Recherche des Grands
                                Brûlés/LOEX and Département
                                de Chirurgie, Université Laval,
                                Hôpital du Saint-Sacrement,
                                1050 Chemin Sainte-Foy,
                                Québec, G1S 4L8, Canada

E. C. Muchaneta-Kubara    Sheffield Kidney Institute,
                          Northern General Hospital,
                          Herries Road, Sheffield S5 7AU,
                          United Kingdom

N. Narani                 MRC Group In Periodontal Physiology,
                          Faculty of Dentistry, Room 4384,
                          Medical Sciences Building,
                          University of Toronto,
                          8 Taddle Creek Road, Toronto, Ontario,
                          M5G 1G6, Canada

V. Neaud                  Groupe de Recherches pour l'Etude du
                          Foie, Université Victor Segalen,
                          146, Rue Léo Saignat, 33076 Bordeaux,
                          France

A. Noel                   Laboratory of Tumor and Developmental
                          Biology, University of Liège,
                          Sart-Tilman, 4000 Liège, Belgium

M. O'Connor-McCourt       Biotechnology Research Institute,
                          Montréal, Québec, Canada

D. Paulin                 Biologie Moléculaire de la Différenciation,
                          Institut Pasteur – Université Paris 7,
                          Case 7136, 2 Place Jussieu,
                          75251 Paris Cedex 05, France

B. Pennington             Department of Pathology,
                          C-3321 MCN, Vanderbilt University
                          School of Medicine, Nashville,
                          TN 37232 – 2561, USA

S. H. Phan                Department of Pathology,
                          University of Michigan Medical School,
                          Ann Arbor, MI 48109 – 0602, USA

J. Rosenbaum              Groupe de Recherches pour l'Etude du
                          Foie, Université Victor Segalen
                          Bordeaux 2, 146, Rue Léo-Saignat,
                          33076 Bordeaux Cedex, France

D. Schuppan               Department of Medicine I,
                          University of Erlangen-Nürnberg,
                          Krankenhausstr. 12, 91054 Erlangen,
                          Germany

W. Schürch                    Département de Pathologie,
                              Centre Hospitalier de l'Université de
                              Montréal, Hôtel-Dieu,
                              3840, Rue St-Urbain, Montréal, Québec,
                              H2W 1T8, Canada,

P. J. Sime                    Department of Pathology, McMaster
                              University, 1200 Main Street West,
                              Hamilton, Ontario, L8N 3Z5, Canada

A. Siméon                     Laboratory of Biochemistry – UPRESA,
                              CNRS 6021, Faculty of Medicine,
                              IFR 53-Biomolécules, 51 Rue Cognacq-Jay,
                              51095 Reims Cedex, France

N. Tamimi                     Sheffield Kidney Institute,
                              Northern General Hospital,
                              Herries Road,
                              Sheffield S5 7AU,
                              United Kingdom

G. M. Tremblay                Department of Pathology,
                              McMaster University,
                              1200 Main Street West,
                              Hamilton, Ontario, L8N 3Z5, Canada

B. Tuchweber                  Département de Nutrition, Université de
                              Montréal, C.P. 6128, Succ. Centre-Ville,
                              Montréal, Québec, H3C 3J7, Canada,

Y. Wegrowski                  Laboratory of Biochemistry – UPRESA,
                              CNRS 6021, Faculty of Medicine,
                              IFR 53-Biomolécules, 51 Rue Cognacq-Jay,
                              51095 Reims Cedex, France

J. S. Whitsitt                Department of Pathology, C-3321 MCN,
                              Vanderbilt University School of Medicine,
                              Nashville, TN 37232 – 2561, USA

Z. Xing                       Department of Pathology,
                              McMaster University,
                              1200 Main Street West,
                              Hamilton, Ontario, L8N 3Z5, Canada

I. M. Yousef                  Département de Pharmacologie,
                              Université de Montréal, Montréal,
                              Québec, H3C 3J7, Canada

H. Y. ZHANG          Department of Pathology,
                     University of Michigan Medical School,
                     Ann Arbor, MI 48109 – 0602, USA

K. ZHANG             Department of Pathology,
                     University of Michigan Medical School,
                     Ann Arbor, MI 48109 – 0602, USA

# Preface

This volume contains the papers presented at the meeting on "Mechanisms involved in tissue repair and fibrosis: role of the myofibroblast (differentiation and apoptosis)," which took place in Lyon, December 1997, on the occasion of the tenth "Entretiens du Centre Jacques Cartier."

During the three-days meeting, about 25 conferences reviewed the knowledge accumulated on the myofibroblast, a cell first described in 1971 by Gabbiani et al. in *Experientia*. From the content of the book, it is evident that the topic has been discussed by specialists from diverse disciplines and that the myofibroblast is implicated in many diverse disease processes.

Myofibroblastic differentiation appears temporarily during cutaneous repair when the damage is moderate. However, in some organs, after injury, specialized cells cannot regenerate and myofibroblasts appear permanently, becoming involved in the excessive deposition of extracellular matrix components. Thus, myofibroblasts play an important role in restitutive repair, after which they disappear by apoptosis, and in pathological repair, where they expand and participate in the development of the fibrotic lesion. Furthermore, myofibroblasts are the main components of the stromal reaction developing around tumors.

During the first day of the meeting, the molecular and cellular biology of the myofibroblast was reviewed. Of major interest was the role played by myofibroblasts in contraction. Indeed, myofibroblasts show smooth muscle differentiation and express $\alpha$-smooth muscle actin, the actin isoform typical of contractile vascular smooth muscle cells.

The second day of the meeting was devoted to the in vitro and in vivo models available for the study of the myofibroblast. In culture conditions and upon serum-induced stimulation, normal fibroblasts acquire myofibroblastic features; cytokines, growth factors and extracellular matrix components modulate this phenotypic differentiation. In vivo, it has become evident that different fibroblastic subpopulations can undergo myofibroblastic differentiation and participate in development of fibrosis in various organs.

Finally, the last day of the meeting was focused on the involvement of the myofibroblast in diverse disease processes. The role of the stromal reaction to tumors was debated. For example, one question was whether the stromal reaction is an attempt by the organism to encapsulate the tumor or a reaction to facilitate the development of the lesion.

The possibility of the myofibroblast as a neoplastic cell was also raised. In addition, not only the mechanisms involved in the development of the fibrotic lesion were discussed but also the possibility of reversibility. A round table discussion highlighted the conclusion of the symposium and pointed to the need to better define this cell and develop better markers of differentiation.

In conclusion, it is encouraging and exciting to see the diversity and extent of interests that were brought to this area of cell biology. In this rapidly developing field, research of the myofibroblast will lead to a better understanding and treatment of many different pathological processes.

Lyon/Montréal                                        ALEXIS DESMOULIÈRE
Spring 1999                                           BEATRIZ TUCHWEBER

# Contents

# Some Historical and Philosophical Reflections on the Myofibroblast Concept

G. Gabbiani

## 1 Development of the Myofibroblast Concept

The phenomena of wound contraction and scar retraction have been known since the old ages (for review see [29]). In the first part of our century, the work of A. Carrel and P. Lecomte du Noüy contributed to the notion that the forces producing wound contraction are generated within the granulation tissue itself [5]. These forces were generally considered to depend on extracellular-matrix re-arrangements; however, M. Abercrombie and coworkers reported in the 1950s that fibroblasts exert tractional forces in vitro [1]. Similarly, H. Hoffmann-Beerling showed that the addition of adenosine triphosphate (ATP) to permeabilized fibro-blasts in culture produces the contraction of their cytoplasm [22]. In this context, and in the context of emerging work on cytoskeleton morphology and function [4], the ultrastructural observation made in our laboratory in 1971 showed that during granulation tissue evolution, fibroblasts acquire smooth-muscle (SM) cell features, such as the presence of cytoplasmic microfilament bundles [17], allowing the pro-position that these cells are the source of the force producing wound contraction, and probably connective-tissue retraction during a fibrotic phenomena. Shortly there-after, it was shown that strips of granulation tissue isolated and placed in a pharma-cological bath would contract and relax under the influence of substances that are notoriously capable of contracting and relaxing SM cells [18, 28]. It is noteworthy (particularly because this observation has never been developed) that granulation tissues from different locations respond differently to the same agonist or antagonist stimulus, suggesting that the capacity of reacting with contraction to a given stimulus by fibroblastic cells depends on their location [18]. The term myofibroblast was suggested for this modified and possibly contractile fibroblast [28].

During the next few years, several laboratories reported, by means of ultra-structural techniques, the presence of myofibroblasts in several lesions charac-terized by fibrosis and retraction, such as fibromatoses [19], liver cirrhosis [30], pulmonary [2] and renal [23] fibrosis. The presence of myofibroblasts was also shown in normal tissues in a location in which a certain degree of tension was needed for function, such as the theca externa of the ovary [9], the alveolar septum [24] and the intestinal pericriptal cells [32]. Hence, the concept was developed that

Current Topics in Pathology, Volume 93
A. Desmoulière, B. Tuchweber (Eds.)
© Springer-Verlag Berlin Heidelberg 1999

in both normal and pathological situations, myofibroblasts develop in response to traction stimuli and may exert a force producing tissue resistance and, particularly in pathological cases, tissue deformation (for review see [11]).

Because of the emerging concept that non-muscle cells contain contractile proteins, which up to that time had been considered typical of muscle cells, and because of the description of other cytoskeletal structures, such as microtubules and intermediate filaments, an important effort was placed by our laboratory and a few other laboratories in the characterization of contractile and cytoskeletal elements present in myofibroblasts (for review see [33]). It was shown that myofibroblasts contain higher amounts of polymerized actin compared with normal fibroblasts in vivo [27]. It was also shown that normal tissues containing myofibroblasts, such as the lung alveolus, would produce contraction upon the stimulus of agents contracting SM cells [15]. A significant advance was allowed by the production of an antibody against $\alpha$-SM actin [38], one of the six actin isoforms present in mammalian tissues and considered typical of vascular SM cells [21]. The use of this antibody showed that $\alpha$-SM actin is expressed temporarily in granulation tissue of an experimental wound and disappears when the scar develops [10]. Thus, an actin isoform typical of SM cells is expressed during wound healing in granulation-tissue fibroblasts; this expression coincides with the phenomenon of wound contraction. Studies by several laboratories demonstrated the presence of $\alpha$-SM actin in myofibroblastic cells present in fibrotic tissues of different organs, such as the liver [16, 34], the lung [25], the kidney [13], the heart [3, 39] and the breast [26, 31, 36]; moreover, $\alpha$-SM actin was suggested as the most significant marker of myofibroblastic cells, at least in pathological settings [33].

Further work demonstrated that myofibroblasts, according to the pathological situation, may express other markers of SM cells, such as SM myosin heavy chains and desmin, the intermediate filament protein characteristic of muscle cells [11, 33]. Other muscular proteins described in myofibroblasts were caldesmon, SM22 and tropomyosin [26]. $\alpha$-SM actin is the SM-cell marker generally present in myofibroblasts of normally healing granulation tissue; other markers appear in more permanent fibrotic situations, such as liver cirrhosis, and become importantly expressed in the stroma reaction to epithelial tumors, e.g., breast cancer [8, 26, 31, 35]. Thus, it is possible to conclude that, during the evolution of fibrosis, fibroblasts acquire SM cell features; these appear temporarily in normal wound healing and more permanently in irreversible fibrotic situations. The presence of myofibroblasts was shown to coincide with collagen type-III expression in Dupuytren's nodules [20]; this collagen isoform is known to be present in remodeling connective tissue. In addition to these early biochemical observations, more precise in situ hybridization studies showed that myofibroblasts, characterized by the expression of $\alpha$-SM actin, were the cells responsible for collagen type-I messenger RNA (mRNA) production in pulmonary fibrosis [40].

Studies aimed at the elucidation of the mechanisms regulating the transition between granulation tissue and scar formation demonstrated that apoptosis is the mechanism through which myofibroblasts disappear during this transition [12]. This observation clarified an important aspect of wound healing and suggested that hypertrophic scar formation may be the consequence of a lack of myofibroblast apoptosis at the appropriate time of healing.

The role of myofibroblasts in wound contraction was confirmed by work show-ing that during fetal wound healing, when regeneration phenomena rather than scarring predominate, there is no appearance of myofibroblasts [14].

## 2 How Is a Discovery Made?

In the following few paragraphs I would like to summarize some considerations I have put together about the mechanisms of emergence of a discovery.

I fully agree with H. SELYE's statement that it is not to see something first, but to establish solid connections between the previously known and the hitherto un-known that constitutes the essence of scientific discovery [37]. When this is achiev-ed and a new concept develops, one can speak of a cultural mutation [7].

Generally, a discovery derives from one or a series of observations, which in experimental sciences are the products of carefully planned experiments. However, it is well accepted that logic, in Latin "ratio", is not the main reason for the actual process of discovery, just as it is not the main reason for the process of artistic creation. The process of discovery has been described as a sort of "illumination", as it appears to take place suddenly and sometimes even unexpectedly, although the future discoverer is generally driven by an intense and sometimes obsessive interest for the problem he or she studies.

My purpose is to suggest the essential role of imagination in the process of making a discovery. Imagination was initially discussed and defined by Aristotle as "phantasia", then considered, albeit not very extensively, by several philosophers and, in the second half of our century, rediscovered and highlighted, also on the basis of psychoanalytical studies, by CORNELIUS CASTORIADIS [6].

CASTORIADIS defined imagination as the capacity of creating representations, whether or not proceeding from perceptions due to external stimuli. In this way, the brain integrates sensorial perceptions derived from the external environment in order to allow the emergence and the representation of sounds, colors, odors, etc. Moreover, and probably more importantly, imagination allows the emergence of the same representations without any external stimulus, such as in the process of artistic creation. This integrative activity is compatible on the one hand with the fact that the same external phenomena are perceived and represented in a compar-able way by different individuals, thus making communication possible, and on the other hand with the notion that perception is very personal, accounting for highly varying interpretations of the same phenomenon. According to CASTORIADIS, the difference between animal and human imagination is that animal imagination is bound to functional goals, while human imagination is absolutely free and creates forms and contents that are not bound to any physiological need. Obviously, how-ever, the imaginative activity elicited by a given perception depends strictly on the actual status of the recipient's mind.

It is well accepted that a discovery allows the development of a representation or of a concept, which then becomes obvious (although slowly) to other individuals and eventually to everybody. I suggest that the discoverer uses imagination in order to find a new solution, a new interpretation or a new theoretical approach; then, using possibly logic or "ratio", the discoverer first realizes by himself and then shows to other individuals that the imagined solution explains the reality better than the previous concept, up to the point that the new approach or solution becomes gradually accepted by the scientific community. With this interpretation, the process of discovery and the process of artistic creation would share common physiological mechanisms.

The logical or rational consequence of the present suggestion about the role of imagination is that efforts should be placed on the understanding of the biological mechanisms involved in the interpretation of perception and in the functioning of imagination. This will allow a better understanding, not only of the production of representations, but also of the production of new concepts and correlations.

## References

1. Abercrombie M, Flint MH, James DW (1956) Wound contraction in relation to collagen formation is scorbutic guinea pigs. J Embryol Exp Morphol 4:167–175
2. Adler KB, Low RB, Leslie KO, Mitchell J, Evans JN (1989) Biology of disease. Contractile cells in normal and fibrotic lung. Lab Invest 60:473–485
3. Blankesteijn WM, Essers-Janssen YPG, Verluyten MJA, Daemen MJA, Smits JFM (1997) A homologue of Drosophila tisse polarity gene frizzled is expressed in migrating myofibroblasts in the infarcted rat heart. Nat Med 3:541–544
4. Bray D (1973) Cytoplasmic actin: a comparative study. In: Gordon J (ed) Cold Spring Harbor symposia on quantitative biology: the mechanisms of muscle contraction, vol 37. Cold Spring Harbor Laboratory Press, Cold Spring Harbor, pp 567–571
5. Carrel A, Hartmann A (1916) Cicatrization of wounds. I. The relation between the size and the rate if its cicatrization. J Exp Med 24:429–450
6. Castoriadis C (1997) Fait et à Faire. Les Carrefours du Labyrinthe V, Seuil, Paris, pp 233
7. Cavalli-Sforza LF (1997) Qui sommes-nous? Flammarion, Paris, pp 295–296
8. Chiavegato A, Bochaton-Piallat ML, D'Amore E, Sartore S, Gabbiani G (1995) Expression of myosin heavy chain isoforms in mammary epithelial cells in myofibroblasts from different fibrotic settings during neoplasia. Virchows Arch 426:77–86
9. Czernobilsky B, Shezen E, Lifschitz-Mercer B, Fogel M, Luzon A, Jacob N, Skalli O, Gabbiani G (1989) Alpha smooth muscle actin ($\alpha$-SM actin) in normal human ovaries, in ovarian stromal hyperplasia and in ovarian neoplasma. Virchows Arch B Cell Pathol 57:55–61
10. Darby I, Skalli O, Gabbiani G (1990) $\alpha$-smooth muscle actin is transiently expressed by myofibroblasts during experimental wound healing. Lab Invest 63:21–29
11. Desmoulière A, Gabbiani G (1994) Modulation of fibroblastic cytoskeletal features during pathological situations: the role of extracellular matrix and cytokines. Cell Motil Cytoskeleton 29:195–203
12. Desmoulière A, Redard M, Darby I, Gabbiani G (1995) Apoptosis mediates the decrease in cellularity during the transition between granulation tissue and scar. Am J Pathol 146:56–66
13. Diamond JR, van Goor H, Ding G, Engelmyer E (1995) Myofibroblasts in experimental hydronephrosis. Am J Pathol 146:121–129
14. Estes JM, Vande Berg JS, Adzick NS, MacGillivray TE, Desmoulière A, Gabbiani G (1994) Phenotypic and functional features of myofibroblasts in sheep fetal wounds. Differentiation 56:173–181
15. Evans JN, Adler KB (1981) The lung strip: evaluation of a method to study contractility of pulmonary parenchyma. Exp Lung Res 2:187–195
16. Friedman SL (1993) The cellular basis of hepatic fibrosis. Mechanisms and treatment strategies. N Engl J Med 328:1828–1835
17. Gabbiani G, Ryan GB, Majno G (1971) Presence of modified fibroblasts in granulation tissue and their possible role in wound contraction. Experientia 27:549–550
18. Gabbiani G, Hirschel BJ, Ryan GB, Statkov PR, Majno G (1972) Granulation tissue as a contractile organ. A study of structure and function. Exp Med 135:719–734

19. Gabbiani G, Majno G (1972) Dupuytren's contracture: fibroblast contraction. Am J Pathol 66:131–146
20. Gabbiani G, Le Lous M, Bailey AJ, Bazin S, Delaunay A (1976) Collagen and myofibroblasts of granulation tissue. A chemical, ultrastructural and immunologic study. Virchows Arch B Cell Pathol 21:133–145
21. Gabbiani G, Schmid E, Winter S, Chaponnier C, de Chastonay C, Vandekerckhove J, Weber K, Franke WW (1981) Vascular smooth muscle cells differ from other smooth muscle cells: predominance of vimentin filaments and a specific $\alpha$-type actin. Proc Natl Acad Sci U S A 78:298–302
22. Hoffmann-Beerling H (1954) Adenosintriphosphat als betriebsstoff von zellbewegungen. Biochim Biophys Acta 14:182–194
23. Johnson RJ, Iida H, Alpers CE, Majesky MW, Schwartz SM, Pritzl P, Gordon K, Gown AM (1991) Expression of smooth muscle cell phenotype by rat mesangial cell sin immune complex nephritis. J Clin Invest 87:847–858
24. Kapanci Y, Assimacopoulos A, Irlé C, Zwahlen A, Gabbiani G (1974) "Contractile interstitial cells" in pulmonary septa. J Cell Biol 60:375–392
25. Kapanci Y, Ribaux C, Chaponnier C, Gabbiani G (1992) Cytoskeletal features of alveolar myofibroblasts and pericytes in normal human and rat lùng. J Histochem Cytochem 40:1955–1963
26. Lazard D, Sastre X, Frid MG, Glukhova MA, Thiery JP, Koteliansky VE (1993) Expression of smooth muscle-specific proteins in myoepithelium and stromal myofibroblasts of normal and malignant human breast. Proc Natl Acad Sci U S A 90:999–1003
27. Low RB, Chaponnier C, Gabbiani G (1981) Organization of actin in epithelial cells during regenerative and neoplastic conditions. Correlation of morphologic, immunofluorescent, and biochemical findings. Lab Invest 44:359–367
28. Majno G, Gabbiani G, Hirschel BJ, Ryan GB, Statkov PR (1971) Contraction of granulation tissue in vitro: similarity to smooth muscle. Science 173:548–550
29. Majno G (1975) The healing hand: man and wound in the ancient world. Harvard University Press, Cambridge
30. Ramadori G, Veit T, Schwögler S, Dienes HP, Knittel T, Rieder H, Meyer KH (1990) Expression of the gene of $\alpha$-smooth muscle-actin isoform in rat liver and in rat fat-storing (Ito) cells. Virchows Arch B Cell Pathol 59:349–357
31. Ronnov-Jessen L, Petersen OW, Koteliansky VE, Bissell MJ (1995) The origin of the myofibroblasts in breast cancer. J Clin Invest 95:859–873
32. Sappino AP, Dietrich PY, Widgren S, Gabbiani G (1989) Colonic pericryptal fibroblasts. Differentiation pattern in embryogenesis and phenotypic modulation in epithelial proliferative lesions. Virchows Arch A Pathol Anat 415:551–557
33. Sappino AP, Schürch W, Gabbiani G (1990) Differentiation repertoire of fibroblastic cells: expression of cytoskeletal proteins as marker of phenotypic modulation. Lab Invest 63:144–161
34. Schmitt-Gräff A, Krüger S, Bochard F, Gabbiani G, Denk H (1991) Modulation of alpha smooth muscle actin and desmin expression in perisinusoidal cells of normal and diseased human livers. Am J Pathol 138:1233–1242
35. Schmitt-Gräff A, Desmoulière A, Gabbiani G (1994) Heterogeneity of myofibroblast phenotypic features: an example of fibroblastic cell plasticity. Virchows Arch 425:3–24
36. Schürch W, Seemayer TA, Lagacé R (1981) Stromal myofibroblasts in primary invasive and metastatic carcinoma. A combined immunological, light and electron microscopic study. Virchows Arch A 391:125–139
37. Seyle H (1964) From dream to discovery. Mc Gow-Hill, New York. pp 89
38. Skalli O, Ropraz P, Trzeciak A, Benzonana G, Gillessen D, Gabbiani G (1986) A monoclonal antibody against $\alpha$-smooth muscle actin: a new probe for smooth muscle differentiation. J Cell Biol 103:2787–2796
39. Sun Y, Weber KT (1996) Angiotensin converting enzyme and myofibroblasts during tissue repair in the rat heart. J Mol Cell Cardiol 28:851–858
40. Zhang K, Rekhter MD, Gordon D, Phan SH (1994) Myofibroblasts and their role in lung collagen gene expression during pulmonary during pulmonary fibrosis. A combined immunohistochemical and in situ hybridization study. Am J Pathol 145:114–125

# Transcriptional Regulation of the Desmin and SM22 Genes in Vascular Smooth Muscle Cells

M. Mericskay, Z. Li, D. Paulin

## 1 Introduction

There are several stages in the differentiation of smooth-muscle cells (SMCs) (embryonic, fetal, prenatal and adult) and a number of genes are specifically activated at each stage. The factors regulating myogenesis in skeletal muscle responsible for determination and differentiation, members of the MyoD family, have been identified [23]. However, the transcriptional mechanisms regulating the various stages of determination and differentiation in vascular SMCs are still unknown. Our studies over the past few years have focused on the regulation of genes linked to the differentiation of this tissue.

It is generally agreed that the mature, differentiated cells are produced and maintained by regulation that depends on factors inside and outside the cell. Thus, the intrinsic genetic programs regulate differentiation to form a mature cell. In recent years, many gene knock-outs have been made in different groups, resulting in mutants displaying various phenotypes in the vascular system (Table 1).

The phenomena of proliferation, migration and dedifferentiation of SMCs during neointimal hyperplasia following the appearance and development of atheromatous plaques have been described and analyzed in great detail in man and a number of animals. They indicate that several growth factors, including basic fibroblast growth factor (bFGF), platelet-derived growth factor (PDGF), transforming growth factor $\beta$ (TGF$\beta$), etc., and the dysfunction of the vascular endothelium that occurs either during these disorders or following a lesion caused by the balloon catheters used in angioplasty [22], are responsible. There also appears to be no doubt that the vascular SMCs proliferate in response to these stimuli. The vascular SMCs proliferate, migrate and become dedifferentiated to form secretory SMCs (loss of myofilaments, and great development of the endoplasmic reticulum and Golgi apparatus) by changes in their program of gene expression. Knowledge of how the genes are regulated in SMCs is, therefore, essential for a clear understanding of the point at which it is possible to intervene to stop the process of neointimal hyperplasia.

Current Topics in Pathology, Volume 93
A. Desmoulière, B. Tuchweber (Eds.)
© Springer-Verlag Berlin Heidelberg 1999

**Table 1.** Phenotypes of vascular system mutants obtained by gene knockout in mice

| Target gene Structure | Family | Phenotype[a] | Reference[b] |
|---|---|---|---|
| Desmin | Intermediate filaments | Cardiomyopathy, loss of elasticity in the aorta | [16] |
| Col3α1 | Extracellular matrix | Lethal 48 h, blood vessel break | [26] |
| Fibrillin 1 | Extracellular matrix | Lethal 3w, multiple haemorrhages, aortic wall thinning | [27] |
| **Receptors** | | | |
| α-1 Integrin | Receptor | No apparent vascular phenotype in vivo, in vitro: deficient migration of SMC and fibroblast on collagen IV and fibronectin | [28] |
| V-CAM 1 | Receptor (lig: Int a4) | Lethal E12, deficient coronary arteries, multiple cardiac defects | [29, 30, 31] |
| Flt-1 | TK receptor (lig: VEGF) | Lethal E9–11.5, abnormal angiogenesis (disorganised vessel nettwork) | [32] |
| Flk-1 | TK receptor (lig: VEGF) | Lethal E8.5–9.5, absence of yolk sac and embryonnic vasculogenesis due to loss haemangioblast precursor cells. | [33] |
| Tie1 | TK receptor | Lethal neonatal, deficient endothelial cell differentiation, haemorrhages | [34] |
| Tie2/Tek | TK receptor (lig: angiopoïetin) | Lethal E10.5, deficient angiogenesis, abnormal endocardium | [34] |
| PDGFR β | TK receptor (lig: PDGF) | Lethal neonatal, haemorrhages | [35] |
| Gna13 | Membrane G- protein | Lethal E10.5, absence of yolk sac vasculogenesis, cephalic vessels dilatation | [36] |
| **Growth factors** | | | |
| VEGF-A | Angiogenic factor | Lethal heterozygous E11–12, deficient vasculogenesis and angiogenesis | [37, 38] |
| Angiopoietin 1 | Angiogenic factor | Lethal E12.5, abnormal angiogenesis due to deficient SMCs and pericytes recruitment to the vascular wall | [39] |
| TGF β | Growth factor | 50 % Lethal E10.5, deficient yolk sac vasculogenesis and angiogenesis | [40] |
| PDGF B | Growth factor | Lethal neonatal, haemorrhages, heart and large arteries dilatation, absence of pericytes | [41] |
| **Coagulation factors** | | | |
| Tissue factor | Membrane receptor | Lethal E9.5, deficient yolk sac angiogenesis | [42, 43] |
| Factor V | Coagulation factor | Lethal 50 % E9.5–50 % perinatal, deficient yolk sac vasculature | [44] |
| CF7 | Coagulation factor | Lethal neonatal, intracranial and abdominal haemorrhages | [45] |
| Plasminogen | Plasmin precursor | Non-lethal, deficient SMC migration in vascular lesions | [46] |

**Table 1** (continued)

| Target gene Structure | Family | Phenotype[a] | Reference[b] |
|---|---|---|---|
| Nuclear factors | | | |
| LKF | Zn-finger factor | Lethal E12.5–14.5, haemorrhages, dedifferentiation of the SMC from the media | [47] |
| MEF-2 | MADS box factor | Lethal E10.5, absence of right ventricle, vascular defects | [48] |
| Vhlh | Nuclear protein | Lethal E8.5–12.5, deficient vasculogenesis of the placenta | [49] |
| Lipoproteins | | | |
| ApoE | Lipoprotein | Non-lethal, atherosclerotic lesions | [50] |
| ApoA1 | Lipoprotein | Non-lethal, potential model for coronary diseases | [51] |

*E* Embryonic day; *li* ligand; *TK* tyrosine kinase; *MEF* myocyte-specific enhancer-binding factor; *TGF* transforming growth factor; *VEGF* vascular endothelial growth factor; *PDGF* platelet-derived growth factor

[a] Only the phenotype concerning the vascular system and eventually the cardiac system is mentioned.

[b] Recent publication on the mutant, see reference therein.

These programs of dedifferentiation within the cell following arterial diseases, such as atherosclerosis or restenosis after angioplasty, will be modulated by extrinsic factors, which will cause cell dedifferentiation and proliferation. There are three types of factors: (1) soluble substances of plasma or parietal origin, (2) cell–matrix interactions, and (3) cell–cell interactions.

We have studied the regulation of two genes expressed in the vascular system, one encoding the intermediate filament protein, desmin, and the other encoding the calponin-like protein, SM22. Our findings indicate that the regulatory sequences from these genes may be used to control the synthesis of proteins of therapeutic interest. We have isolated and characterized two types of sequence for this purpose. Sequences derived from the desmin gene can be used to make skeletal muscle produce factors that are secreted into the circulation. More recently, we have obtained sequences from the SM22 gene that allow specific targeting of the arterial SMC (Fig. 1).

# 2 Regulation of the SM22 Gene

SM22 is a 22-kDa protein that has the same domains as calponin, particularly in the calcium-binding region [5]. The exact function of this protein is not yet known, but its abundance and specificity for smooth muscle cells in the adults of several species (man, mouse, rat, chicken) and its very early production in the embryo make it most attractive for studies on transcriptional regulation of a promoter specific to SMCs. This work was carried out in collaboration with the group of. SMALL et al. (Salzburg, Austria), who have cloned the mouse SM22 gene.

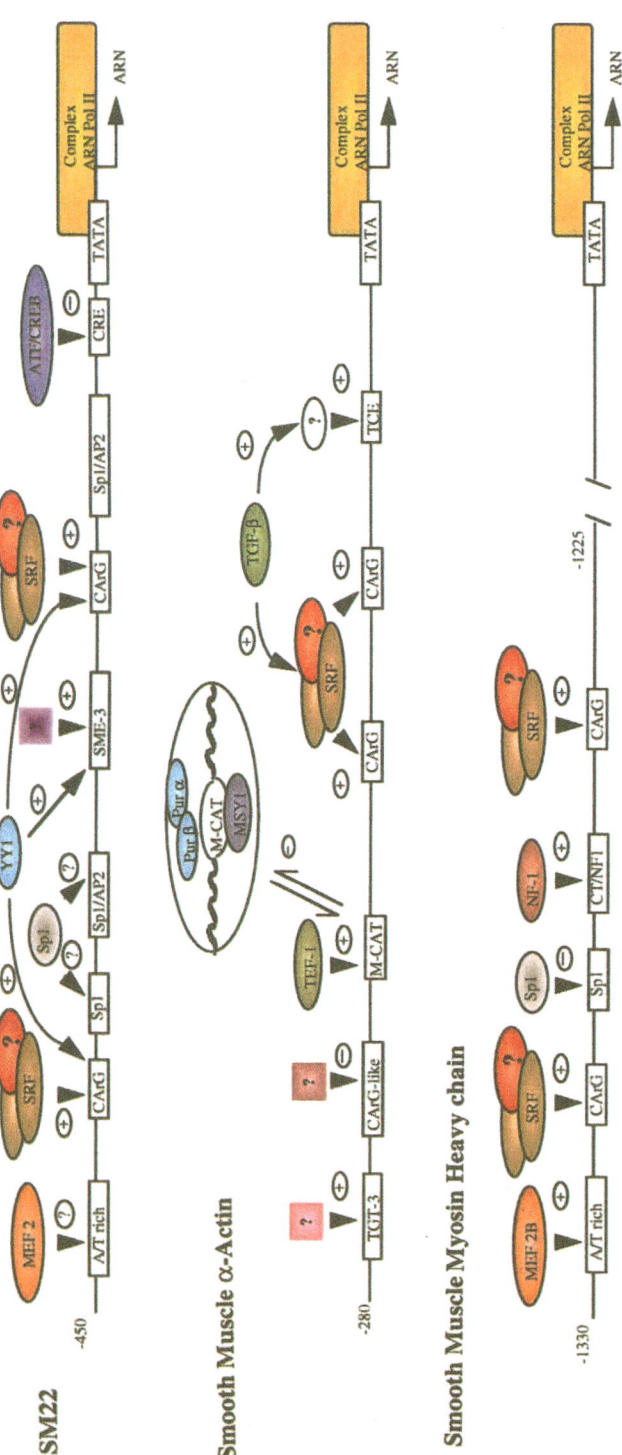

**Fig. 1.** Promoter regulatory sequences of genes expressed in smooth muscle. The transcription factors are shown above the binding sites and their action as transcription activators (+), inhibitors (−), or whose action is unknown (?) are shown. All promoters generally have binding sites for a specific factor, but only those that have been shown to bind factors are indicated. The *M-CAT* site for the actin-a promoter may be either a double strand and recognized by transactivator enhancing factor (*TEF*)-1 or as a single strand, with the strand sense being recognized by Pur a/b and the complementary strand by *MSY1*. The co-factor(s) of serum response factor (*SRF*) specific for smooth muscle cells (*SMC*) are still unknown. All these factors interact with the transcription initiation *complex of Pol II*. Data are compiled from references cited in the text for each gene and references therein

The SM22 gene is active in the mouse embryo from the initial stages of muscle-cell differentiation in the somite myotomes (E9), the right ventricle of the heart (E8.5) and the vascular (E9) and visceral (E13.5) smooth muscle. The range of tissues in which it is active is gradually reduced to the smooth muscle during development, and it is restricted to this tissue after stage E14.5 in the adult. The regulatory sequences in the *cis* promoter of the SM22 gene have been studied in vivo in transgenic mice.

The results obtained for two independent lines indicated that a fragment from position −2126 bp to +65 bp in exon 1 directs the transient expression of the lacZ gene in the somites and the right ventricle in the embryo, with a temporal profile identical to that of the endogenous gene. The expression of the lacZ gene is specific for arterial smooth muscle, and does not occur in the venous or visceral systems, where there is also the endogenous protein. Adding the 4000 bp of intron 1 to the start of exon 2 does not alter the profile of transgene expression. Finally, we have analyzed first generation (FO) transgenic embryos and shown that the region responsible for the arterial specificity lies between positions −445 and +65, with increased sensitivity at the integration site, which results in ectopic expression in other tissues in certain individuals [18]. These results were independently confirmed by another group [11].

The study shows that there are different regulatory programs in the various types of SMC (arterial, venous vascular cells and visceral SMC).

## 3  Regulation of the Desmin Gene

Desmin is the constituent of the intermediary filament network specific to muscle cells. Gene-knockout studies have shown that it contributes to resistance and tissue elasticity [15, 16, 24]. Desmin is synthesized as soon as each type of muscle cell begins to differentiate in the embryo, starting with the precardiac areas (E7.5 in mice), followed by skeletal muscle (E9 in somitic myotomes) and last in smooth muscle (E9 in arteries) [12]. It continues to be produced there throughout adult life. Studies on the regulation of the human desmin gene have shown that the amplifier situated between −900 bp and −700 bp positions is important for its specific activity in skeletal muscle [13, 14].

The regulatory sequences of the mouse desmin gene were analyzed in vivo by transgenesis (Fig. 2). Initial results showed that 4004 bp upstream of the desmin gene targeted expression of the lacZ reporter gene in the three muscle tissues (heart, vascular smooth muscle and skeletal muscle) with the same temporal and spatial patterns as the endogenous gene product. However, the regulatory regions for visceral smooth muscle lay outside this region. The transgenic mice were subjected to detailed histological and immunocytochemical analyses to identify the blood vessels in which the transgene was expressed, as little work has yet been done on this in mice. Considerable data was obtained on the vasculogenesis and angiogenesis in the mouse embryo. It was shown that the transgene was activated later in veins than in arteries in a given organ, emphasizing the difference in activation of the transcription programs in the vein and artery SMCs. This was reminiscent of the findings for the SM22 gene, showing that the regulatory programs for these two

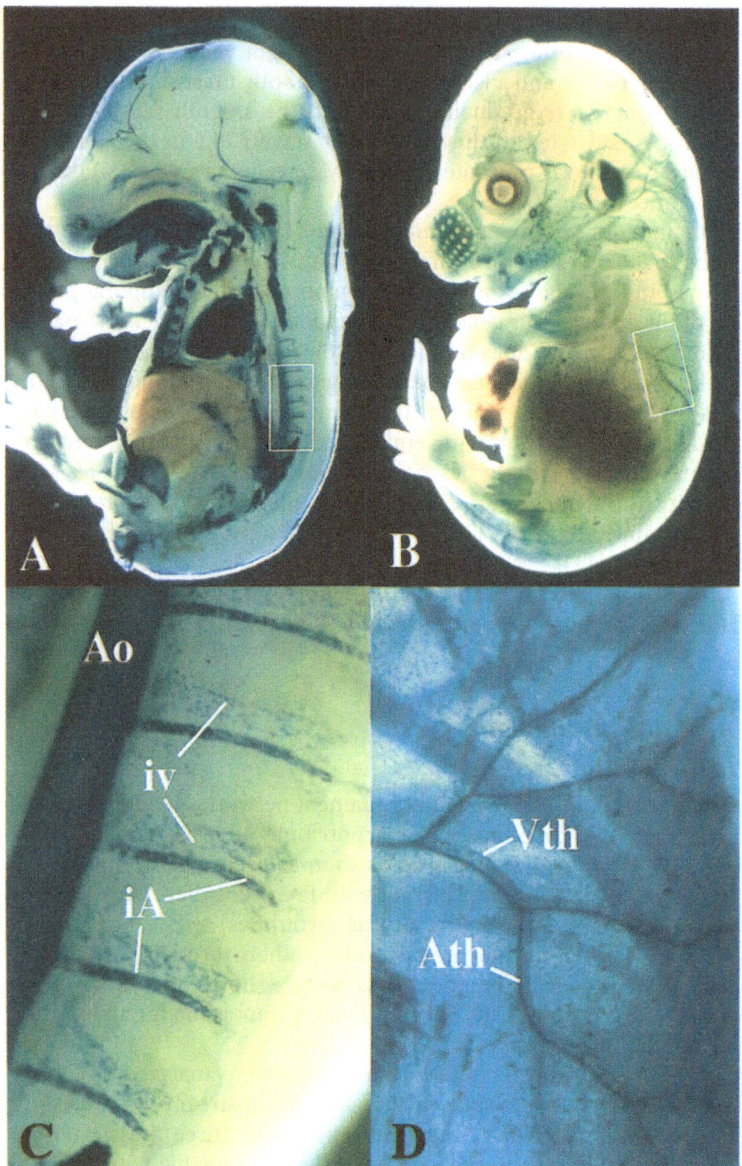

**Fig. 2A–D.** Expression of the desmin–lacZ transgene in blood vessels of the mouse embryo. A 15-day embryo stained to show the activity of the reporter gene lacZ. Sagittal sections of the internal (**A, C**) and external (**B, D**) surfaces. The regulatory region contains the regulatory elements needed for gene expression in the arteries, veins and heart. The enlargement shows the networks of arteries (*Ao,* aorta; *ia,* intercostal arteries; *Ath,* external thoracic artery) and veins (*iv,* intercostal veins; *Vth,* external thoracic veins)

subtypes of vascular SMC are independent. The group of PARMACEK et al. [9] recently extended our observations on the SM22 promoter and showed that activation of the 450 bp promoter of SM22 is mainly due to two CArG sequences. They also found that the transgene is no longer activated in vivo when these sequences are made incapable of binding serum response factor (SRF) by directed mutagenesis.

These observations led to the definition of specific amplifier sequences that may constitute a paradigm for the regulation of transcription in arterial smooth muscle, much like the specific amplifiers in skeletal muscle linking the myogenic regulation factors of the MyoD family and the myocyte-specific enhancer-binding factors-2 (MEF-2).

A human SMC line immortalized with the T antigen of SV40 has several attractive features for this work; it is stable and expresses the desmin gene as well as several other markers of advanced SMC differentiation, such as SM-myosin heavy chain (MHC) or caldesmon, which are generally inactive in most cell lines derived from SMCs, or are very rapidly lost in primary culture because of the capacity for phenotypic modulation that is characteristic of these cells. Several criteria (structural markers, specific receptors) indicate that these cells are one of the best in vitro models of differentiated SMC available today (Dandré, unpublished data). The effects of point mutations on the activity of the desmin promoter were analyzed in transfection studies. Deletion mutants were also analyzed in vivo by transgenesis in mice to confirm the in vitro findings.

The results obtained with the human gene indicating that only skeletal muscle is specified in the regulatory elements up to – 1000 bp [13, 14] have shown that this is also true for the murine gene, with the possible addition of the right ventricle [10]. We also know that desmin gene expression in vein SMCs regulated in the fragment – 4004 bp, but does not involve the region – 4004 to – 2500 (to be confirmed). This suggests that the regions responsible for gene transcription in venous SMCs are likely to lie between positions – 2500 and – 1000. This region was first examined by in vivo transgenesis studies and the potential sites were then analyzed using the methods described for the genes in arterial SMC.

# 4 Conclusion

There are CArG sites that bind the SRF factors in the promoters of several of the genes expressed in smooth muscle, such as the gene for telokine, a protein which is the C-terminal part of the smooth-muscle myosin light-chain kinase (SM-MLCK), and with messenger RNA (mRNA) that is transcribed from an alternative promoter in an intron of SM-MLCK [7], and the caldesmon [20] and integrin $\alpha$1 genes [21] and the SM-MHC [17] and the SM $\alpha$ actin [6] genes. If the gene is expressed in more than one cell type, such as the desmin or integrin $\alpha$1 genes, it is the interaction between the CArG sequence and factor SRF that is responsible for activating transcription in the SMCs. The CArG sequence can direct the expression of a reporter gene under the control of a heterologous promoter, specifically in smooth muscle. These results showing the importance of SRF in the control of specific transcription in smooth muscle are somewhat surprising, as SRF is also implicated in the regulation of genes specific to the heart, such as cardiac actin [4] or skeletal muscle, such as the gene for the myosin 1A light chain [2]. Initial studies on SRF have also been carried out on HeLa cells and fibroblasts using serum response elements to the c-fos promoter [25]. They suggest that SRF has a ubiquitous role, although expression of the factor in vivo seemed to be restricted to muscle tissues [1, 4]. The studies done on SRF to date suggest that the transcriptional activity of the factor is made specific by association with a cell-specific co-factor. MEF2, a member of the MCM1-agamous-ARG80-deficiens-SRF (MADS) family, like SRF, can associate with the MyoD transcription factor in skeletal muscle [19]. MyoD is a member of the helix/loop/helix family of muscle regulators responsible for the determination and differentiation of skeletal muscle cells in the embryo. SRF is associated with the homobox gene, Nkx 2.5, for transactivation of the cardiac actin promoter in the heart. This gene is essential for cardiac development [3]. Many co-factors have been identified that interact with SRF in the response to serum and growth factors; these include transcription factors such as SRF-associated protein (SAP1), ELK1, Net/Erp of the erythroblastoid factor (ets) family and the cellular enhancer binding protein (C/EBP) or activating transcription factors (ATFs). The transcriptional activities of all of these complexes are modified by phosphorylation due to the activation cascades of signal transduction tyrosine kinases or serine/threonine kinases transmitting stimuli from the environment [25]. Thus, it appears that SRF can associate with co-factors of a wide variety of families, including ets, homobox and zinc finger, which enables it to act on the multimeric complex of transcription machinery for RNA polymerase II in the context of specific cells.

Thus, it is perhaps significant that we have consensus sequences that are potential binding sites in the sequences that are contiguous with, or overlap, the CArG sites in the SM22 genes. These include GGAA for Ets proteins, E boxes; CANNTG for bHLH factors and ATGCWAAT for binding octamer-type factors. The most interesting hypothesis is that the specific activity of the CArG sequences in SMCs involves co-factors specific to SMCs, which bind to SRF depending on their specific activity.

# References

1. Belaguli N, Schildmeyer LA, Schwartz RJ (1997) Organization and myogenic restricted expression of the murine serum response factor gene – a role for autoregulation. J Biol Chem 272:18222–18231
2. Catala F, Wanner R, Barton P, Cohen A, Wright W, Buckingham M (1995) A skeletal muscle-specific enhancer regulated by factors binding to E and CArG boxes is present in the promoter of the mouse myosin light-chain 1A gene. Mol Cell Biol 15:4585–4596
3. Chen CY, Schwartz RJ (1996) Recruitment of the tinman homolog Nkx-2.5 by serum response factor activates cardiac α-actin gene transcription. Mol Cell Biol 16:6372–6384
4. Croissant JD, Kim J, Eichele G, Goering L, Lough J, Prywes R, Schwartz RJ (1996) Avian serum response factor expression restricted primarily to muscle cell lineages is required for α-actin gene transcription. Dev Biol 177:250–264
5. Duband JL, Gimona M, Scatena M, Sartore S, Small JV (1993) Calponin and SM22 as differentiation markers of smooth muscle: spatiotemporal distribution during avian embryonnic development. Differentiation 55:1–11
6. Hautman MB, Owen GK (1997) A transforming growth factor β (TGFβ) control element drives TGFβ-induced stimulation of smooth muscle α-actin gene expression in concert with two CArG elements. J Biol Chem 272:10948–10956

7. Herring BP, Smith AF (1996) Telokin expression is mediated by a smooth muscle cell-specific promoter. Am J Physiol 270:C1656–1665
8. Kelm RJ, Siquan S Jr, Strauch AR, Gtz MJ (1996) Repression of transcriptional enhancer factor-1 and activator protein-1-dependent enhancer activity by vascular actin single stranded DNA-binding factor 2. J Biol Chem 271:24278–24285
9. Kim S, Ip HS, Lu MM, Clendenin C, Parmacek MS (1997) A serum response factor-dependent transcriptional regulatory program identifies distinct smooth muscle cell lineages. Mol Cell Biol 17:2266–2278
10. Kuisk IR, Li H, Tran D, Capetanaki Y (1996) A single MEF2 site governs desmin transcription in both heart and skeletal muscle during mouse embryogenesis. Dev Biol 174: 1–13
11. Li L, Miano JM, Mercer B, Olson EN (1996) Expression of the SM22a promoter in transgenic mice provides evidence for distinct transcriptional regulatory programs in vascular and visceral smooth muscle cells. J Cell Biol 132:849–859
12. Li Z, Lillienbaum A, Butler-Browne G, Paulin D (1989) Human desmin coding gene: complete nucleotide sequence, characterization and regulation of expression during myogenesis and development. Gene (Amst) 78:243–254
13. Li Z, Paulin D (1993) Different factors interact with myoblast-specific and myotube-specific enhancer regions of the human desmin gene. J Biol Chem 268:10403–10415
14. Li Z, Marchand P, Humber J, Babinet C, Paulin D (1993) Desmin sequence elements regulating skeletal muscle-specific expression in transgenic mice. Development 117: 947–959
15. Li Z, Collucci-Guyon E, Pinçon-Raymond M, Mericskay M, Pournin S, Paulin D, Babinet C (1996) Cardiovascular lesions and skeletal myopathy in mice lacking desmin. Dev Biol 175:362–366
16. Li Z, Mericskay M, Agbulut O, Butler-Browne G, Carlsson L, Thornell L-E, Babinet C, Paulin D (1997) Desmin is essential for the tensile strength and integrity of myofibrils but not for myogenic commitment, differentiation and fusion of skeletal muscle. J Cell Biol 139: 129–144
17. Madsen CS, Regan CP, Owens GK (1997) Interaction of CArG elements and a GC-rich repressor element in transcriptional regulation of the smooth muscle myosin heavy chain in vascular smooth muscle cells. J Biol Chem 272:29842–29851
18. Moessler H, Mericskay M, Li Z, Nagl S, Paulin D, Small JV (1996) The SM22 promoter directs tissue-specific expression in arterial but not venous nor visceral smooth muscle cells in transgenic mice. Development 122:415–425
19. Molkentin JD, Black BL, Martin JF, Olson EN (1995) Cooperative activation of muscle gene transcription by MEF2 and myogenic bHLH proteins. Cell 83:1125–1136
20. Momiyama T, Hayashi K, Obata H, Chimori Y, Nishida T, Kamiike W, Matsuda H, Sobue K (1998) Functional involvement of serum response factor in the transcriptional regulation of caldesmon gene. Biochem Biophys Res Commun 242:429–435
21. Obata H, Hayashi K, Nishida W, Momiyama T, Uchida A, Ochi T, Sobue K (1997) Smooth muscle cell phenotype-dependent transcriptional regulation of the a1 integrin gene. J Biol Chem 272:26643–26652
22. Schwartz SM, deBlois D, O'Brien ERM (1995) The intima: soil for atherosclerosis and restenosis. Circ Res 77:445–465
23. Tajbakhsh S, Cossu G (1997) Establishing myogenic identity during somatogenesis. Curr Opin Genet Dev 7:634–641
24. Thornell L-E, Carlsson L, Li Z, Mericskay M, Paulin D (1997) Null mutation in the desmin gene gives rise to a cardiomyopathy. J Mol Cell Cardiol 29:2107
25. Treisman R (1994) Ternary complex factors: growth factor regulated transcriptional activators. Curr Biol 4:96–101
26. Liu X, Wu H, Byrne M, Krane S, Jaenisch R (1997) Type III collagen is crucial for collagen I fibrillogenesis and for normal cardiovascular development. Proc Natl Acad Sci U S A 94:1852–1856
27. Pereira L, Andrikopoulos K, Tian J, Lee SY, Keene DR, Ono R, Reinhardt DP, Sakai LY, Biery NJ, Bunton T, Dietz HC, Ramirez F (1997) Targetting of the gene encoding fibrillin-1 recapitulates the vascular aspect of Marfan syndrome. Nat Genet 17:218–222

28. Gardner H, Kreidberg J, Koteliansky V, Jaenisch R (1996) Deletion of integrin alpha 1 by homologous recombination permits normal murine development but gives rise to a specific deficit in cell adhesion. Dev Biol 175:301–313

29. Gurtner GC, Davis V, Li H, McCoy MJ, Sharpe A, Cybulsky MI (1995) Targeted disruption of the murine VCAM1 gene: essential role of VCAM-1 in chorioallantoic fusion and placentation. Genes Dev 9:1–14

30. Kwee L, Baldwin HS, Shen HM, Stewart CL, Buck C, Buck CA, Labow MA (1995) Defective development of the embryonic and extraembryonic circulatory systems in vascular cell adhesion molecule (VCAM-1) deficient mice. Development 121:489–503

31. Yang JT, Rayburn H, Hynes RO (1995) Cell adhesion events mediated by alpha 4 integrins are essential in placental and cardiac development. Development 121:549–560

32. Fong GH, Rossant J, Gertsenstein M, Breitman ML (1995) Role of the Flt-1 receptor tyrosine kinase in regulating the assembly of vascular endothelium. Nature 376:66–70

33. Shalaby F, Ho J, Stanford WL, Fischer KD, Schuh AC, Schwartz L, Bernstein A, Rossant J (1997) A requirement for Flk1 in primitive and definitive hematopoiesis and vasculogenesis. Cell 89:981–990

34. Sato TN, Tozawa Y, Deutsch U, Wolburg-Buchholz K, Fujiwara Y, Gendron-Maguire M, Gridley T, Wolburg H, Risau W, Qin Y (1995) Distinct roles of the receptor tyrosine kinases Tie-1 and Tie-2 in blood vessel formation. Nature 376:70–74

35. Soriano P (1994) Abnormal kidney development and hematological disorders in PDGF beta-receptor mutant mice. Genes Dev 8:1888–1896

36. Offermanns S, Mancino V, Revel JP, Simon MI (1997) Vascular system defects and impaired cell chemokinesis as a result of Galpha13 deficiency. Science 275:533–536

37. Carmeliet P, Ferreira V, Breier G, Pollefeyt S, Kieckens L, Gertsenstein M, Fahrig M, Vandenhoeck A, Harpal K, Eberhardt C, Declercq C, Pawling J, Moons L, Collen D, Risau W, Nagy A (1996) Abnormal blood vessel development and lethality in embryos lacking a single VEGF allele. Nature 380:435–439

38. Ferrara N, Carver-Moore K, Chen H, Dowd M, Lu L, O'Shea KS, Powell-Braxton L, Hillan KJ, Moore MW (1996) Heterozygous embryonic lethality induced by targeted inactivation of the VEGF gene. Nature 380:439–442

39. Suri C, Jones PF, Patan S, Bartunkova S, Maisonpierre PC, Davis S, Sato TN, Yancopoulos GD (1996) Requisite role of angiopoietin-1, a ligand for the TIE2 receptor, during embryonic angiogenesis. Cell 87:1171–1180

40. Dickson MC, Martin JS, Cousins FM, Kulkarni AB, Karlsson S, Akhurst RJ (1995) Defective haematopoiesis and vasculogenesis in transforming growth factor-beta 1 knock out mice. Development 121:1845–1854

41. Lindahl P, Johansson BR, Leveen P, Betsholtz C (1997) Pericyte loss and microaneurysm formation in PDGF-B-deficient mice. Science 277:242–245

42. Bugge TH, Xiao Q, Kombrinck KW, Flick MJ, Holmback K, Danton MJ, Colbert MC, Witte DP, Fujikawa K, Davie EW, Degen JL (1996) Fatal embryonic bleeding events in mice lacking tissue factor, the cell-associated initiator of blood coagulation. Proc Natl Acad Sci U S A 93:6258–6263

43. Carmeliet P, Mackman N, Moons L, Luther T, Gressens P, Van Vlaenderen I, Demunck H, Kasper M, Breier G, Evrard P, Muller M, Risau W, Edgington T, Collen D (1996) Role of tissue factor in embryonic blood vessel development. Nature 383:73–75

44. Cui J, O'Shea KS, Purkayastha A, Saunders TL, Ginsburg D (1996) Fatal haemorrhage and incomplete block to embryogenesis in mice lacking coagulation factor V. Nature 384:66–68

45. Rosen ED, Chan JC, Idusogie E, Clotman F, Vlasuk G, Luther T, Jalbert LR, Albrecht S, Zhong L, Lissens A, Schoonjans L, Moons L, Collen D, Castellino FJ, Carmeliet P (1997) Mice lacking factor VII develop normally but suffer fatal perinatal bleeding. Nature 390:290–294

46. Carmeliet P, Moons L, Ploplis V, Plow E, Collen D (1997) Impaired arterial neointima formation in mice with disruption of the plasminogen gene. J Clin Invest 99:200-208

47. Kuo CT, Veselits ML, Barton KP, Lu MM, Clendenin C, Leiden JM (1997) The LKLF transcription factor is required for normal tunica media formation and blood vessel stabilization during murine embryogenesis. Genes Dev 11:2996–3006

48. Lin Q, Schwarz J, Bucana C, Olson EN (1997) Control of mouse cardiac morphogenesis and myogenesis by transcription factor MEF2C. Science 276:1404–1407
49. Gnarra JR, Ward JM, Porter FD, Wagner JR, Devor DE, Grinberg A, Emmert-Buck MR, Westphal H, Klausner RD, Linehan WM (1997) Defective placental vasculogenesis causes embryonic lethality in VHL-deficient mice. Proc Natl Acad Sci USA 94:9102–9107
50. Smith JD, Breslow JL (1997) The emergence of mouse models of atherosclerosis and their relevance to clinical research. J Internal Med 242:99–109
51. Williamson R, Lee D, Hagaman J, Maeda N (1992) Marked reduction of high density lipoprotein cholesterol in mice genetically modified to lack apolipoprotein A-I. Proc Natl Acad Sci U S A 89:7134–7138

# Modulation of Myofibroblast and Smooth-Muscle Phenotypes in the Lung

R. B. Low

## 1 Introduction

The lung contains a full complement of vascular and visceral smooth-muscle cells (SMCs) [2, 16, 18]. Additionally, in the normal alveolar wall, there are contractile interstitial cells that contribute to normal function [10, 12] as well as to alveolar remodeling seen in such disorders as pulmonary hypertension and interstitial fibrosis [11, 21]. This review will present three topics: (1) the differentiation of these cells during normal lung development, (2) the phenotypic changes that occur during pulmonary interstitial remodeling, including the appearance of alveolar and interstitial myofibroblasts during pulmonary fibrosis, and (3) the regulation of cell phenotype by transforming growth factor-$\beta$ (TGF-$\beta$). Other chapters in this volume also are particularly relevant to what is covered here (Chaps. 1, 5, 6, 15, 18).

## 2 Lung Development

Lung development is characterized by a series of morphological transitions that typify the process of branching morphogenesis [3]. Prenatal stages are characterized by a fractal-like pattern of epithelial tube branching morphogenesis within a tissue-specific mesenchyme. Early in this process, the pattern of smooth-muscle $\alpha$-actin (SMA) antibody reactivity is intermediate between that for a general mesenchymal marker, e. g., vimentin, and that of fully differentiated smooth muscle [16, 20]. $\alpha$-Actin antibody reactivity extends into areas of mesenchymal condensation, indicating SMC differentiation from the loose mesenchyme. At this point, these cells do not react with antibodies against smooth-muscle myosin heavy chains (SMMHCs). Noteworthy is the appearance of SMA-positive cells in the cleft that forms between branching epithelial tubes, raising the possibility that branching morphogenesis and the induction of smooth-muscle differentiation are

Current Topics in Pathology, Volume 93
A. Desmoulière, B. Tuchweber (Eds.)
© Springer-Verlag Berlin Heidelberg 1999

related processes. A cell in the region of cleft formation and capable of contraction or perhaps serving as a tether, may play a role in directing the complex three-dimensional growth that is occurring at this time. An analogue of this branch point specialization also occurs during later phases of development; new septa are "capped" with $\alpha$-actin-positive cells and the septal interstitium and enclosing epithelium grow away from this cap [3].

SMA antibody reactivity in cells that are desmin- and smooth-muscle-myosin negative remains prominent as lung development proceeds still further [20]. These cells may be precursors to vascular pericytes during this period in which a double capillary bed exists [3]. Reduction in the double capillary bed, together with continued lung growth and expansion and possibly apoptosis [12] (Chaps. 1 and 18) may provide the explanation for the much simpler $\alpha$-actin pattern of reactivity seen in the adult lung [16,20] (Table 1). Finally, studies of SMA localization indicate that differentiation of airway smooth muscle precedes that of the vasculature and that differentiation of arterial precedes venous elements.

Antibody reactivity against SMMHCs begins much later in lung development than for SMA [29]. Reactivity is first observed in fetal lung tissue during the glandular and canalicular phases of development, with a general MHC antibody that recognizes the SMMHC isoforms, SM-1 and SM-2 [1], which differ in the tail region of the molecule [1], as well as the non-muscle MHC-B (NM-B) that is present in developing smooth muscle [14]. NM-B reactivity is prominent in the SMC of larger airways and around the larger pulmonary arteries that parallel the lobar and sub-segmental bronchi. Following this, SM-1 begins to appear, with reactivity initially restricted to the larger airway elements. Reactivity with vascular tissues remains absent through the saccular phase of development, before appearing first in larger vascular elements and, then, last in venous smooth muscle. SM-2 reactivity first appears during the process of alveolarization and occurs again,

**Table 1.** Distribution of contractile proteins in lung cells

| Lung cells | Smooth muscle $\alpha$-actin | Smooth-muscle myosin heavy chain isoform | | |
|---|---|---|---|---|
| | | SM-1 | SM-2 | SM-B |
| Arterial SMC | | | | |
|   Large | Yes | Yes | Yes | No |
|   Small | Yes | Yes | No | No/yes[b] |
| Venous SMC | Yes | Yes | No | No/yes[b] |
| Airway | Yes | Yes | Yes | Yes |
| Septal tip | Yes | Yes | No | Yes |
| CIC[c] | No | No | No | No |
| Myofibroblast | | | | |
|   Type V[d] | No | No | No | No |
|   Type VA[d] | Yes | No | No | No |

*SMC*, smooth-muscle cell; *CIC*, contractile interstitial cells.
[a] Many of these cells also contain smooth-muscle gamma-actin.
[b] Some small vessels do not contain SM-B antibody-reactive cells; in other vessels, some but not all SMC are SM-B positive.
[c] CIC express smooth-muscle $\alpha$-actin in some forms of pulmonary hypertension [11].
[d] See Skalli et al. [26] for discussion of myofibroblast subtypes.

first in airway elements. The adult pattern of reactivity appears at the end of the alveolar maturation process, e. g., after postnatal day 20 in the rat (Table 1).

Two additional SMMHC isoforms recently have been identified that are due to an alternative splice site in the head region of the molecule and that occur in both the SM-1 and SM-2 isoforms [28]. There is strong evidence that the SM-B isoforms possess a higher actin-activated ATPase activity and a higher rate of in vitro and in vivo contractile velocity [6, 13, 25]. SM-B is not found in the larger blood vessels of the lung, but is prominent in many smaller resistance vessels. This isoform is found throughout the airways (Table 1). Of note is that SM-B appears to be present in some individual SMC in vessels in which it is found [17].

KAPANCI et al. [10, 12] were the first to describe another contractile cell type in mammalian lung. Located within the thick portion of the air-blood barrier, these "contractile interstitial cells" (CIC) contain prominent actin microfilaments unlike conventional fibroblasts and are thought to play an important role in the regulation of alveolo-capillary perfusion. CICs do not normally contain SMA [10, 12] (Table 1).

# 3 Interstitial Fibrosis

The myofibroblast was first discovered in the context of wound repair [7] (Chap. 1). Later, it became apparent that such cells are found in a wide variety of pathological conditions [26] (Chap. 1). In some of these circumstances, these cells express smooth-muscle contractile proteins such as SMA.

The existence of myofibroblasts in human lung disease as well as in animal models of airway and interstitial disease has been appreciated for some time [12]. MITCHELL, et al. [21] were the first to demonstrate that these cells often contain SMA. For example, in bleomycin-induced fibrosis in the rat, prominent SMA antibody reactivity is observed in areas of parenchymal damage within days of bleomycin instillation [12, 21] (see chapter by Phan, this volume). Staining is most intense in the focal fibrotic lesions characteristic of this animal model and is especially noted in airspace lesions (Fig. 1). An important factor is that these cells do not express smooth-muscle myosin or desmin.

SMA-positive myofibroblasts also occur in other forms of lung disease, including hypersensitivity pneumonitis, idiopathic bronchiolitis obliterans with organizing pneumonia (BOOP) and idiopathic pulmonary fibrosis (IPF) [15]. In a recent study, PACHE, et al. [23] carried out a systematic study of SMA-containing myofibroblasts in cases of human diffuse alveolar damage (DAD), which in its severest forms is manifest as Acute Respiratory Distress Syndrome (ARDS). In the exudative phase of DAD, there appear numerous SMA-positive interstitial cells. Cells interspersed within hyaline membranes at this stage rarely are SMA-positive. In the proliferative phase of the disease, many interstitial fibroblasts and, now, alveolar cells are SMA-positive, especially in areas of fibroplasia. These cells continue to be prominent in the fibrotic phase, when normal peripheral lung structure has been replaced by compact areas of fibrosis. Characteristically, these SMA myofibroblasts contain vimentin, but contain desmin only very rarely. They also do not express smooth-muscle myosin.

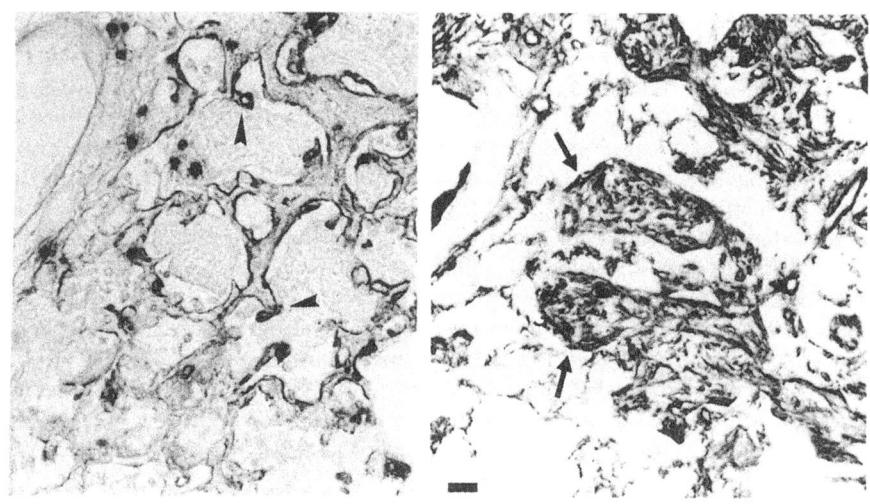

a                                                                          b

Fig. 1 a, b. Immunoperoxidase staining of serial sections of fibrotic rat lung with antibodies against epithelial keratins and smooth-muscle actin (SMA) (see Mitchell et al. [21] for details). Keratin staining (a) shows the location of alveolar epithelial cells around the periphery of alveolar spaces filled with fibroblasts and matrix. In serial section, the airspace fibroblasts are highly SMA-reactive (b)

The important observation that CICs, which normally do not express SMA, can be induced to do so in human cases of pulmonary hypertension was first made by KAPANCI et al. [11]. Importantly, this occurs with post-, but not with pre-capillary hypertension, suggesting a possible role for mechanical forces as an inductive signal.

The question as to origin of these SMA-positive cells remains unanswered. The absence of desmin and smooth-muscle myosin might suggest these cells do not come from vascular or airway smooth muscle; however, this is not certain given the known phenotypic plasticity of SMC [4, 22]. Indeed, in bleomycin fibrosis, the SMCs of both vascular and airway elements show evidence of loss of smooth-muscle markers, as well as present the appearance that SMA-positive cells are migrating into the surrounding tissue. CIC could also clearly be contributors, given that they can acquire SMA [11] (see above). The SMA-negative interstitial fibroblast is also a possible, even likely, source based on what is observed as SMA-positive cells begin to appear [2], and on their likely conversion to a smooth-muscle phenotype in pulmonary hypertension [9].

## 4 Regulation of Smooth-Muscle $\alpha$-Actin Expression by TGF-$\beta$

What is known regarding the regulation of expression of smooth-muscle contractile proteins recently has been reviewed [4, 18, 22]. Based on the known roles of TGF-$\beta$ in development and tissue remodeling [24], it was entirely logical to suspect that this cytokine might well be involved in the regulation of lung mesenchymal cell phenotype. Particularly noteworthy is the role of TGF-$\beta$ in the evolution of

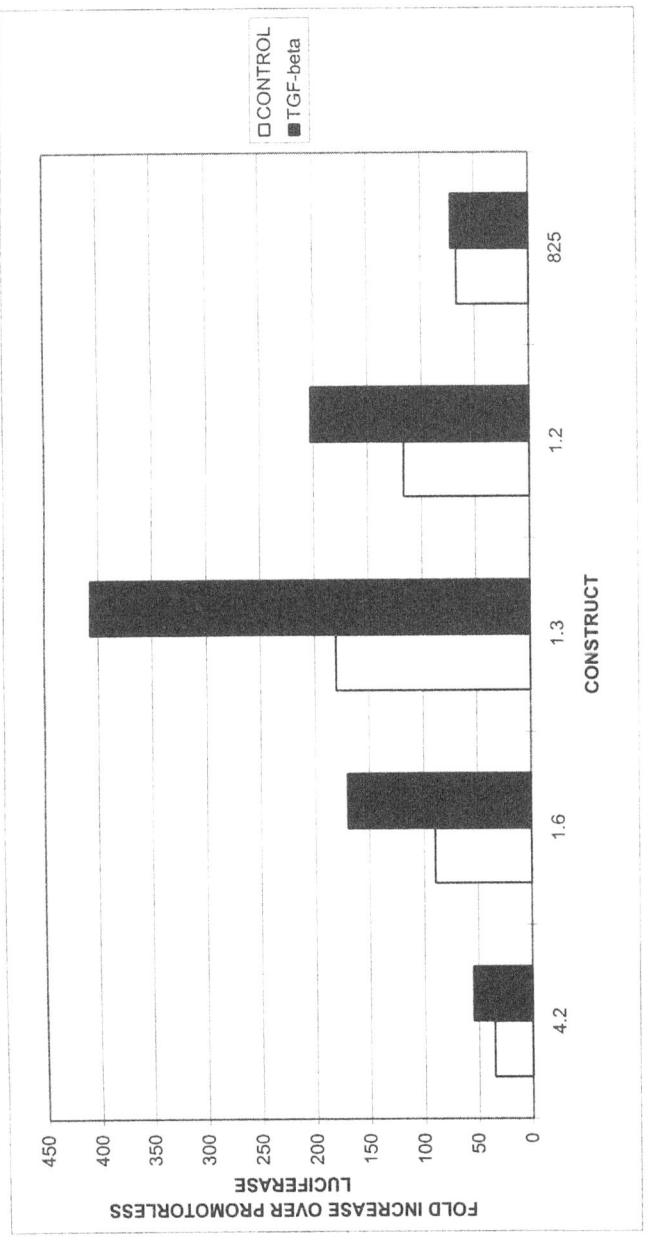

**Fig. 2.** Transfection analysis of lung mesenchymal cells (see White and Low [27] for details). Confluent cells were transfected with smooth-muscle myosin heavy chain (SMMHC) promoter constructs and then cultured with or without TGF-$\beta$ (10 ng/ml) in the absence of serum. Data represent means of duplicate measurements which varied by 20%. Transforming growth factor-$\beta$ (TGF-$\beta$) causes increased expression of the 4.2, 1.6 and 1.2-kb constructs, but not the 602-bp construct. All but the 602-bp construct contain TGF-$\beta$ response elements similar to those known to be involved in TGF-$\beta$ regulation of smooth-muscle actin (SMA) [8]

interstitial and airspace fibrosis in lung [2] (Chap. 18). This led to the observation, by DESMOULIERE et al. [5], that TGF-$\beta$ is an important regulator of fibroblast SMA expression both in vivo and in vitro. Thus, subcutaneous administration of TGF-$\beta$ increases SMA protein and messenger RNA (mRNA) in granulation tissue fibroblasts. The cytokine also increases SMA protein and mRNA in growing and in quiescent human or rat subcutaneous fibroblasts in culture. Simultaneously, MITCHELL et al. [19] showed that TGF-$\beta$ selectively increases SMA content and synthesis by cultured lung mesenchymal cells. This appears to be due to increases in SMA in cells in which SMA already is present. Though total actin mRNA was increased, TGF-$\beta$ did not change the proportion of SMA to total actin mRNA.

The molecular basis of these actions of TGF-$\beta$ on SMA expression has been further explored in studies of the SMA gene promoter in cultured systemic vascular SMCs [8]. Three *cis* elements, two highly conserved CArG boxes, plus a novel TGF-$\beta$ control element are necessary and sufficient to bestow TGF-$\beta$ sensitivity. Similar elements, including the TGF-$\beta$ control element are found as well in the promoter for SMMHC; thus, it should not be surprising that SMMHC expression also is induced by TGF-$\beta$ [8, 27]. Indeed, TGF-$\beta$ also increases SMMHC expression in cultured lung mesenchymal cells and it would appear that the same promoter regulatory elements are involved (Fig. 2). If TGF-$\beta$ is an important initiating signal in conditions of lung remodeling, such as seen in interstitial fibrosis, the important issue remains as to why the myofibroblast in these circumstances expresses SMA, but not SMMHC. Clues as to how this might occur have come from recent studies of the dependency of TGF-$\beta$ induction on altered matrix production (see the chapter by Gauldie et al., this volume) and the finding that the effects of TGF-$\beta$ on SMA expression is dependent on the three-dimensional nature of the matrix used to culture target cells (see the chapter by Narani et al., this volume).

## 5 Summary

Considerable progress has been made in defining the phenotype of contractile cells of the lung during development, in the adult and during the remodeling process. The high degree of phenotypic heterogeneity of subgroups of these cells, such as SMCs, is appreciated. Recent studies also have explored the relationship between phenotype and cell function, though this remains an important area for research in the coming years. Similarly, though our understanding of the regulation of cell phenotype is expanding rapidly, much remains to be done, particularly at the level of gene regulation. New transgenic models, coupled with gene-promotor analyses in transgenic animals and in cultured cells should allow rapid progress. Studies of the regulation of specific contractile and cytoskeletal proteins at the gene level by specific cytokines and extracellular-matrix elements will be particularly important.

# References

1. Babij P, Periasamy M (1989) Myosin heavy chain isoform diversity in smooth muscle is produced by differential RNA processing. J Mol Biol 210:673–679
2. Broekelman, TJ, Limper AH, Colby TV, McDonald JA (1991) Transforming growth factor-$\beta$1 is present at sites of extracellular matrix gene expression in human pulmonary fibroblasts. Proc Natl Acad Sci U S A 88:6642–6646
3. Burri PH (1985) Development and growth of the human lung. In: Fishman AP, Fisher AB (eds) Handbook of physiology: the respiratory system. American Physiological Society, Bethesda, pp 1–46
4. Desmouliére A, Gabbiani G (1995) Smooth muscle cell and fibroblast biological and functional features: similarities and differences. In: Schwartz S, Mecham R (eds) The vascular smooth muscle cell. Academic Press, New York, pp 329–359
5. Desmouliere A, Geinoz A, Gabbiani F, Gabbiani G (1993) Transforming growth factor-$\beta$1 induces alpha-smooth muscle actin expression in granulation tissue myofibroblasts and in quiescent and growing cultured fibroblasts. J Cell Biol 122:103–111
6. DiSanto ME, Cox RH, Wang Z, Chacko S (1997) NH2-terminal inserted myosin II heavy chain is expressed in smooth muscle of small muscular arteries. Am J Physiol 272: C1532–C1542
7. Gabbiani G, Ryan GB, Majno G (1971) Presence of modified fibroblasts in granulation tissue and their possible role in wound contraction. Experimentia 27:549–550
8. Hautmann MB, Madsen CS, Owens GK (1997) A transforming growth factor-$\beta$ (TGF-$\beta$) control element drives TGF-$\beta$-induced stimulation of smooth muscle alpha-actin expression in concert with two CArG elements. J Biol Chem 272:10948–10956
9. Jones R (1992) Ultrastructural analysis of contractile cell development in lung microvessels in hyperoxic pulmonary hypertension. Am J Pathol 141:1491–1505
10. Kapanci Y, Assimacopoulos I, Irle C, Zwahlen A, Gabbiani G (1974) "Contractile interstitial cells" in pulmonary alveolar septa: a possible regulator of ventilation/perfusion ratio? Ultrastructural, immunofluorescence and in vitro studies. J Cell Biol 60:375–392
11. Kapanci Y, Burgan S, Pietra GG, Conne B, Gabbiani G (1990) Modulation of actin isoform expression in alveolar myofibroblasts (contractile interstitial cells) during pulmonary hypertension. Am J Pathol 136:881–889
12. Kapanci Y, Gabbiani G (1997) Contractile cells in pulmonary alveolar tissue. In: Crystal RG, West JB (eds) The lung: scientific foundations. Lippincott-Raven, Philadelphia, pp 697–707
13. Kelley CA, Takahashi M, Yu JH, Adelstein RS (1993) An insert of seven amino acids confers functional differences between smooth muscle myosins from the intestines and vasculature. J Biol Chem 268:12848–12854
14. Kuro-O M, Nagai R, Buchimodu H, Katoh M, Yazaki Y, Ohkubo A, Takadu F (1989) Developmentally regulated expression of vascular smooth muscle myosin heavy chain isoforms. J Biol Chem 264:18272–18275
15. Leslie K, King TE Jr, Low R (1991) Smooth muscle actin is expressed by airspace fibroblast-like cells in idiopathic pulmonary fibrosis and hypersensitivity pneumonitis. Chest 99:47s–48s
16. Leslie KO, Mitchell J, Low RB (1992) Lung myofibroblasts. Cell Motil Cytoskel 22:92–98
17. Low RB, White SL (1998) Myosin heavy chain (SMHC) SM-B isoform is differentially expressed in developing and adult smooth muscle tissues of the rat. Chest 114:31s–33s
18. Low RB, White SL (1998) Lung smooth muscle differentiation. Int J Biochem Cell Biol (in press)
19. Mitchell JJ, Woodcock-Mitchell J, Perry L, Low RB, Baldor L, Absher M (1993) In vitro expression of the alpha-smooth muscle actin isoform by rat lung mesenchymal cells: regulation by culture conditions and transforming growth factor-$\beta$. Am J Respir Cell Mol Biol 9:10–18
20. Mitchell JJ, Reynolds SE, Leslie KO, Low RB, Woodcock-Mitchell J (1990) Smooth muscle cell markers in developing rat lung. Am J Respir Cell Mol Biol 3:515–523
21. Mitchell J, Woodcock-Mitchell J, Reynolds S, Low R, Leslie K, Adler K, Gabbiani G, Skalli O (1989) Alpha-smooth muscle actin in parenchymal cells of bleomycin-injured rat lung. Lab Invest 60:643–650

22. Owens G (1995) Regulation of differentiation of vascular smooth muscle cells. Physiol Rev 75:487–517
23. Pache J-C, Christakos PG, Gannon DE, Mitchell JJ, Low RB, Leslie, KO (1998) Myofibroblasts in diffuse alveolar damage of the lung. Mod Pathol (in press)
24. Roberts AB, Flanders KC, Heine UI, Jakowlew S, Kondaiah P, Kim SJ, Sporn MB (1990) Transforming growth factor-$\beta$: multifunctional regulator of differentiation and development. Philos Trans R Soc Lond B Biol Sci 327:145–154
25. Rovner AS, Freyzon Y, Trybus KM (1997) An insert in the motor domain determines the functional properties of expressed smooth muscle myosin isoforms. J Muscle Res Cell Motil 18:103–110
26. Skalli O, Schurch W, Seemayer T, Lagace R, Montandon D, Pittet B, Gabbiani G (1989) Myofibroblasts from diverse settings are heterogeneous in their content of actin isoorms and intermediate filament proteins. Lab Invest 60:275–285
27. White SL, Low RB (1996) Identification of promoter elements involved in cell-specific regulation of rat smooth muscle myosin heavy chain gene transcription. J Biol Chem 271:15008–15017
28. White S, Martin A, Periasamy M (1993) Identification of a novel smooth muscle myosin heavy chain cDNA: isoform diversity in the S1 head region. Am J Physiol 264:C1252–C1255
29. Woodcock-Mitchell J, White S, Stirewalt W, Periasamy M, Mitchell J, Low RB (1993) Myosin isoform expression in developing and remodeling rat lung. Am J Respir Cell Mol Biol 8:617–625

# Role of Platelet-Derived Growth Factors in Angiogenesis and Alveogenesis

P. Lindahl, H. Boström, L. Karlsson, M. Hellström, M. Kalén,
C. Betsholtz

## 1 Background

Platelet-derived growth factors (PGDFs) are 30-kDa dimeric proteins that exert their functions by binding to and activating PDGF receptors in the cell membrane [12, 22]. Two different PDGF monomers exist; the A chain and the B chain, and these may assemble into AA and BB homodimers as well as AB heterodimers. The two known PDGF-receptor proteins, the PDGF-$\alpha$ receptor (PDGF-R$\alpha$) and the $\beta$ receptor (PDGF-R$\beta$) are both receptor tyrosine kinases and interact differentially with the PDGF molecules; PDGF-R$\beta$ binds only the PDGF B chain with high affinity, whereas PDGF-R$\alpha$ binds both chains with high affinity. Accordingly, the different PDGF dimers may bind to, dimerize and signal through different receptor pairs. Dimerization of the receptors is a prerequisite for signaling, since it allows for tyrosine phosphorylation of the intracellular part of the receptor molecules [11]. The resulting phosphotyrosine residues constitute binding sites for molecules carrying src-homology-2 (SH2) and other phosphotyrosine-binding domains. Their association with the PDGF receptor is a critical step in downstream signaling [5, 13].

PDGF receptors are usually localized to connective-tissue cells, which may respond to PDGF through several activities – mitogenesis, migration, contraction, extracellular-matrix synthesis, cytokine production and others [1].

## 2 PDGF and PDGF Receptor Knockout Mice

The two PDGF chains and the two PDGF receptors are encoded with different chromosomal locations. The two PDGF ligand genes, PDGF-A and PDGF-B, as well as the two receptor genes, PDGF-R$\alpha$ and PDGF-R$\beta$, have all been inactivated in the mouse by homologous recombination in embryonic stem cells [2, 14, 28, 29]. All four mutations are lethal, although at different stages of embryonic and early post-

Current Topics in Pathology, Volume 93
A. Desmoulière, B. Tuchweber (Eds.)
© Springer-Verlag Berlin Heidelberg 1999

natal development. PDGF-B- and -R$\beta$-null embryos die at late gestation (E16–19) and display indistinguishable phenotypes [14, 28]. Since there is generally a risk that certain phenotypes seen in mutant mice generated by gene targeting do not occur as a result of loss of the targeted gene, but as a result of effects on neighboring loci (neighborhood effects) [21], the high degree of similarity between the PDGF-B- and -R$\beta$-null mice strongly suggests that the phenotypes are caused by the absence of PDGF-B and PDGF-R$\beta$, respectively. The similarity further suggests that the major ligand for R$\beta$ is PDGF-B, which is consistent with in vitro data, and that the major receptor for PDGF-B is R$\beta$, although in vitro data have suggested that R$\alpha$ is also a major receptor for PDGF-B.

PDGF-A knockouts show a spectrum of viability restriction points [2]. A large proportion of these embryos die at approximately E10, whereas those surviving this period develop until term with minor problems. Postnatal development of several organ systems is, however, compromised in PDGF-A knockouts and these mutants normally die from severe pulmonary disease at the age of 2–6 weeks. PDGF-R$\alpha$ knockouts appear to die uniformly at E14–16 [29]. There are several possible explanations for the difference between the phenotypes of PDGF-A and R$\alpha$ knockouts. As indicated above, one or several of the phenotypes described for these mice (see below for further details) may not relate to the absence of PDGF-A or -R$\alpha$, respectively, but to neighborhood effects. There is only limited information available on the organization of the PDGF-A and -R$\alpha$ in relation to neighboring loci. The KIT locus, which is located in the vicinity of PDGF-R$\alpha$ [3, 27, 30], is not likely to be affected by the targeted PDGF-R$\alpha$ mutation, since these mice do not display the pigmentation defects typical of KIT mutants. Another explanation for discrepancies between PDGF-A and -R$\alpha$ knockouts is the possibility that PDGFB may partially substitute for the loss of PDGF-A since it can bind to R$\alpha$. Other explanations involve the transfer of gene product from the mother to the embryo. This may occur for PDGF-A, but is not likely for PDGF-R$\alpha$, unless soluble forms of the receptor exist and may cross the placenta. In summary, the reason(s) for the different phenotypes between PDGF-A- and -R$\alpha$-null embryos remains to be explored.

## 3  Role of PDGF-B and -R$\beta$ in the Recruitment of the Vascular Wall

PDGF-B- and -R$\beta$-null embryos die at late gestation from widespread vascular leakage and hemorrhage. They show cardiac defects consisting primarily of a hypotrophic myocardium. They also show abnormal kidney glomeruli resulting from the absence of mesangial cells [14, 28]. The vascular leakage and hemorrhage is most likely caused by pericyte deficiency [16]. Pericytes are mesenchymal smooth-muscle-cell-like cells that encase capillaries and locate within the capillary endothelial basement membrane [26]. When new blood vessels form through an angiogenic process (sprouting of new vessels from preexisting ones) [10], vascular-wall cells have to be recruited. Two models have been presented for such recruitment, one proposing that undifferentiated mesenchymal cells surrounding the endothelium are induced to undergo smooth-muscle-cell differentiation [9], and the other proposing that pericytes from the preexisting vessel wall migrate on the basal side of the endothelium from the root to the tip of the angiogenic sprout [19]. The pericyte deficiency in PDGF-B- and -R$\beta$-null embryos appears to result from deficient spreading of pericyte precursors along angiogenic sprouts [16]. The endothelial cells of the sprout express PDGF-B and the pericyte precursors express PDGF-R$\beta$, implying that this spreading of pericyte progenitors is controlled through paracrine signaling. It is not possible to conclude from these observations that migration is the cellular function controlled by PDGF-B. The data are equally consistent with the possibility that proliferation of the pericyte progenitors is driven by PDGF-B. Pericyte proliferation would be a prerequisite for the spreading and coverage of a rapidly expanding vascular network, such as the one in the developing embryo, if a limited number of pericyte progenitors are available for the earliest stages of co-recruitment. This issue needs further study.

The pericyte loss in PDGF-B- and -R$\beta$-null embryos is not uniform. Organs such as liver contain a normal number of specialized liver pericytes (ito- or fat-storing cells), whereas organs such as the brain and the heart show an almost complete loss of pericytes. This implies that the development of vascular-wall cells occurs by different mechanisms at different sites and that both PDGF-dependent and PDGF-independent pericyte development exists [16] (Hellström et al, unpublished results).

The lack of glomerular mesangial cells in PDGF-B- and -R$\beta$-null embryos is principally and mechanistically similar to the loss of pericytes at other sites, and appears to be a result of failure of comigration of mesangial cells with the endothelial sprout entering into the developing glomerulus. Glomerular endothelial cells express PDGF-B and mesangial cells express PDGF-R$\beta$, again implying that a paracrine PDGF-B signal is vital for the recruitment of mesangial cells into the developing glomerular tuft [18].

The extensive hemorrhaging seen in late-stage PDGF-B- and -R$\beta$-null embryos is preceded by microaneurysm formation [16]. A correlation between pericyte dropout from the capillary wall and microaneurysm formation has been pointed out before, in conjunction with diabetic retinopathy [4, 6]. In this disease, however, it has not been clear whether pericyte dropout causes microaneurysm formation or occurs as a result of microaneurysm formation. In the PDGF-B and PDGF-R$\beta$ mutant mouse embryos, it is highly likely that the absence of pericytes causes microaneurysms. In this instance, pericytes, but not endothelial cells, carry PDGF-R$\beta$ and are, therefore, the primary targets for PDGF-B or -R$\beta$ deficiency. Any effects on the endothelial cells, such as microaneurysm formation, should be secondary.

Microaneurysm formation secondary to pericyte loss may relate to a reduced capacity of the capillary to withstand high blood pressure. The onset of hemorrhage in PDGF-B and -R$\beta$ mutant embryos occurs close to birth and may correlate with the increase in systemic blood pressure expected to occur at this time. The pericytes may, thus, have a role in providing mechanical support to small blood vessels. However, it is becoming increasingly apparent that signaling from periendothelial cells to endothelial cells is critical in the control of endothelial-cell proliferation, differentiation and function. In this context, the angiopoietins, which bind to the endothelial tie-2 receptor molecule, are of particular interest, since they are expressed by periendothelial cells and appear to have a critical role in the maturation of the vascular endothelium [7]. Lack of tie-2 or angiopoietin-1 results in embryonic death [8, 25, 31]. The vascular phenotype of these mutants include lack of endothelial integrity and reduction in the amount of vascular-wall cells. The latter is also seen in human venous malformation, a inheritable syndrome caused by a mutation in the tie-2 locus [32]. It is likely that the vascular-wall defects of tie-2 and Ang-1 mutants occur indirectly, since the vascular-wall cells are devoid of tie-2 receptors, and it has been proposed that these defects may result from altered PDGF-B expression in endothelial cells [32]. However, the vascular phenotype of tie-2 and ang-1 knockouts is far more severe than in PDGF-B and -R$\beta$ knockouts, arguing that endothelial functions other than PDGF-B expression, which are important for vascular-wall recruitment, have to be regulated by the ang-1/tie-2 system. Similar to the microanerysms in PDGF-B and -R$\beta$ mutants, these defects highlight the important reciprocal signaling between vascular endothelium and periendothelial support cells, such as pericytes and vascular smooth muscle cells.

In summary, the phenotypes of PDGF-B- and -R$\beta$-null mouse embryos suggest a role for this ligand-receptor pair in blood-vessel formation, particularly in the recruitment of smooth muscle cells and pericytes to newly formed vessels.

## 4  Role of PDGF-A and R$\alpha$ in the Recruitment of Alveolar Smooth-Muscle Cell

PDGF-A-null mice die at pre- or early postnatal periods [2]. Although the reason for the variability in survival capacity is unclear at the moment, there are reasons to believe that genetic background may play a role. Postnatally surviving PDGF-A-null mice develop a severe pulmonary emphysema, which is also the likely cause of death. The emphysema reflects the complete lack of alveolar septa but, rather than occurring as a result of septal destruction as in human emphysema, the PDGF-A-null phenotype results from the failure of alveolar septum formation. This process normally begins around 1 week of age and is completed by 3 weeks of age. Septum formation correlates with pronounced deposition of elastin in the developing septal wall and it has been proposed that elastin deposition is a driving force in septation [20]. Using different types of markers for developing lungs, we studied alveolar septation in normal mice and its failure in PDGF-A-null mice [17]. We found that normal alveolar septa contains smooth muscle cells (alveolar SMC) which were positive for $\alpha$-smooth-muscle actin (ASMA), whereas PDGF-A-null mice lacked such cells [2]. The alveolar SMC appears to stem from a population of PDGF-R$\alpha$-positive mesenchymal cells residing at the buds of the epithelial branches at the pseudoglandular stage of lung development (until approximately E16.5). Next, at the canalicular and saccular stages (E16.5 to birth), these cells spread along the distal tubules to position as singular cells in the walls of the alveolar saccules. The multiplication and spreading of the PDGF-R$\alpha$-positive cells failed in PDGF-A-null lungs; instead, the cells remained at more proximal locations surrounding the terminal bronchioles [17]. The developing respiratory epithelium expresses PDGF-A, suggesting that paracrine signaling promotes the proliferation and distal spreading of PDGF-R$\alpha$-positive cells in the lung. In conjunction with alveogenesis, a scattered cell type with a similar location to the PDGF-R$\alpha$-positive cells begins to express tropoelastin very strongly. This expression lasts as long as alveogenesis proceeds. Lack of temporal overlap in expression makes it difficult to formally prove that the PDGF-R$\alpha$-positive cells and the later tropoelastin-positive cells belong to the same lineage. However, both types are lost in PDGF-A knockouts, as are the later occurring ASMA-positive alveolar SMCs. This, combined with the fact that electron microscopy failed to reveal the lack of any other cell type in the lung apart from the alveolar SMCs, strongly suggests that PDGF-R$\alpha$ and tropoelastin are both early, but temporally separate markers for the alveolar SMC lineage.

## 5 Functional Analogies

The analysis of PDGF-A- and PDGFB-null mice reveal different levels of the analogies between PDGF functions, which were recently discussed [15]. First, both PDGF-A and PDGF-B appear to drive the development of certain types of smooth muscle cells. In the case of PDGF-A, the ligand is produced by epithelial cells, and the smooth muscle cells affected are spatially closely associated with the epithelium, as in the case of alveolar SMCs, which are in close contact with the respiratory epithelium. PDGF-B is produced by vascular endothelial cells and act on vascular smooth muscle progenitors, and promote their corecruitment along capillary sprouts. Thus, a generic function of PDGF-family ligands is to control the development of distal or "secondary" populations of smooth muscle cells.

Another level of analogy relates to the functions of the cells controlled by PDGFs. The lung emphysema in PDGF-A knockouts reveals a critical role for the alveolar SMC in alveolar septum formation, a process which leads to folding of the respiratory epithelium and the generation of a substantially increased area involved in gas exchange. A similar role may be proposed for the glomerular mesangial cells controlled by PDGF-B. In the absence of PDGF-B and mesangial cells, a glomerular tuft of capillaries is not formed. Rather, a single capillary loop fills the Bowman's space. Clearly, folding of the glomerular basement membrane and branching of glomerular capillaries is under the influence of mesangial cells. This leads to enlargement of the active surface involved in filtration of the blood and primary urine production. The SMC types also appear critical in providing structural support to the respiratory units and the capillaries. Absence of the alveolar SMC leads to dilation and the subsequent rupture of the peripheral lung tissue, causing pneumothorax. Absence of pericytes and mesangial cells leads to microaneurysm formation and the subsequent vessel rupture and hemorrhage.

## 6 Perspectives

A number of phenotypes in PDGF and PDGF-receptor knockouts are still unexplored at the level of cellular interactions, and the analysis of these phenotypes will undoubtedly challenge the hypothesis presented above concerning generic functions for PDGFs and PDGF-dependent cells in embryonic development. Genetic analysis of PDGF functions in the adult life and in disease is not straightforward, since all mutants are lethal. However, refined gene-targeting technologies, such as conditional mutagenesis, the introduction of small mutations and the generation of chimeras between mutant and wild-type cells by, e.g., tissue transplantation, may potentially circumvent these problems. In the near future, it should, therefore, be possible to experimentally test existing hypotheses concerning the involvement of PDGF in diseases such as atherosclerosis, rheumatoid disease, cancer and other conditions in which pathogenic roles of PDGFs have been implicated [23, 24, 33, 34].

# References

1. Betsholtz C, Raines E (1997). Platelet-derived growth factor: a key regulator of connective tissue cells in embryogenesis and pathogenesis. Kidney Int. 51:1361–1369
2. Boström H, Willetts K, Pekny M, Levéen P, Lindahl P, Hedstrand H, Pekna M, Hellström M, Gebre-Medhin S, Schalling M, Nilsson M, Kurland S, TörnellJ, Heath JK, Betsholtz C (1996) PDGF-A signaling is a critical event in lung alveolar myofibroblast development and alveogenesis. Cell 85:863–873
3. Brunkow ME, Nagle DL, Bernstein A, Bucan M (1995) A 1.8-Mb YAC contig spanning three members of the receptor tyrosine kinase gene family (Pdgfra, Kit and Flk-1) on mouse chromosome 5. Genomics 25:421–432
4. Buzney SM, Frank RN, Varma SD, Tanishima T, Gabbay KH (1977) Aldose reductase in retinal mural cells. Invest Ophthalmol Vis Sci 16:392–396
5. Claesson-Welsh L (1994) Platelet-derived growth factor receptor signals. J Biol Chem 269: 32023–32026
6. Cogan DG, Toussaint D, Kuwabara T (1961) Retinal vascular patterns. IV. Diabetic retinopathy. Arch Ophthalmol 66:366–378
7. Davis S, Aldrich TH, Jones PF, Acheson A, Compton DL, Jain V, Ryan TE, Bruno J, Radziejewski C, Maisonpierre PC, Yancopolous GD (1996) Isolation of angiopoietin-1, a ligand for the TIE2 receptor by secretion-trap expression cloning. Cell 87:1161–1169
8. Dumont D. Gradwohl JG, Fong GH, Puri MC, Gertsenstein M, Auerbach A, Breitman ML (1994) Dominant-negative and targeted null mutations in the endothelil receptor tyrosin kinase tek, reveal a critical in vasculogenesis of the embryo. Genes Dev 8:1897–1909
9. Folkman J, D'Amore PA (1996) Blood vessel formation: what is its molecular basis? Cell 87:1153–1155
10. Folkman J, Shing Y (1992) Angiogenesis. J Biol Chem 267:10931–10934
11. Heldin CH (1995) Dimerization of cell surface receptors in signal transduction. Cell 80: 213–223
12. Heldin CH (1992) Structural and functional studies of platelet-derived growth factor. EMBO J 11:4251–4259
13. Kazlauskas A (1994) Receptor tyrosine kinases and their targets. Curr Opin Genet Dev 4:5–14
14. Levéen P, Pekny M, Gebre-Medhin S, Swolin B, Larsson E, Betsholtz C (1994) Mice deficient for PDGF B show renal, cardiovascular, and hematological abnormalities. Genes Dev 8:1875–1887
15. Lindahl P, Betsholtz C (1998) Not all myofibroblasts are alike: revisiting the role of PDGF-A and PDGF-B using PDGF-targeted mice. Curr Opin Nephrol Hypert 7:21–26
16. Lindahl P, Johansson B, Levéen P, Betsholtz C (1997) Pericyte loss and microaneurysm formation in PDGF-B-deficient mice. Science 277:242–245
17. Lindahl P, Karlsson L, Hellström M, Gebre-Medhin S, Willetts K, Heath JK, Betsholtz C (1997) Alveogenesis failure in PDGF-A deficient mice is coupled to lack of distal spreading of alveolar smooth muscle cell progenitors during lung development. Development 124:3943–3953
18. Lindahl P, Hellström M, Kalén M, Karlsson L, Pekny M, Pekna M, Soriano P, Betsholtz C (1998) Paracrine PDGF-B/PDGF-R$\beta$ signaling controls mesangial cell development in kidney glomeruli. Development 125:3313–3322

19. Nicosia RF, Villaschi S (1995) Rat aortic smooth muscle cells become pericytes during angiogenesis in vitro. Lab Invest 73:658–666
20. Noguchi A, Samaha H (1991) Developmental changes in tropoelastin gene expression in the rat lung studied by in situ hybridization. Am J Respir Cell Mol Biol 5:571–578
21. Olson EN, Arnold HH, Rigby PWJ, Wold BJ (1996) Know your neighbors: three phenotypes in null mutants of the myogenic bHLH gene MRF4. Cell 85:1–4
22. Raines EW, Bowen-Pope DF, Ross R (1990) Platelet-derived growth factor. In: Sporn MB, Roberts AB (eds) Peptide growth factors and their receptors. Springer-Verlag, Berlin Heidelberg New York, pp 173–262 (Handbook of Experimental Pharmacology, vol 95 part I)
23. Ross R (1993) The pathogenesis of atherosclerosis: a perspective for the 1990s. Nature 362:801–809
24. Ross R, Raines EW, Bowen-Pope DF (1986) The biology of platelet-derived growth factor. Cell 46:155–169
25. Sato TN, Tozawa Y, Deutch U, Wolburg-Buchholz K, Fujiwara Y, Gendron-Maguire M, Gridley T, Wolburg H, Risau W, Qin Y (1995) Distinct roles of the receptor tyrosine kinases Tie-1 and Tie-2 in blood vessel formation. Nature 376:70–74
26. Sims DE (1986) The pericyte – a review. Tissue Cell 18:153–174
27. Smith EA, Seldin MF, Martinez L, Watson ML, Choudhury GG, Lalley PA, Pierce J, Aaronson SA, Barker J, Naylor SL, Sakaguchi AY (1991) Mouse platelet-derived growth factor receptor a gene is deleted in W19H and patch mutations on chromosome 5. Proc Natl Acad Sci U S A 88:4811–4815
28. Soriano P (1994) Abnormal kidney development and hematological disorders in PDGF beta-receptor mutant mice. Genes Dev 8:1888–1896
29. Soriano P (1997) The PDGF alpha receptor is required for neural crest cell survival and for normal patterning of the somites. Development 124:2691–2700
30. Stephenson DA, Mercola M, Anderson E, Wang C, Stiles CD, Bowen Popc DF, Chapman VM (1991) Platelet-derived growth factor receptor a-subunit gene (PDGFra) is deleted in the patch (Ph) mutation. Proc Natl Acad Sci U S A 88:6–10
31. Suri C, Jones PF, Patan S, Bartunkova S, Maisonpierre PC, Davis S, Sato TN, Yancopolous GD (1996) Requisite role of angiopoietin-1, a ligand for the TIE2 receptor, during embryonic development. Cell 87:1171–1180
32. Vikkula ML, Boon M, Carraway KL III, Calvert JT, Diamonti AJ, Goumnerov B, Pasyk KA, Marchuk DA, Warman ML, Cantley LC, Mulliken JB, Olsen BR (1996) Vascular dysmorphogenesis caused by an activating mutation in the receptor tyrosine kinase TIE2. Cell 87:1181–1190
33. Westermark B, Heldin CH (1991) Platelet-derived growth factor in autocrine transformation. Cancer Res 51:5087–5092
34. Westermark B, Sorg CE (1993) Biology of platelet-derived growth factor, vol 5, Karger, Basel

# Transforming Growth Factor-$\beta$ Gene Transfer to the Lung Induces Myofibroblast Presence and Pulmonary Fibrosis

J. Gauldie, P. J. Sime, Z. Xing, B. Marr, G. M. Tremblay

## 1 Introduction

Many cytokines have been implicated in the initiation or propagation of fibrogenesis. In particular, the early-phase inflammatory cytokines, interleukin (IL) and tumor necrosis factor (TNF), and members of the chemokine families, including IL and monocyte chemotactic peptide (MCP-1) are known to be present in inflamed tissue, both at the beginning and at advanced stages of fibrosis. In addition, growth and differentiating factors, such as the fibroblast growth factors (FGFs), transforming growth factors (TGFs) and platelet-derived growth factors (PDGFs) are all implicated in the pathogenesis of fibrosis through their putative mode of action and demonstrated presence in fibrotic tissue. Most data implicating the various cytokines arises from studies involving immunohistochemistry or detection of gene expression within fibrotic tissue and from in vitro experiments showing activity on matrix formation by structural cells (fibroblasts, smooth-muscle cells, etc.).

In addition to the presence of enhanced-matrix deposition, the presence of myofibroblasts within the fibrotic tissue is an additional component of fibrogenesis. Some fibrogenic cytokines, including TGF$\beta$ and granulocyte macrophage-colony stimulating factor (GM-CSF), are known to induce myofibroblast differentiation in vivo and/or in vitro [5, 7, 8, 12, 22–24, 32]. Whether the presence of myofibroblasts in fibrotic tissue arises as a result of differentiation from fibroblasts or other precursor cells is not known. However, the conceptual process of fibrogenesis involves the presence of tissue injury, the release of fibrogenic cytokines, the induction of myofibroblasts and enhanced-matrix deposition, all within the context of chronic tissue remodelling with resultant organ dysfunction [3, 10, 14, 31, 28, 37].

There are limiting factors when exploring the specific role of any single cytokine in the fibrogenic process. Available in vivo systems are limited by the fact that most cytokines have very short half-lives in circulation (in the order of 20 – 30 min) and the delivery of recombinant protein to mimic the sustained presence of raised

Current Topics in Pathology, Volume 93
A. Desmoulière, B. Tuchweber (Eds.)
© Springer-Verlag Berlin Heidelberg 1999

levels of these individual factors within the tissue is limited to only a few accessible tissue sites. We have had a long-standing interest in pursuing the pathogenesis of pulmonary fibrosis and have developed an approach that allows investigation of the in vivo function of single-cytokine genes when present at raised levels over an extended, but not permanent period of time. These approaches have allowed us to define the role of some significant factors in inducing myofibroblast presence and fibrotic-tissue changes within the lung.

## 2 Cytokine-Gene Transfer with Adenovirus Vectors

In order to mimic the conditions related to a prolonged inflammatory response, which is thought to be a precursor to the fibrogenic outcome, we have developed a series of replication-deficient adenoviral vectors expressing cytokine genes to accomplish the transient, but sustained release of the individual gene product (in this case the cytokine) within lung tissue [2, 29, 33]. Adenoviral vectors are the most efficient for transient transfer of genes, particularly to epithelial cells. The intratracheal instillation of a vector results in the transfer of the gene with an expression driven by a high-efficiency promoter, such as the cytomegalovirus (CMV) promoter, to the airway's epithelial cells. As a result, the gene product is expressed at high levels, both within the lumen of the lung and within the paren-chymal tissue. The marked expression begins within 24 h of the administration of the vector, resulting in raised levels of the cytokine present in lung washings [bronchoalveolar lavage fluid (BAL)] as well as in serum over a 7-day to 10-day period [29, 34, 36]. The use of a high-efficiency promoter allows us to deliver a low load of viral vector, which results in only low-background inflammation. Sub-sequently, we can interpret the changes seen as being the result of biological effects by the transgene product and this overexpression can be instituted on either a mouse or rat with a normal adult background. Moreover, it has the ability to be initiated on any background of choice, such as in neonatal stages or in a series of knockout mouse models.

The work described below restricts itself to interpretation of cytokine-gene func-tion within the lung, but the same approach can be applied to a number of other tissues, since adenovirus vectors can infect a wide variety of cell types without inte-gration into the genome. Furthermore, "transient transgenic expression" within the tissue can be accomplished in a reasonably organ-restrictive manner [2, 33, 36].

Using this approach, we have shown that members of the various chemokine families can be expressed, resulting in pulmonary accumulation of a spectrum of inflammatory cells. However, as the expression of the gene product terminates, the cells recede from the lung (possibly by apoptosis) and the lung returns to normal function over a period of 7–21 days [1, 9]. This is also the case for a number of other cytokines such as IL-6 [36]. However, several cytokines have led to more pro-found tissue reactions with fibrogenic sequelae in the lung and these will be de-scribed below.

## 3 Tumor Necrosis Factor $\alpha$

TNF$\alpha$ has been implicated in the fibrogenic process as demonstrated in several studies. Certainly, it is a well-accepted concept that TNF$\alpha$ is a highly inflammatory cytokine, capable of eliciting a wide variety of tissue responses [19,20,21,31]. Studies have shown that TNF-neutralizing antibodies given prior to the administration of either bleomycin or silica to the lung results in abrogation of fibrotic responses, even though administration of recombinant TNF$\alpha$ alone under those conditions did not initiate a fibrogenic process [21]. Further studies using a tissue-specific promoter of the surfactant protein C (SPC) driving transgenic expression of TNF have shown the presence of marked inflammatory changes to the transgenic lung and the induction of a fibrogenic response, somewhat limited in nature, however, clearly developing complications of the prolonged expression of TNF [18].

We have constructed an adenoviral vector expressing the murine TNF$\alpha$ gene driven by the murine CMV promoter and instilled this into the lung of Sprague-Dawley rats (P.J. Sime et al., unpublished observations). Over the course of the tissue expression, TNF$\alpha$ levels in lavage fluid were detected as high as 150 ng/ml, which represents exceptionally high levels of TNF$\alpha$ within the lung tissue. The extent of expression was over 7 days or 8 days. Tissue-morphology examination has shown extensive inflammatory changes to the lung as early as 3 days, with accumulation of inflammatory cells and some structural alterations to the lung. The inflammatory changes continue to be present over 7–10 days, but there was a remarkable lack of evidence of tissue destruction (P. J. Sime et al., unpublished observations). Given the very high amounts of TNF and the presence of inflammatory cells, this was contrary to what was expected. However, there was limited evidence of matrix deposition in scattered areas throughout the lung and, as the inflammation resolved, these scarring areas remained. There was a marked presence of myofibroblasts, as detected by the immunohistochemical localisation of smooth-muscle actin-positive cells [5, 22, 24, 25, 27], in the early stages of inflammation, which slowly resolved. However, residual presence of these cells remained, consistent with the limited fibrotic changes seen, up to 60 days.

When the lavage fluid was examined for the presence of other cytokines, the most significant change seen was the presence of raised levels of TGF$\beta$, consistent with the timing of the presence of myofibroblasts and the onset of the fibrogenic

**Table 1.** Cytokines that induce smooth muscle actin

| | Hu Lung Fbl recombinant protein in vitro | Ad Vector gene transfer in vivo |
|---|---|---|
| Tumor necrosis factor $\alpha$ | (–) | + |
| Granulocyte macrophage-colony stimulating factor | (–) | ++ |
| Transforming growth factor $\beta$1 | +++ | ++++ |
| Connective-tissue growth factor | ? | ? |

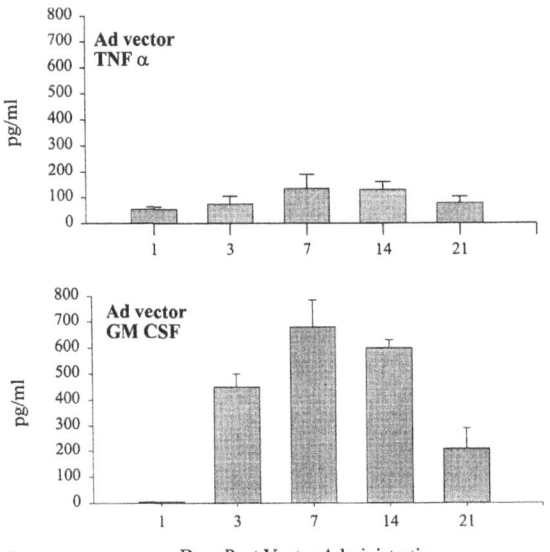

**Fig. 1 a, b.** Total TGF levels in bronchoalveolar lavage (BAL) fluids after administration of fibrogenic cytokines through use of adenovirus vectors

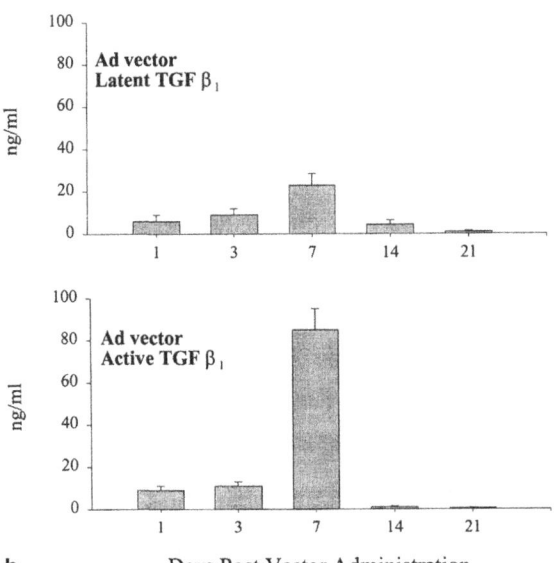

process (Fig. 1a; Tables 1, 2). As a result, it can be concluded that TNFα over-expression in such a tissue-restricted and prolonged manner can result in a dramatic inflammatory response; the induction of myofibroblasts and TGFβ, and the onset of fibrogenesis. Of note, the extent and intensity of fibrosis were limited, which was inconsistent with high levels of TNF present in the tissue (P. J. Sime et al., unpublished observations).

Table 2. Transforming growth factor (TGF), myofibroblasts and fibrosis after cytokine gene transfer in vivo (Ad Vector in vivo)

| | Levels of TGF-$\beta_1$ in BAL | Smooth muscle actin myofibroblasts | Fibrosis |
|---|---|---|---|
| Tumor necrosis factor $\alpha$ | 150 pg/ml | + | + |
| GM–CSF | 600 pg/ml | ++ | ++ |
| TGF-$\beta_1$ | >50 ng/ml | ++++ | ++++ |
| Chemokines | n.d. | (–) | (–) |

## 4 Granulocyte Macrophage-Colony Stimulating Factor

Another factor which has been implicated in the fibrogenic process is GM-CSF. While this cytokine has been found upregulated in a number of lung diseases, it is particularly associated with chronic allergic airways eosinophilic inflammation. The capacity for GM-CSF to influence stromal-cell differentiation is less well documented, although GM-CSF has been shown to modify fibroblast-colony formation in at least one in vitro assessment [6]. One further study with chronic administration of GM-CSF through a mini-osmotic pump in a subcutaneous site implied that it may contribute to fibrogenesis, although possibly in an indirect manner [24].

We created a vector that expressed murine GM-CSF and instilled this into the trachea of rats [33–35]. GM-CSF is known to be species specific; however, rodents respond equally well to the murine cytokine. Once again, the expression of the cytokine was evident within 24 h and remained raised over a period of 7–10 days and was detectable both in the lavage fluid and in the serum. The levels of GM-CSF were considerably higher (up to 30 ng/ml BAL fluid) than those seen in a model of lung transgenic overexpression of GM-CSF [11].

As a result of the extended expression of this cytokine, chronic tissue eosinophilia was seen throughout the lung parenchyma. This eosinophilia lasted for up to 12 days and was the expected result commensurate with the known function of GM-CSF in hemopoietic differentiation. However, two further changes occurred over the subsequent period of examination. The first was evidence of macrophage granuloma formation with multinucleate giant cells apparent within the parenchyma of the lung, and the emergence of areas of scar formation and an intermediate level of fibrotic tissue generation. There were expanded areas of myofibroblast present within the tissue and the distribution of these smooth-muscle actin (SMA)-positive cells was consistent with the patchy distribution of fibrosis that was seen. These tissue changes were more extensive than those seen with the TNF model (above) and were present until the termination of the experiment (40 days). Similar to our study with TNF, we measured other cytokines in the lung and found that there were no detectable levels of TNF generated throughout the experiment, thereby ruling out a role for TNF in this direct initiation of fibrogenesis. At the same time, we found raised levels of TGF with concentrations up to 600 pg/ml of BAL fluid and a time frame of presence consistent with the onset of the fibrogenic process. The level of TGF in BAL was greater than that seen in the TNF model, as was the presence of the myofibroblast and the extent of the fibrotic changes seen in the lung [30, 33–35].

## 5 Transforming Growth Factor β

Considering the details described above, it was necessary to determine the effects of expressing TGFβ within the lung parenchyma, as this cytokine has been implicated from extensive in vitro studies in regulating matrix formation [7, 22, 23]. In addition, we have shown that TGFβ can directly induce SMA expression in pulmonary fibroblasts in culture (Fig. 2). Moreover, in vivo delivery of recombinant protein through the use of mini-osmotic pumps induced marked fibrogenic changes in subcutaneous tissue, along with the induction of myofibroblasts [7, 8].

TGFβ is one of a family of proteins with synthesis that involves the initial release of a large propeptide made up of one component representing the active fragment and another larger component (the latency associated peptide), which is cleaved prior to releasing the active fragment. On cleavage, two molecules of the active fragment associate through disulphide-bond interaction and two molecules of the latency-associated peptide also associate themselves through disulphide-bond formation. These two dimers then become associated through non-covalent interaction, resulting in a latent form of TGFβ, which requires activation to release the active form of TGFβ [16, 17]. This activation process is not fully known in vivo, but may involve the action of enzymes such as plasmin [15–17, 26]. The molecule is also known to contribute to autoactivation, giving rise to prolonged expression of the TGFβ gene in stromal cells such as fibroblasts stimulated with active TGFβ. The product from these cells is primarily the latent form, while the product from activated myeloid cells such as macrophage appears to be in the active form [13, 15, 16].

Recently, a mutated form of TGFβ was described in which point mutations were introduced to change the cysteine code to serine, resulting in the latency-associated peptides no longer being able to form a dimer through disulphide-bond interaction and, therefore, no longer being able to bind to and inhibit the active form of TGFβ [4]. The use of this mutated form of TGFβ would result in the release of fully active TGFβ.

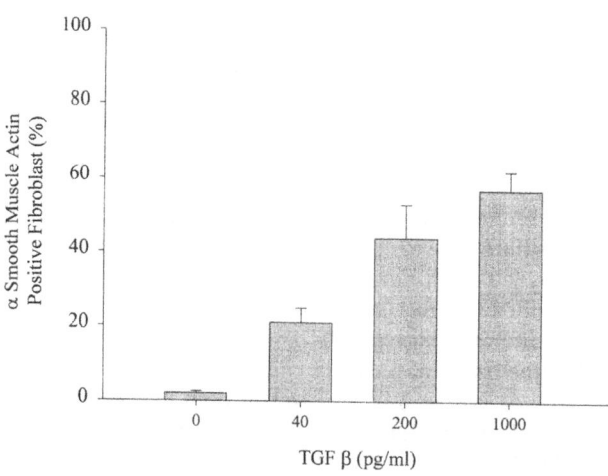

Fig. 2. Smooth muscle actin induction in human lung fibroblasts by treatment (24 h) with purified transforming growth factor

We constructed two separate adenoviral vectors, one encoding the full length latent form of TGF$\beta$ and one encoding the full length, but mutated (active) form of TGF$\beta$ [29]. Instillation of the vector encoding the latent form caused prolonged presence of markedly raised levels of latent TGF$\beta$ over a 10-day period, but little detectable levels of active TGF$\beta$ in the BAL fluid (Fig. 1b). Histologic examination showed the accumulation of mononuclear cells over 3–5 days of maximum expression, with little evidence of tissue destruction (Fig. 3). This inflammatory cell accumulation subsequently resolved as the expression of TGF$\beta$ waned and, by 21 days, the lung showed no evidence of residual inflammatory changes and no evidence of fibrogenesis [29]. However, when the vector that expressed the spontaneously active form of TGF$\beta$ was instilled intratracheally, a drastically different pattern of responses emerged. Within 24 h there was evidence of raised levels of total TGF$\beta$ in the BAL fluid accompanied by raised active levels (up to 12 ng/ml BAL), which persisted over a number of days, with a dramatically increased level of latent TGF$\beta$ seen at 7 days (Fig. 1b). Subsequently, the levels of both active and latent TGF$\beta$ became undetectable in the lavage fluid from about 10 days onward. The raised level of latent TGF$\beta$ detected at 7 days most likely was the result of autocrine stimulation due to the presence of active TGF$\beta$, achieved by gene transfer, causing the upregulation of the endogenous TGF$\beta$ gene. These findings may give some hint as to mechanisms associated with chronic tissue stimulation.

On examination of morphologic changes, there was ample evidence of fibroblast accumulation and scar formation in the lung and, within 3 days, evidence of accumulation of mononuclear cells and polymorphonuclear cells throughout the lung (Fig. 3). Despite the dramatic evidence of inflammation, there was little evidence of actual tissue destruction, rather remodelling was more evident. Scar formation continued over the extent of the experiment (60 days). Gene expression was no longer evident at 10 days, yet scar formation at 7 days and 14 days showed an increasing deposition of matrix. An examination for myofibroblast content showed a steadily increased presence of myofibroblasts throughout the lung parenchyma with a dramatic spread of scar tissue evident throughout the lung. The fibrogenic response continued, until by day 60 the lung was shrunken on gross examination. Most striking were changes seen in the pleural surface of the lung, where there was gross thickening and deposition of matrix proteins which appeared within 14 days and were still present at 60 days (Fig. 3). This surprising element, also seen in idiopathic pulmonary fibrosis, was evident even though the gene was delivered only to the bronchial luminal surface of the lung, yet manifest itself at a distal tissue site by modifying the structure of the pleural surface of the lung.

The levels of detection of active and/or total TGF$\beta$ and the extensive presence of myofibroblasts and fibrosis would appear to be closely related. On examination of a number of other cytokine-gene products, there was no evidence of TNF$\alpha$, bFGF or PDGF, which were some of the cytokines thought to be involved in the fibrogenic process. We did, however, see expression of connective-tissue growth factor (CTGF), a factor known to be activated downstream from TGF$\beta$ and thought to be involved in matrix formation through stimulation of fibroblasts and other stromal cells.

Thus, the presence of the latent gene product of TGF$\beta$ by itself was not fibrogenic. However, the activation of that gene product and release of active TGF$\beta$ are clearly required for the initiation of the fibrogenic response. The level of expression

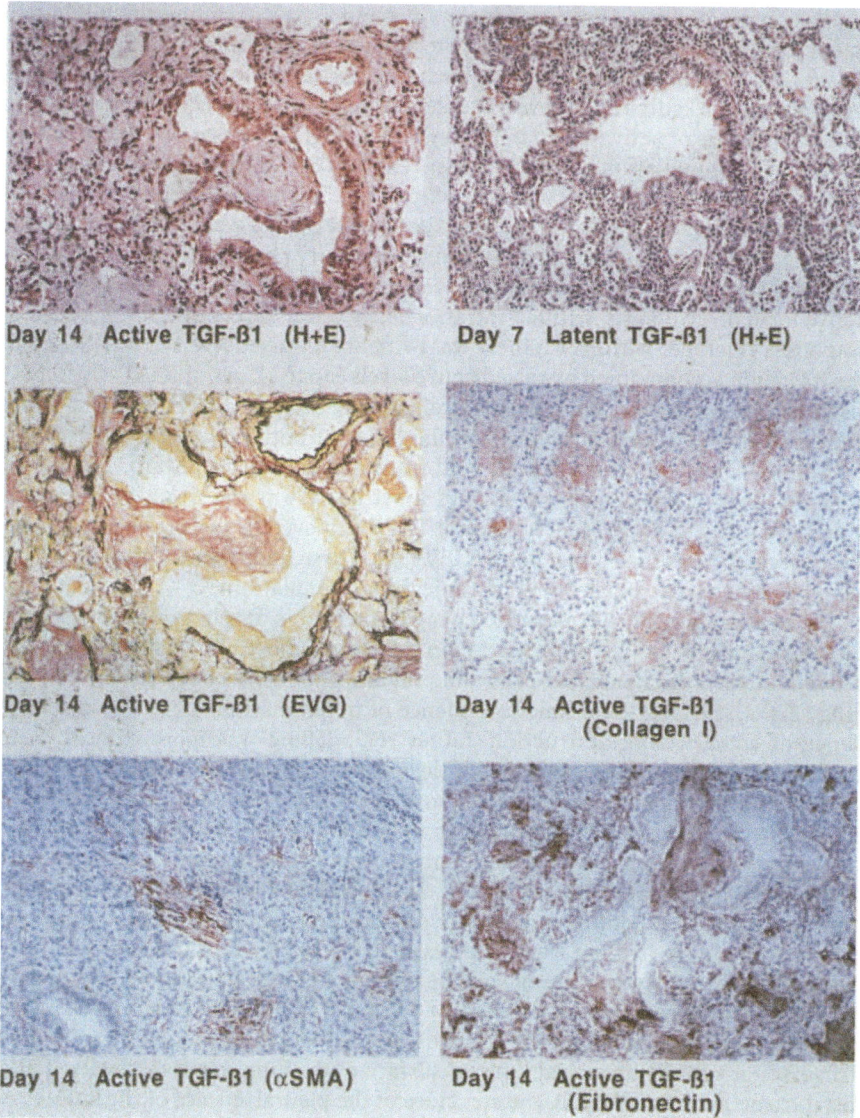

**Fig. 3.** Morphologic examination of rat lung after instillation of adenovirus vector expressing mutant (active) transforming growth factor. Stains include hematoxylin and eosin (*H&E*), elastic Van Geeson for matrix (*EVG*), smooth muscle actin for myofibroblasts (*SMA*), collagen and fibronectin deposition by immunohistochemistry with specific antibodies

of TGF$\beta$ and extent of fibrogenesis, along with the extent of myofibroblasts present, imply that episodes that generate the active TGF$\beta$ molecule are important in fibrogenesis. In the GM-CSF model, we were able to show that the alveolar macrophage removed from the animals that over-expressed GM-CSF in the lung spontaneously released TGF$\beta$. This, presumably, is the mechanism whereby GM-CSF exerts its fibrogenic activities [13]. How TNF induces the release of TGF$\beta$ and what cells release this factor are still unclear at this point.

## 6 Conclusions

By the use of transient gene transfer to the airways of the lung, we have been able to examine the role of individual cytokines in inducing myofibroblast expression and initiating their fibrogenic activities (Table 1). It would appear that TNF$\alpha$, while not showing a direct effect in vitro on myofibroblast differentiation, may induce limited presence of myofibroblasts and initiate fibrosis, probably through the activation and expression of TG$\beta$F. GM-CSF, however, activates macrophages to release TGF$\beta$, and the level of TGF$\beta$ in this model was higher than that seen with TNF as was the extent of myofibroblast accumulation and fibrosis. The greatest extent of fibrosis and myofibroblast accumulation was seen in the model with active-TGF$\beta$ vector. Thus, it seems likely that the most crucial element in inducing myofibroblasts and fibrogenesis is the process whereby TGF$\beta$ is either overexpressed and activated or is released in a spontaneously activated form (Table 2). This suggests several therapeutic intervention strategies for fibrosis, such as processes designed to interfere with the activation of TGF$\beta$ and those designed to interfere with the upregulation of this same molecule. The role that CTGF may play is unknown, but it is interesting to note that this molecule is found within the same system after TGF$\beta$ expression. One can now speculate that CTGF may be a future target for therapeutic intervention if, indeed, it by itself can induce myofibroblast expression and augment the matrix deposition associated with fibrosis.

**Acknowledgements.** This work was supported through grants from the Medical Research Council of Canada and Astra Draco AB, Sweden. PJS is a Parker Francis Fellow and ZX is an MRC Scholar.

## References

1. Braciak TA, Bacon K, Xing Z et al. (1996) Overexpression of RANTES using a recombinant adenovirus vector induces the tissue-directed recruitment of monocytes to the lung. J Immunol 157:5076–5084
2. Bramson JL, Graham FL, Gauldie J (1995) The use of adenoviral vectors for gene therapy and gene transfer in vivo. Curr Opin Biotechnol 6:590–595
3. Broekelmann TJ, Limper AH, Colvy TV, McDonald JA (1991) Transforming growth factor 1 is present at sites of extracellular matrix gene expression in human pulmonary fibrosis. Proc Natl Acad Sci U S A 88:6642–6646
4. Brunner Am, Marquardt H, Malacko AR, Lioubin MN, Purchio AF (1989) Site-directed mutagenesis of cysteine residues in the pro region of the transforming growth factor 1 precursor: expression and characterization of mutant proteins. J Biol Chem 264:13660–13664

 5. Darby I, Skalli O, Gabbiani G (1990) Smooth muscle actin is transiently expressed by myo-
    fibroblasts during experimental wound healing. Lab Invest 63:21–29
 6. Dedhar S, Gaboury L, Galloway P, Eaves C (1988) Human granulocyte-macrophage colony-
    stimulating factor is growth factor active on a variety of cell types of non-hemopoietic origin.
    Proc Natl Acad Sci U S A 85:9253–9257
 7. Desmouliere A (1995) Factors influencing myofibroblast differentiation during wound
    healing and fibrosis. Cell Biol Int 19:471–476
 8. Desmoulière A, Geinoz A, Gabbiani F, Gabbiani G (1993) Transforming growth factor-β1
    induces α-smooth muscle actin expression in granulation tissue myofibroblasts and in
    quiescent and growing cultured fibroblasts. J Cell Biol 122:103–111
 9. Foley R, Driscoll K, Wan Y, Braciak T, Howard B, Xing Z, Graham F, Gauldie J (1995) Adeno-
    viral gene transfer of macrophage inflammatory protein-2 in rat lung. Am J Pathol 149:
    1395–1403
10. Gauldie J, Jordana M, Cox G(1993) Cytokines and pulmonary fibrosis. Thorax 48:931–935
11. Glasser SW, Korfhagen TR, West SE, Whitsett JA (1994) Transgenic models for study of pul-
    monary development and disease. Am J Physiol 267:L489–L497
12. Kapanci Y, Desmouliere A, Pache J-C, Redard M, Gabbiani G (1995) Cytoskeletal protein
    modulation in pulmonary alveolar myofibroblasts during idiopathic pulmonary fibrosis:
    possible role of TGF-β and TNF-α. Am J Respir Crit Care Med 152:2163–2169
13. Khalil N, Whitman C, Danielpour D, Greenberg A (1993) Regulation of alveolar macrophage
    transforming growth factor-β secretion by corticosteroids in bleomycin-induced pul-
    monary inflammation in the rat. J Clin Invest 92:1812–1818
14. Khalil N, O'Conner RN, Flanders KC, Umruh H (1996) TGF-β1, but not TGF-β2 or TGF-β3,
    is differentially present in epithelial cells of advanced pulmonary fibrosis: an immuno-
    histochemical study. Am J Respir Cell Mol Biol 14:131–138
15. Khalil N, Corne S, Whitman C, Yacyshyn H (1996) Plasmin regulates the activation of cell-
    associated latent TGF-β1 secreted by rat alveolar macrophages after in vivo bleomycin
    injury. Am J Respir Cell Mol Biol 15:252–259
16. Lyons RM, Keski-Oja J, Moses HL (1988) Proteolytic activation of latent transforming
    growth factor-β from fibroblast-conditioned medium. Eur J Biochem 1990:1659–1665
17. Lyons RM, Gentry LE, Purchio AF et al. (1990) Mechanism of activation of latent recom-
    binant TGFβ1 by plasmin. J Cell Biol 110:1361–1367
18. Miyazaki Y, Araki K, Vesin C, Garcia I, Kapanci Y, Whitsett JA, Piguet P-F, Vassalli P (1995)
    Expression of a tumor necrosis factor- transgene in murine lung causes lymphocytic and
    fibrosing alveolitis. J Clin Invest 96:250–259
19. Phan SH, Kunkel SL (1992) Lung cytokine production in bleomycin-induced pulmonary
    fibrosis. Exp Lung Res 18:29–43
20. Piguet P-F. Cytokines involved in pulmonary fibrosis. Int Rev Exp Pathol 34B:173–181
21. Piguet PF, Collart MA, Grau GF, Kapanci Y, Vassalli P (1989) Tumor necrosis factor-α cachectin
    plays a key role in bleomycin-induced pneumopathy and fibrosis. J Exp Med 170:655–663
22. Rønnov-Jessen L, Petersen OW (1993) Induction of -smooth muscle actin by transforming
    growth factor-β1 in quiescent human breast gland fibroblasts. Implications for myofibro-
    blast generation in breast neoplasia. Implications for myofibroblast generation in breast
    neoplasia. Lab Invest 68:696–707
23. Roberts AB, Sporn MB, Assoian RK, Smith JM, Roche NS, Wakefield LM, Heine UI, Liotta LA,
    Falanga V, Kehrl JH, Fauci AS (1986) Transforming growth factor type β: rapid induction of
    fibrosis and angiogenesis in vivo and stimulation of collagen formation in vitro. Proc Natl
    Acad Sci U S A 83:4167–4171
24. Rubbia-Brandt L, Sappino A-P, Gabbiani G (1991) Locally applied GM-CSF induces the
    accumulation of smooth muscle actin containing myofibroblasts. Virchows Arch B Cell
    Pathol 60:73–82
25. Sappino AP, Schürch W, Gabbiani G (1990) Differentiation repertoire of fibroblastic cells:
    expression of cytoskeletal proteins as marker of phenotypic modulations. Lab Invest 63:
    144–161
26. Sato Y, Rifkin DB (1989) Inhibition of endothelial cell movement by pericytes and smooth
    muscle cells: activation of a latent transforming growth factor-β – like molecule by plasmin
    during co-culture. J Cell Biol 109:309–315

27. Schmitt-Graff A, Desmouliere A, Gabbiani G (1994) Heterogeneity of myofibroblast phenotypic features: an example of fibroblastic cell plasticity. Virchows Arch 425:3–24
28. Schürch W, Seemayer TA, Gabbiani G (1992) Myofibroblast. In: Sternberg SS (ed) Histology for pathologists. Raven Press, New York, pp 109–144
29. Sime PJ, Xing Z, Graham FL, Csaky KG, Gauldie J (1997) Adenovector-mediated gene transfer of active TGF-$\beta$1 induces prolonged severe fibrosis in rat lung. J Clin Invest 100:768–776
30. Sime PJ, Marr RA, Gauldie D, Xing Z, Hewlett BR, Graham FL, Gauldie J (1998) Transfer of TNF$\alpha$ to rat lung induces severe pulmonary inflammation and patchy interstitial fibrogenesis with induction of TGF-$\beta$1 and myofibroblasts.
31. Tremblay GM, Jordana M, Gauldie J, Särnstrand B (1995) Fibroblasts as effector cells in fibrosis. In: Phan SH, Thrall RS (eds) Pulmonary fibrosis. Marcel Dekker Inc, New York, pp 541–577
32. Ulich TR (1993) Tumor necrosis factor. In: Kelley J (ed) Cytokines of the lung. Marcel Dekker, New York, pp 307–332
33. Vyalov S, Desmoulière A, Gabbiani G (1993) GM-CSF-induced granulation tissue formation: relationships between macrophage and myofibroblast accumulation. Virchows Arch B Cell Pathol 63:231–239
34. Xing Z, Braciak T, Ohkawara Y, Sallenave J-M, Roley R, Sime PJ, Jordana M, Graham FL, Gauldie J (1996) Gene transfer for cytokine functional studies in the lung: the multifunctional role of GM–CSF in pulmonary inflammation. J Leukocyte Biol 59:481–488
35. Xing Z, Ohkawara Y, Jordana M, Graham FL, Gauldie J (1996) Transfer of granulocyte-macrophage colony-stimulating factor gene to rat lung induces eosinophilia, monocytosis, and fibrotic reactions. J Clin Invest 97:1102–1110
36. Xing Z, Tremblay GM, Sime PJ, Gauldie J (1997) Overexpression of granulocyte-macrophage colony-stimulating factor induces pulmonary granulation tissue formation and fibrosis by induction of transforming growth factor-$\beta$1 and myofibroblast accumulation. Am J Pathol 150:59–66
37. Xing Z, Braciak T, Jordana M, Croitoru K, Graham FL, Gauldie J (1994) Adenovirus-mediated cytokine gene transfer at tissue sites. Overexpression of IL-6 induces lymphocytic hyperplasia in the lung. J Immunol 153:4059–4069
38. Zhan K, Rekhter MD, Gordon D, Phan SH (1994) Myofibroblasts and their role in lung collagen gene expression during pulmonary fibrosis. A combined immunohistochemical and in situ hybridization study. Am J Pathol 145:114–125

# Transforming Growth Factor-β Induction of α-Smooth Muscle Actin Is Dependent on the Deformability of the Collagen Matrix

N. Narani, P. D. Arora, A. Lew, L. Luo, M. Glogauer, B. Ganss, C. A. G. McCulloch

## 1 Introduction

Current evidence suggests that fibroblasts undergo phenotypic modulation during several physiologic and pathologic conditions, such as wound healing and fibro-contractive diseases [29]. These phenotypically altered fibroblasts develop cyto-skeletal features similar to those of smooth muscle cells (SMCs), including the expression of α-smooth muscle actin (α-SMA), which is a contractile isoform of actin and, hence, they have been denoted as myofibroblasts [8]. The myofibroblast is thought to contribute to the process of wound contraction, as well as contractile phenomena observed during fibrotic diseases. However, little is known about the mechanisms responsible for phenotypic modulation of fibroblasts and the expression of α-SMA. Several types of growth factors and cytokines that are locally released from inflammatory and stromal cells at wound sites, as well as components of the extracellular matrix, have been studied to evaluate their role in fibroblastic differentiation. A likely candidate for regulation of α-SMA is transforming growth factor-β (TGF-β) [7], a potent regulator of matrix remodeling. This regulation may be achieved in part by modulation of cell–matrix interactions.

The development of mechanical stress in tissue can be a determinant of cell responsiveness to growth factors [21, 22]. Mechanical stress may also regulate myo-fibroblastic differentiation under certain conditions, such as the repair processes

Current Topics in Pathology, Volume 93
A. Desmoulière, B. Tuchweber (Eds.)
© Springer-Verlag Berlin Heidelberg 1999

in which fibroblasts are involved. Indeed, during wound healing, the rheological properties of the nascent extracellular matrix are modified with wound maturation and the fibroblasts are likely exposed to different levels of both mechanical stress and TGF-$\beta$. Compared with other isoforms, TGF-$\beta_1$ is widely expressed by different cell types and is the most abundant isoform in platelets. Therefore, in this study, we have focused on the effect of TGF-$\beta_1$ on $\alpha$-SMA expression by fibroblasts cultured in collagen matrices of various deformabilities. We used three tissue-culture models with variations of mechanical resistance to deformation, including collagen-coated monolayer cultures, anchored collagen gels and floating collagen gels. We tested the hypothesis that TGF-$\beta_1$-induced regulation of $\alpha$-SMA expression in human gingival fibroblasts is dependent on the deformability of the substrate and on the development of intracellular tension.

# 2 Materials and Methods

Primary cultures of human gingival fibroblasts were obtained from biopsies of normal gingiva in patients aged between 10 years and 16 years as described [20]. Cells at passages 3–12 were used for all experiments.

## 2.1 Collagen Substrates

Collagen solutions were prepared as described [2]. We used type-1 collagen as the substrate for all types of gels to validate comparisons based solely on the mechanical properties of the gels. For rigid collagen substrates and the production of monolayer cultures, films of collagen (~ 10 μm thick) were prepared on tissue-culture plastic and polymerized by neutralizing the collagen films to pH 7.4. Cells were plated subsequently. For anchored or floating gels, a cell suspension in $\alpha$-minimal essential medium (MEM) without serum was added to the solution. The floating gels were of relatively low rigidity, offered little resistance to deformation and could contract in all three dimensions. In contrast, the anchored gels were of moderate rigidity and offered resistance to deformation in the $x$ and $y$ axes. Collagen gels were incubated at 37 °C in 95 % air and 5 % $CO_2$ until polymerization was completed. The gels were covered with growth medium minus serum for 24 h. For TGF-$\beta_1$ treatment, the medium was removed and gels were covered with $\alpha$-MEM with or without TGF-$\beta_1$ (R and D Systems; Minneapolis, Minn.) for 3 days.

## 2.2 Western Blotting

To quantify TGF-$\beta_1$-induced effects on $\alpha$-SMA content, Western-blot analysis was performed on cells in monolayer cultures and in anchored and floating collagen gels. Cells were plated in collagen-coated 35-mm tissue-culture dishes and incubated in $\alpha$-MEM ± serum or TGF-$\beta_1$. Triplicate samples were assayed at 24 h and 72 h after incubating with TGF-$\beta_1$. Cells were scraped from the dishes and lysed with sodium dodecyl sulfate (SDS) sample buffer.

Cells were harvested from gels with trypsin/ethylene diamine tetra-acetate (EDTA) followed by incubation with collagenase. Cells were collected by centrifugation and incubated with extraction buffer. Protein content was assessed by the BioRad assay. Samples were boiled for 3 min at 95 °C and equal amounts of protein were electrophoresed on a 10% SDS gel. Separated proteins were transferred to nitrocellulose filters and probed with the mouse monoclonal antibody for $\alpha$-SMA followed by a horseradish peroxidase (HRP)-conjugated second antibody, and were developed with chemiluminescence reagents. Blots were stripped and probed with a monoclonal antibody for $\beta$-actin (clone AC-15; Sigma) for comparison. Subsequently, films were exposed to the blots.

## 2.3 Integrins

To investigate the effect of TGF-$\beta_1$ on the expression of $\alpha_2$- and $\beta_1$ integrin subunits, immunoblotting for $\alpha_2$- and $\beta_1$ integrins was performed with mouse monoclonal antibodies (clone P1H5; Calbiochem, Temescula, Calif. and 4B4-RD1; Coulter, Burlington, ON, respectively). The importance of the $\alpha_2\beta_1$ integrin on TGF-$\beta_1$-induced expression of $\alpha$-SMA was studied using the same antibodies to block $\beta_1$ and/or $\alpha_2$ integrin subunits. Cells were preincubated with mouse monoclonal antibodies for $\beta_1$ integrin and/or $\alpha_2$ integrin at room temperature. The next day, media were removed, cultures were covered with $\alpha$-MEM containing 10 ng/ml TGF-$\beta_1$ and supplemented with $\beta_1$ integrin (1:30) and/or $\alpha_2$ (1:50) integrin antibodies and incubated for 3 days. The antibodies were replenished once during the 3-day incubation with the same concentrations used for preincubation. Each experimental condition was prepared in triplicate. At the end of treatment, immunoblotting for $\alpha$-SMA was conducted as described before and blot density was normalized to $\beta$-actin.

## 2.4 Flow Cytometry

Cell suspensions were prepared, fixed with formaldehyde, permeabilized in Triton with phosphate-buffered saline (PBS) and stained for $\alpha$-SMA as described [1]. Cells were washed and analyzed on a FACSTAR Plus flow cytometer (Becton-Dickinson, Mississauga, ON). For all flow-cytometry analyses, at least $1 \times 10^4$ cells were assessed in each sample. Mouse monoclonal antibodies for $\alpha_2$ (1:20 dilution, clone P1H5) and $\beta_1$ (undiluted, clone 4B4-RD1) integrins were used for staining.

## 2.5 Northern Analysis

Northern blots were performed on monolayer cultures to determine the effect of TGF-$\beta_1$ on messenger RNA (mRNA) levels for $\alpha$-SMA. Cells were plated on collagen-coated 150-mm dishes in medium without serum. The medium was removed 24 h later, cells were covered with $\alpha$-MEM (no serum), with or without 10 ng/ml TGF-$\beta_1$ and incubated for 3 days. The cells were isolated from gels as described for western blotting and total RNA was isolated. RNA samples were separated in denaturing 1.3% formaldehyde–agarose gels, transferred to a nylon membrane and crosslinked by ultraviolet (UV) $\gamma$-$^{32}$P-ATP-labeled oligonucleotide probes, based on sequences in the untranslated region of $\alpha$-SMA and $\beta$-actin that were used to identify the respective mRNAs and blots that were exposed to film. The blots were stripped and reprobed with $\gamma$-$^{32}$P-ATP-labeled glyceraldehyde phosphate dehydrogenase.

## 2.6 Transforming Growth Factor-$\beta$

The levels of active and total TGF-$\beta_1$ produced by fibroblasts and the effect of exogenous TGF-$\beta_1$ on these levels were measured with a human TGF-$\beta_1$ immunoassay (Quantikine, R and D Systems) with a sensitivity of 5 pg/ml. Cells were incubated with $\alpha$-MEM, with or without 10 ng/ml TGF-$\beta_1$. After 3 days culture, supernatants were collected, and triplicate samples and activated and non-activated forms were assayed. To determine the amount of adherence of TGF-$\beta_1$ to collagen, 10 ng/ml TGF-$\beta_1$ was incubated in collagen-coated plates without cells and the medium was assayed after 3 days.

To determine the specificity of the effect of TGF-$\beta_1$ on $\alpha$-SMA expression, an anti-TGF-$\beta$ neutralizing antibody was used to block the effect of TGF-$\beta_1$. Cells were plated on 35 mm collagen-coated dishes. After 24 h, media were replaced by $\alpha$-MEM, with or without 10 ng/ml TGF-$\beta_1$, with or without anti TGF-$\beta_1$ neutralizing antibody. After 3 days, $\alpha$-SMA content was quantified by means of Western blot.

## 3 Results

In a preliminary experiment, concentrations of 1 ng/ml, 5 ng/ml and 10 ng/ml TGF-$\beta_1$ were tested to study the effect on the expression of $\alpha$-SMA. Cells immunostained for $\alpha$-SMA showed a dose-dependent response to TGF-$\beta_1$ and the optimal intensity of staining was observed with 10 ng/ml TGF-$\beta_1$. As this dosage has also been used in previous experiments to study TGF-$\beta_1$ regulation of $\alpha$-SMA [7] and is similar to levels found in healing wounds [5], we used this dosage for all subsequent experiments.

To determine whether TGF-$\beta_1$ induces changes of $\alpha$-SMA content, Western blotting was performed and $\beta$-actin content was used for comparison and normalization of protein loading.

Cells grown on collagen-coated plastic showed a marked increase in the level of $\alpha$-SMA after TGF-$\beta_1$ treatment in the presence or absence of serum (Fig. 1). This enhancement of $\alpha$-SMA content required 3 days. Indeed, overnight incubation of human gingival fibroblasts (HGFs) on collagen-coated plastic with TGF-$\beta_1$ (10 ng/ml) did not significantly increase $\alpha$-SMA. When cells were grown in three-

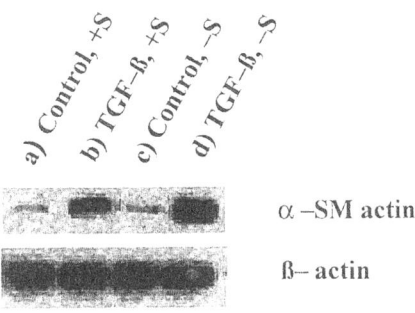

$\alpha$ –SM actin

$\beta$– actin

**Fig. 1.** Cells grown on collagen-coated tissue-culture plastic were incubated with $\alpha$-minimal essential medium ($\alpha$-MEM) in the presence (*a, b*) or absence (*c, d*) of serum, without (*a, c*) or with (*b, d*; 10 ng/ml) transforming growth factor-$\beta_1$ (TGF-$\beta_1$) for 3 days. Three independent samples were assayed for $\alpha$-smooth muscle actin ($\alpha$-SM actin) content using the Western-blot technique. $\beta$-actin content was used for normalization of protein loading

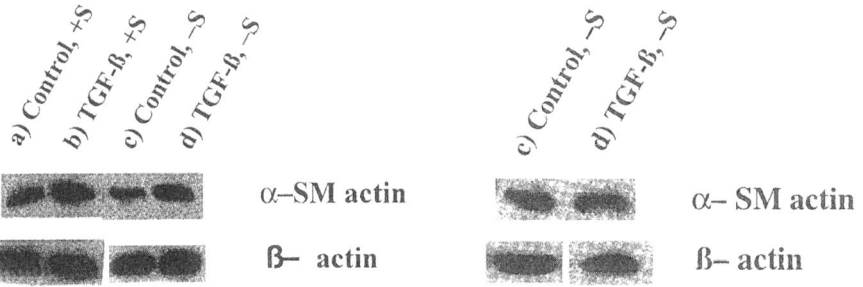

$\alpha$–SM actin

$\beta$– actin

$\alpha$– SM actin

$\beta$– actin

2                                                                                           3

**Fig. 2.** Cells in three-dimensional anchored collagen gels were incubated with $\alpha$-minimal essential medium ($\alpha$-MEM) in presence (*a, b*) or absence (*c, d*) of serum, without (*a, c*) or with (*b, d*; 10 ng/ml) transforming growth factor-$\beta_1$ (TGF-$\beta_1$) for 3 days. Western-blotting analysis was used as described in Fig. 1 for assessment of $\alpha$-smooth muscle actin ($\alpha$-SM actin) and $\beta$-actin content in three independent samples

**Fig. 3.** Cells in floating collagen gels were incubated with $\alpha$-minimal essential medium ($\alpha$-MEM) in presence (*a, b*) or absence (*c, d*) of serum, without (*a, c*) or with (*b, d*; 10 ng/ml) transforming growth factor-$\beta_1$ (TGF-$\beta_1$) for 3 days. Three independent samples were analyzed for $\alpha$-smooth muscle actin ($\alpha$-SM actin) and $\beta$-actin as described in Fig. 1

dimensional anchored collagen gels and treated with TGF-$\beta_1$ (10 ng/ml), $\alpha$-SMA protein content increased by 70% in serum and 90% in serum-free conditions (compared with controls) (Fig. 2). In cells plated in floating gels, TGF-$\beta_1$ (10 ng/ml) induced no significant change in the level of $\alpha$-SMA (with or without serum) (Fig. 3).

## 3.1 Northern-Blot Hybridization

To assess whether TGF-$\beta_1$ induced $\alpha$-SMA at the mRNA level, total RNA from cells in monolayer cultures was separated by electrophoresis, blotted and hybridized with $\alpha$-SMA or $\beta$-actin-specific oligonucleotide probes. For assessment of equal loading, the blots were also sequentially hybridized with a labeled complementary DNA (cDNA) probe for glyceraldehyde-3-phosphate dehydrogenase (GAPDH) (Fig. 4). In

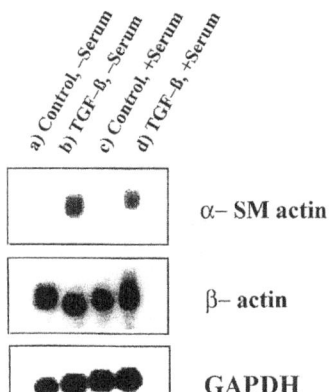

α– SM actin

β– actin

GAPDH

**Fig. 4.** Cells grown on collagen-coated plastic and incubated with α-minimal essential medium (α-MEM) in +serum (*a, b*) or –serum (*c, d*) conditions without (*a, c*) or with (*b, d*; 10 ng/ml) TGF-$\beta_1$ for 3 days were assayed for α-smooth muscle actin (α-SM actin) messenger RNA (mRNA) content. Northern blots were hybridized with oligonucleotide probes specific for either human α-SM actin or β-actin mRNA. For assessment of equal loading, the blots were also hybridized with a labeled complementary DNA (cDNA) probed for glyceraldehyde phosphate dehydrogenase (GAPDH)

cells treated with TGF-$\beta_1$ (10 ng/ml, 3 days), α-SMA bands were markedly increased compared with control cells and this increase was particularly noticeable in serum-free conditions. In contrast, β-actin mRNA levels were unchanged by TGF-$\beta_1$ treatments.

## 3.2 TGF-$\beta_1$ Blockade

Blocking TGF-$\beta_1$ with an anti-TGF-$\beta$ neutralizing antibody that reacted with all TGF-$\beta$ isoforms was conducted to determine the specificity of the TGF-$\beta_1$ effect on the upregulation of α-SMA. A 3-day incubation of cells with α-MEM plus antibody showed a small decrease in α-SMA content compared with controls (α-MEM alone). Incubation of TGF-$\beta_1$-treated cells (monolayer cultures) with the antibody caused a large reduction of α-SMA content compared with controls (Fig. 5). These results not only demonstrated the specificity of TGF-$\beta_1$ in upregulation of α-SMA expression, but also suggested a possible role for endogenous TGF-$\beta_1$ in the induction of α-SMA expression.

For assessing the actual concentrations of active and latent forms of TGF-$\beta_1$, to which the cells were exposed under different culture conditions, enzyme-linked

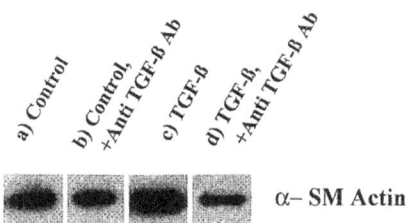

α– SM Actin

**Fig. 5.** Cells grown on collagen-coated plastic were incubated with α-minimal essential medium (α-MEM) (*a, b*) or α-MEM plus transforming growth factor (TGF-$\beta_1$) (*c, d*; 10 ng/ml) without (*a, c*) or with (*b, d*; 15 µg/ml) anti-TGF-$\beta_1$ neutralizing antibody for 3 days. Three independent samples were analyzed for α-smooth muscle actin (α-SM actin) content by Western blot

**Table 1.** Levels of endogenous TGF-$\beta_1$ (in pg/ml). Cells on collagen-coated plastic, anchored and floating gels were incubated with $\alpha$-MEM alone or supplemented with 15% FCS, with or without 10 ng/ml TGF-$\beta_1$ for 3 days. To determine the concentrations of total and active forms of TGF-$\beta_1$ in cell supernatants, ELISA was performed on activated and non-activated samples, respectively. The amount of exogenous TGF-$\beta_1$ was subtracted from the values obtained for TGF-$\beta_1$-treated cultures

| Cell preparation | | + Serum | | – Serum | |
|---|---|---|---|---|---|
| | | Control | TGF-$\beta$ | Control | TGF-$\beta$ |
| Monolayer | Total | $1060 \pm 26.5$[d] | $5473 \pm 44.4$[a,b,c] | $767 \pm 24.9$ | $2276 \pm 110.2$[a] |
| cultures<?1> | Active | $<5$ | $4236 \pm 120$[a,b,c] | $<5$ | $1051 \pm 29.3$[a] |
| Anchored | Total | $728 \pm 37.1$[d] | $4877 \pm 189$[a,b,c] | $752.3 \pm 46.9$ | $2012.3 \pm 117.1$[a] |
| gels<?1> | Active | $<5$ | $3964 \pm 140$[a,b,c] | $<5$ | $1094 \pm 22.8$[a] |
| Floating gels<?1> | Total | $171 \pm 17.5$ | $2714.3 \pm 83.6$[a,b] | $690.6 \pm 28.5$ | $1756 \pm 135.5$[a] |
| | Active | $<5$ | $2557.3 \pm 55.9$[a,b] | $<5$ | $1060 \pm 24.4$[a] |

[a] $p < 0.01$; significantly different from control.
[b] $p < 0.05$; significantly different from TGF-$\beta_1$, – serum.
[c] $p < 0.05$; significantly different from floating gels (TGF-$\beta_1$ treated).
[d] $p < 0.01$; significantly different from floating gels (control).

immunosorbent assays (ELISAs) were performed on three independent activated and non-activated samples, and the mean $\pm$ s.e.m. was computed for each condition (Table 1). Addition of TGF-$\beta_1$ (10 ng/ml) for all three types of collagen substrates led to increased levels of TGF-$\beta_1$, a large proportion of which was in active form. Comparison of serum-containing and serum-free conditions within each model showed that the effect of exogenous TGF-$\beta_1$ was significantly higher in the presence of serum. In serum conditions, the increase of endogenous TGF-$\beta_1$ (total and active) was largest in monolayer cultures (total: 5.5 ng/ml; active: 4.2 ng/ml) and smallest in floating gels (total: 2.7 ng/ml; active: 2.6 ng/ml) both in control and TGF-$\beta_1$-treated cultures. The concentrations for anchored gels were less than monolayer cultures (total: 4.9 ng/ml; active: 4.0 ng/ml) and the difference was statistically significant in controls ($p < 0.05$), but not in TGF-$\beta_1$-treated cultures ($p > 0.2$). In serum-free conditions, there were no significant differences in the total and active levels of endogenous TGF-$\beta_1$ between the three models.

## 3.3 Integrins

The $\alpha_2\beta_1$ integrin is a major collagen adhesion molecule in human gingival fibroblasts and is the most important integrin in cell adhesion and phagocytosis [4, 17]. HEINO et al. [13] demonstrated upregulation of the $\beta_1$ family of integrins in some, but not all human fibroblast lines. Our group determined the effect of TGF-$\beta_1$ on the total content and surface expression of $\alpha_2\beta_1$ integrins. Flow cytometry analysis of cells grown on collagen-coated plastic for $\alpha_2$ and $\beta_1$ integrin subunits showed no significant differences of the mean intensity of staining or the percentage of positive cells between controls and TGF-$\beta_1$-treated cells in either unfixed or fixed

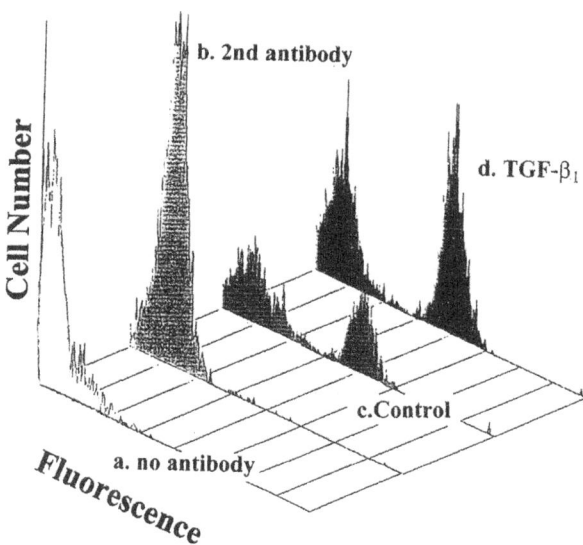

**Fig. 6.** Cells grown on collagen-coated plates were incubated with $\alpha$-minimal essential medium ($\alpha$-MEM) alone (control) or supplemented with 10 ng/ml transforming growth factor-$\beta_1$ (TGF$\beta_1$) for 3 days. Single cell suspensions were stained with either no antibody (*a*) for autofluorescence, only fluorescein isothiocyanate (FITC)-conjugated second antibody (*b*) or primary anti-$\alpha_2$-integrin and FITC-conjugated second antibody (*c, d*). The fluorescence of $\alpha_2$-integrin positive cells was assayed in unfixed cells by flow cytometry to determine the total content or the surface expression of $\alpha$2-integrin subunit, respectively

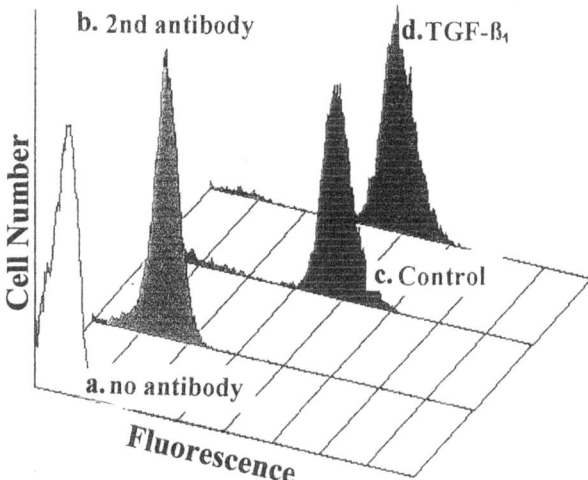

**Fig. 7.** Cells grown on collagen-coated plates were incubated with $\alpha$-minimal essential medium ($\alpha$-MEM) alone (control) or supplemented with 10 ng/ml transforming growth factor (TGF-$\beta_1$) for 3 days. Single cell suspensions were stained with either no antibody (*a*) for autofuorescence, only fluorescein isothiocyante (FITC)-conjugated second antibody (*b*) or primary anti-$\beta_1$-integrin and FITC-conjugated second antibody (*c, d*). Fluorescence staining of $\beta_1$-integrin positive cells was assayed in fixed cells using flow cytometry

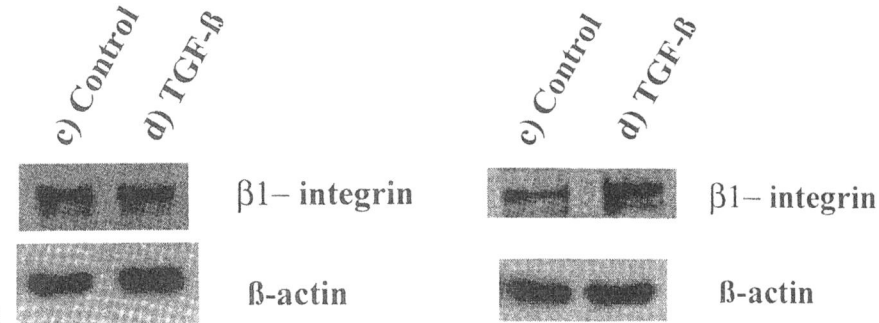

**Fig. 8.** Cells grown on collagen-coated plastic were incubated with $\alpha$-minimal essential medium ($\alpha$-MEM) alone (*a, c*) or supplemented with 10 ng/ml transforming growth factor (TGF-$\beta_1$) (*b, d*) for 24 h. Three independent samples were analyzed for $\alpha_2$-integrin (*a, b*) or $\beta_1$-integrin (*c, d*) protein levels by means of Western blotting, and $\beta$-actin was used for normalization of protein loading

**Fig. 9.** Cells grown on tissue-culture plastic were incubated with $\alpha$-minimal essential medium ($\alpha$-MEM) alone (*a, c*) or supplemented with 10 ng/ml transforming growth factor (TGF-$\beta_1$) (*b, d*) for 24 h. Three independent samples were analyzed for $\alpha_2$-integrin (*a, b*) or $\beta_1$-integrin (*c, d*) protein levels by means of Western blotting. $\beta$-actin was used for normalization of protein loading

samples (Figs. 6 and 7). This result was also confirmed by the immunoblotting of cells (monolayer cultures on collagen) for both subunits (Fig. 8). A possible explanation for these results could be that the collagen coating on the plates induced maximal expression of $\alpha_2\beta_1$ integrin; therefore, further increases induced by TGF-$\beta_1$ would not be detected. Consequently, cells grown on tissue-culture plastic and treated with TGF-$\beta_1$ were probed for $\alpha_2$ and $\beta_1$ subunits. The results showed an approximate twofold increase in the expression level of both subunits after TGF-$\beta$ treatment, compared with controls (Fig. 9).

### 3.4 Integrin Blockade of $\alpha$-Smooth Muscle Actin

Schiro et al. [27] demonstrated a major role for $\alpha_2\beta_1$ integrin in reorganization of a hydrated collagen matrix. Therefore, we considered that the $\alpha_2\beta_1$ integrin is involved in the upregulation of $\alpha$-SMA induced by TGF-$\beta_1$. To test this hypothesis, cells were preincubated with the monoclonal antibodies P1H5 (which blocks the $\alpha_2$ subunit) and/or 4B4 (which blocks the $\beta_1$ subunit) and treated with TGF-$\beta_1$ (10 ng/ml) for 3 days. Western blots for $\alpha$-SMA showed that cells preincubated with both antibodies reduced the effect of TGF-$\beta_1$ to the level of controls (Fig. 10). The decrease in the expression of $\alpha$-SMA in the presence of 4B4 alone or combined with P1H5 was accompanied by cell rounding and apparent loss of intracellular tension. These results were not caused by cell death, as the viability of cells preincubated with antibodies and tested at the end of the incubations exceeded 95%, as measured by trypan blue exclusion.

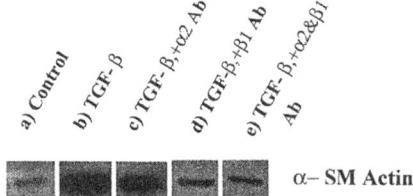

α– SM Actin

**Fig. 10.** Cell suspensions were preincubated with either no antibody (*a, b*), only anti-$\alpha_2$-integrin antibody (*c*), only anti-$\beta_1$-integrin antibody (*d*) or both antibodies (*e*) for 30 min and plated on collagen-coated plastic in the presence of $\alpha$-minimal essential medium ($\alpha$-MEM) (*a*) or supplemented with 10 ng/ml transforming growth factor (TGF-$\beta_1$) (*b, c, d, e*) for 3 days. Antibodies were replenished once during the incubation period. Three independent samples were assayed for the expression of $\alpha$-smooth muscle actin ($\alpha$-SM actin)

## 4 Discussion

Our central finding is that the ability of TGF-$\beta_1$ to increase $\alpha$-SMA expression in fibroblasts is determined by the physical resistance of the substrate to cell-generated forces. $\alpha$-SMA is an abundant actin isoform in vascular smooth muscle cells [26] and is a prominent smooth muscle-cell marker expressed by myofibroblastic populations [6]. The presence of $\alpha$-SMA expressing myofibroblasts in a tissue, such as granulation tissue, is accompanied by rapid matrix remodeling and is also characterized by the development of tension [27]. Indeed, in granulation tissue, increased tension leads to wound contraction, a critical process for mammalian survival. While the modulatory role of TGF-$\beta$ on myofibroblast differentiation and expression of $\alpha$-SMA has been studied previously in monolayer cultures [3, 7, 23], there are no reports on the study of cells responding to TGF-$\beta$ under different levels of tension. Therefore, it was of interest to determine the role of tension in TGF-$\beta$-induced $\alpha$-SMA expression.

In this study, we used three different tissue-culture systems with variations in substrate deformability to provide study models in which cells would be exposed to different levels of mechanical stress. These models included monolayer cultures of fibroblasts on collagen-coated plastic (high tension), three-dimensional anchored (moderate tension) and floating (low tension) collagen gels. The models demonstrated different levels of resistance to the tractional forces exerted by fibroblasts. Collagen-coated plastic is a rigid substrate in which there is no observable alteration of the dimensions of the gel and in which there is high resistance against deformation.

Indeed rhodamine-phalloidin staining of cells for actin filaments showed that cells on rigid collagen-coated surfaces exhibited prominent stress fibers, whereas these were not detected in floating collage gels. Furthermore, based on results of $^3H_2O$ exclusion (data not shown), anchored gels showed a slower contraction rate than floating gels. Thus, deformability was highest in floating gels and lowest in monolayer cultures. We assume, on the basis of these data, that the deformability of anchored gels lies somewhere between floating gels and monolayer cultures, and that different substrate deformability translates into different levels of intracellular tension. Indeed, fibroblasts grown on rigid substrates acquire characteristics of myofibroblasts and develop prominent stress fibers [28]. We suggest that there is an inverse relationship between the degree of substrate deformability and the development of intracellular tension.

## 4.1 Effect of Tension and TGF-$\beta_1$ on $\alpha$-SMA Expression and Localization

The results of immunoblotting for $\alpha$-SMA showed the maximal regulatory effect of TGF-$\beta_1$ on $\alpha$-SMA expression in monolayer cultures, an intermediate effect in anchored gels and no detectable effect in floating gels. To assess whether TGF-$\beta_1$ affects mRNA levels of $\alpha$-SMA and $\beta$-actin, Northern-blot analyses were performed on monolayer cultures. Compared with $\beta$-actin mRNA levels, which were unaltered, the density of the bands for $\alpha$-SMA were markedly increased after treatment with TGF-$\beta_1$ for 72 h compared with controls. In these experiments, cells were exposed to TGF-$\beta_1$ for 3 days; however, incubations of cells for 24 h with TGF-$\beta_1$ did not induce any detectable change in the protein level of $\alpha$-SMA in monolayer cultures. This observation raised the question of how direct the effect of TGF-$\beta_1$ on $\alpha$-SMA expression was. If 24-h incubation of cells with TGF-$\beta_1$ was not long enough to increase $\alpha$-SMA levels, then it might act indirectly, perhaps by inducing the production of other growth factors, such as platelet-derived growth factor (PDGF). Although TGF-$\beta$ can regulate the synthesis of PDGF in some cell types, e.g., endothelial cells [25], this cytokine is unable to induce $\alpha$-SMA expression in dermal fibroblasts in vitro [27].

To determine whether the effect of TGF-$\beta_1$ observed in these experiments was specific, a neutralizing antibody was used to block its action. Compared with controls, there was a significant reduction in $\alpha$-SMA content when TGF-$\beta_1$ treated cells were incubated with the antibody. Furthermore, control cells (no TGF-$\beta_1$ treatment) showed a reduction of $\alpha$-SMA content.

These observations indicate not only the specificity of TGF-$\beta_1$ in mediating an increase of $\alpha$-SMA content, but also a possible role for endogenous TGF-$\beta_1$. Therefore, it was of considerable interest to determine the actual concentrations of TGF-$\beta_1$ to which the cells were exposed in the different models. Previous studies have shown that TGF-$\beta$ is present in the extracellular matrix, both in active and latent forms, but only the active form is able to bind to TGF-$\beta$ receptors [32]. As the latent form can be activated in vitro by acidification [16], we quantified both active and latent forms of TGF-$\beta_1$ in culture medium using an ELISA. The data indicated that exogenous TGF-$\beta_1$ stimulates the cells to produce TGF-$\beta_1$, the majority of which is in an active form. These results are consistent with the findings of Lin et al. [18], showing that TGF-$\beta_1$ amplifies its own production.

## 4.2 Integrins

The $\beta_1$ family of integrins are the major adhesion molecules that mediate fibroblastic interactions with collagen [33]. These interactions play an important role in collagen matrix remodeling, since antibodies against $\beta_1$-containing integrins inhibit contraction of fibroblast-populated collagen lattices [11, 14]. Among the members of the $\beta_1$ family of integrins, $\alpha_2\beta_1$ is believed to play a pivotal role in re-organization of collagen matrices, as it is selectively upregulated on fibroblasts grown in three-dimensional collagen gels [14]. Furthermore, cells expressing low levels of $\alpha_2\beta_1$ are unable to contract collagen gels [27]. Moreover, Heino et al. [13] have shown that TGF-$\beta_1$ upregulation of $B_1$ is cell-type specific. These data led us to question whether TGF-$\beta_1$ upregulates $\alpha_2\beta_1$ in gingival fibroblasts and whether the increased expression of $\alpha_2\beta_1$ is involved in the $\alpha$-SMA modulation induced by TGF-$\beta_1$. Flow cytometric and Western-blot analyses of $\alpha_2\beta_1$ in fibroblasts grown on collagen-coated plastic showed no effect of TGF-$\beta_1$ on both cell-surface expression and the total content of $\alpha_2$ and $\beta_1$ subunits. The data from suspended cells and cells remaining attached to the substrate were similar, showing that cell detachment did not affect expression levels as it did for $\alpha$-SMA. Thus, the increased $\alpha$-SMA levels induced by TGF-$\beta_1$ is not because of increased integrin expression and the presence of more adhesive contacts into which $\alpha$-SMA-containing filaments could insert.

To assess whether $\alpha_2\beta_1$ is involved in the process of TGF-$\beta_1$-induced regulation of $\alpha$-SMA, $\alpha_2$ and $\beta_1$ subunits were blocked with monoclonal antibodies. Western-blot analyses revealed a large decrease in the level of $\alpha$-SMA after $\beta_1$ antibody incubation, and a smaller reduction with $\alpha_2$ antibody, compared with samples treated only with TGF-$\beta_1$. Combined treatment with the two antibodies reduced $\alpha$-SMA content to the level of controls. The reduced $\alpha$-SMA content was accompanied by a change in cell morphology from well spread to rounded. The altered cell morphology was more noticeable toward the end of the incubation with TGF-$\beta_1$, when the maximum effect on the expression of $\alpha$-SMA was expected. These results from blockade of the $\alpha_2\beta_1$ integrin further support the suggestion that the generation of intracellular tension is a requirement for the regulation of $\alpha$-SMA by TGF-$\beta_1$. Inhibition of cell spreading and development of stress fibers through the use of blocking antibodies against $\alpha_2$ and $\beta_1$ subunits significantly reduced the effect of TGF-$\beta_1$ on $\alpha$-SMA expression.

## 4.3 Mechanocoupling and Transcriptional Control

Currently, it is unknown how variations in intracellular tension result in variations in the levels of $\alpha$-SMA mRNA and protein in response to TGF-$\beta_1$. TGF-$\beta$ can increase $\alpha$-SMA expression in SMCs and this requires binding of an unknown factor to a TGF-$\beta$ control element along with the binding of serum response factors to two CArG elements in the promoter region [12]. Conceivably, a number of mechanical signaling systems serve to restrict either TGF-$\beta_1$ binding, signal transduction, transcription-factor binding to the $\alpha$-SMA promoter or transcription of $\alpha$-SMA mRNA to only those cells that have developed significant intracellular tension. As the mechanical features of the extracellular matrix (such as its resistance to cell-generated tensile forces) can influence the biological activity of cells by altering their signal transduction machinery or modulating the cytoskeleton, we speculate below on a possible mechanotransduction model that might be involved in the tension-dependent regulation of $\alpha$-SMA induced by TGF-$\beta_1$.

Mechanosensitive ion channels have been demonstrated in different cell types. These include stretch-activated ion channels in skeletal muscle cells [10], vascular endothelial cells [15] and fibroblasts [31]. Cell shape and the degree of cell spreading have been shown to influence the intracellular $Ca^{2+}$ concentration in endothelial cells [30]. Moreover, changes in cell shape and reorganization of cell-matrix adhesion sites in contracting fibroblasts induce the formation of membrane passages that might be involved in $Ca^{2+}$ uptake [19]. Alterations of intracellular $Ca^{2+}$ concentration are an important signaling mechanism and may dramatically regulate a variety of downstream events. For example, the activity of some transcriptional factors, such as the activator protein AP-1, depends on increased $Ca^{2+}$ [9]. Furthermore, AP-1 binding is involved in the activation of the $\alpha$-skeletal-actin promoter in myocytes [24]. However, this has not been shown for $\alpha$-SMA gene expression. Therefore, tension-induced changes of intracellular ion levels may be involved in TGF-$\beta_1$-induced expression of $\alpha$-SMA, possibly by regulating the activity of signaling molecules involved in this pathway.

In the context of wound healing in vivo, the results of this study support the idea that, in certain situations, e.g., periodontal or skin wound healing, myofibroblast differentiation is modulated locally by microenvironmental, interactive stimuli, including growth factors and mechanical stress. Therefore, it is conceivable that further studies along these lines may lead to more efficient therapeutic strategies for enhancement of wound healing and prevention of pathologic scarring.

**Acknowledgements.** MRC of Canada Group Grant to CAGM.

# References

1. Arora PD, McCulloch CAG (1994) Dependence of collagen remodeling on $\alpha$-smooth muscle actin expression by fibroblasts. J Cell Physiol 159:161–175
2. Bellows CG, Melcher AH, Aubin JE (1981) Contraction and organization of collagen gels by cell cultured from periodontal differences between cell types. J Cell Sci 50:299–314
3. Bjorkerud S (1991) Effects of transforming growth factor-$\beta$1 on human arterial smooth muscle cells in vitro. Arterioscler Thromb 11:892–902
4. Chou DH, Lee W, McCulloch CAG (1996) TNF-alpha inactivation of collagen receptors: implications for fibroblast function and fibrosis. J Immunol 156:4354–4362
5. Cromack DT, Sporn MB, Roberts AB, Merino MJ, Dart LL, Norton JA (1987) Transforming growth factor $\beta$ levels in rat wound chambers. J Surg Res 42:622–628
6. Desmouliere A, Gabbiani G (1994) Modulation of fibroblastic cytoskeletal features during pathological situations: the role of extracellular matrix and cytokines. Cell Motil Cytoskel 29:195–203
7. Desmouliere A, Geiniz A, Gabbiani F, Gabbiani G (1993) Transforming growth factor-$\beta_1$ induces $\alpha$-Smooth muscle actin expression in granulation tissue myofibroblasts and in quiescent and growing cultured fibroblasts. J Cell Biol 122:103–111
8. Gabbiani G, Ryan GB, Majno G (1971) Presence of modified fibroblasts in granulation tissue and their possible role in wound contraction. Experientia 27:549–550
9. Ghosh A, Greenberg ME (1988) Calcium signaling in neurons: molecular mechanisms and cellular consequences. Science 268:239–247
10. Guhary F, Sachs F (1985) Mechanotransducer ion channels in chick skeletal muscle: the effect of extracellular pH. J Physiol 363:119–134
11. Gullberg D, Tingstrom A, Thuresson AC, Olsson L, Terracio L, Borg TK, Rubin K (1990) $\beta_1$ Integrin-mediated collagen gel contraction is stimulated by PDGF. Exp Cell Res 186:264–272

12. Hautmann MB, Madsen CS, Owens GK (1997) A transforming growth factor $\beta$ (TGF-$\beta$) control element derives TGF-$\beta$-induced stimulation of smooth muscle $\alpha$-actin gene expression in concert with two CArG elements. J Biol Chem 272:10948–10956

13. Heino J, Ignotz RA, Hemler ME, Crouse C, Massague J (1989) Regulation of cell adhesion receptors by transforming growth factor-$\beta$. Concomitant regulation of integrins that share a common $\beta_1$ subunit. J Biol Chem 264:380–388

14. Klein CE, Dressel D, Steinmayer T, Mauch C, Eckes B, Krieg T, Bankert RB, Weber L (1991) Integrin $\alpha_2\beta_1$ is up-regulated in fibroblasts and highly aggressive melanoma cells in three-dimensional collagen lattices and mediates the reorganization of collagen I fibrils. J Cell Biol 115:1427–1436

15. Lansman JB, Hallam TJ, Rink TJ (1987) Single stretch-activated ion channels in vascular endothelial cells as mechanotransducers? Nature 325:811–813

16. Lawrence DA, Pircher R, Kryceve-Martinerie C, Jullien P (1984) Normal embryo fibroblasts release transforming growth factors in a latent form. J Cell Physiol 121:184–188

17. Lee W Sodek J McCulloch, CAG (1996) Role of integrin in regulation of collagen phagocytosis by human fibroblasts. J Cell Physiol 168:695–704

18. Lin RY, Sullivan KM, Argenta PA, Meuli M, Lorenz HP, Adzick, NS (1995) Exogenous transforming growth factor-beta amplifies its own expression and induces scar formation in a model of human fetal skin repair. Ann Surg 222:146–154

19. Lin Y-C, Ho C-H, Grinnell F (1997) Fibroblasts contracting collagen matrices form transient plasma membrane passages through which the cells take up fluorescein isothiocyanate-dextran and Ca$^{2+}$. Mol Biol Cell 8:59–71

20. McCulloch CAG, Knowles GC (1993) Deficiencies in collagen phagocytosis by human fibroblasts in vitro: a mechanism for fibrosis? J Cell Physiol 155:461–471

21. Nakagawa S, Pawelek P, Grinnell F (1989a) Extracellular matrix organization modulates fibroblast growth factor responsiveness. Exp Cell Res 182:572–582

22. Nakagawa S, Pawelek P, Grinnell F (1989b) Long-term culture of fibroblasts in contracted collagen gels: effect on cell growth and biosysthetic activity. J Invest Dermatol 93:792–798

23. Orlandi A, Roppaz P, Gabbiani G (1994) Proliferative activity and $\alpha$-smooth muscle actin expression in cultured rat aortic smooth muscle cells are differently modulated by transforming growth factor-$\beta_1$ and heparin. Exp Cell Res 214:526–536

24. Paradis P, MacLellan WR, Belaguli NS, Schwartz RJ, Schneider MD (1996) Serum response factor mediates AP-1-dependent induction of the skeletal $\alpha$-Actin promoter in ventricular myocytes. J Biol Chem 271:10827–10833

25. Roberts AB, Sporn MB (1989) Regulation of endothelial cell growth, architecture and matrix synthesis by TGF-$\beta$. Am Rev Respir Dis 140:1126–1128

26. Rubenstein PA (1990) The functional importance of multiple actin isoforms. Bioessays 12:309–315

27. Sappino AP, Schurch W, Gabbiani G (1990) Biology of disease, differentiation repertoire of fibroblastic cells: expression of cytoskeletal proteins as marker of phenotypic modulations. Lab Invest 63:144–161

27. Schiro JA, Chan BMC, Roswit, WT, Kassner PD, Pentland AP, Hemler ME, Eisen AZ, Kupper TS (1991) Integrin $\alpha_2\beta_1$ (VLA-2) mediates reorganization and contraction of collagen matrices by human cells. Cell 67:403–410

28. Schmitt-Graff A, Desmouliere A, and Gabbiani G (1994) Heterogenity of myofibroblast phenotypic features: an example of fibroblastic cell plasticity. Virchows Arch 425:3–24

29. Schurch W, Seemayer TA, Gabbiani G (1992) The myofibroblast. In: SS Sternbery (ed) Histology for pathologists. New York, Raven, pp 109–144

30. Schwartz MA (1993) Spreading of human endothelial cells on fibronectin or vitronectin triggers elevation of intracellular Ca$^{2+}$. J Cell Biol 120:1003–1010

31. Stockbridge LL, French AS (1988) Stretch-activated cation channels in human fibroblasts. Biophys J 54:187–190

32. Wakefield LM, Smith DM, Masui T, Harris CC, Sporn MB, (1987) Distribution and modulation of the cellular receptor for transforming growth factor-beta. J Cell Biol 105:965–975

33. Wayner EA, Carter WG (1987) Identification of multiple cell adhesion receptors for type VI collagen and fibronectin in human fibrosarcoma cells possessing unique $\alpha$ and common $\beta$-subunits. J Cell Biol 105:1873–1884

# Signal Transduction Pathways Activated During Fibroblast Contraction of Collagen Matrices

F. Grinnell

## 1 Introduction

Fibroblasts cultured in collagen matrices have been used to develop in vitro models of the wound contraction process. Contraction of floating matrices resembles initial wound contraction, contraction of attached matrices resembles granulation tissue formation, and contraction of stressed matrices resembles granulation tissue contraction and regression at the end of repair. Studies in our laboratory have focused on contraction of stressed matrices. The basal component of stressed matrix contraction results in plasma-membrane ectocytosis, actin cytoskeletal disruption, $Ca^{2+}$ uptake, stimulation of cyclic adenosine monophosphate (cAMP) and mitogen-activated protein (MAP) kinase signaling pathways, and transcriptional activation of c-fos and other immediate early genes. The stimulated component of stressed matrix contraction (stimulated by serum or lysophosphatidic acid) results in actin cytoskeletal retraction and growth-factor desensitization. Subsequently, the cells become quiescent and regress through apoptosis.

## 2 Wound Contraction and Myofibroblasts

Closure of cutaneous wounds involves three processes: epithelization, connective tissue deposition, and contraction. The contribution of each process varies according to the type of wound. In general, epithelization results in resurfacing of the wound, connective tissue deposition results in replacement of damaged dermis, and contraction brings the margins of open wounds together [10,63]. In mammals

Current Topics in Pathology, Volume 93
A. Desmoulière, B. Tuchweber (Eds.)
© Springer-Verlag Berlin Heidelberg 1999

with loose skin (loosely attached to the underlying tissue layer), contraction leads to wound closure with little scarring or loss of function. In humans, whose skin is more firmly attached to underlying tissues, the consequences of contraction are often less beneficial, ranging from minimal cosmetic scarring in some cases to loss of joint motion or major body deformation in others [47, 88, 92].

Twenty-five years ago, GABBIANI et al. [29] identified cells in wound granulation tissue that exhibit some ultrastructural features of smooth-muscle cells. Although these cells, called myofibroblasts, express $\alpha$-smooth muscle actin and occasionally other smooth-muscle cytoskeletal components, they are derived from (as yet unidentified) fibroblast precursor cells adjacent to the wound margins that proliferate and migrate into the wound region during granulation tissue formation [12, 21, 101]. No unique immunological markers have been identified, as yet, that are specific to myofibroblasts, therefore, most investigators classify cells as myofibroblasts based on their overall morphology and the presence of $\alpha$-smooth-muscle actin. At the end of wound healing, granulation tissue regresses and the myofibroblast population diminishes markedly. Cellular apoptosis has been implicated in disappearance of myofibroblasts from granulation tissue [17, 30], but the signals that trigger apoptosis after wound closure are unknown.

In general, it is believed that myofibroblasts play a major role in wound contraction [15]. These cells also may contribute to the pathology of fibrotic diseases in such diverse tissues as heart, liver, lung, kidney and tumor stroma [14, 85]. However, myofibroblasts are absent from embryonic wounds, which do not scar [26, 75]. Transforming growth factor-$\beta$1 (TGF-$\beta$1) promotes tissue fibrosis and scarring [83], and also promotes fibroblast differentiation into myofibroblasts [16, 85]; whereas $\gamma$-interferon decreases the fibrotic response and the appearance of myofibroblasts [18, 79].

Under some conditions, wound contractile activity can be attributed to cells at the wound margins rather than to myofibroblasts in granulation tissue [36]. It seems likely that a critical factor in appearance of myofibroblasts is tissue resistance to contractile force. In the absence of resistance, migrating fibroblasts at the wound margins can generate sufficient force to reorganize the tissue. As the cells encounter resistance, they differentiate into myofibroblasts [33].

## 3 In Vitro Models of Wound Contraction

Understanding the interrelated features of cell signaling, contractility and apoptosis during wound contraction is an essential step in the search for therapeutic strategies to control contraction and scarring. Toward this end, we and others have developed several variations of an in vitro model of wound contraction that takes advantage of the ability of fibroblasts cultured within a collagen matrix to reorganize the collagen fibril network into a dense, tissue-like structure [25].

Figure 1 illustrates three variations of in vitro contraction using collagen matrices. No standard terminology has yet evolved for naming these variations. Different authors refer to in vitro contraction as compaction, retraction, condensation or tractional remodeling, and to collagen matrices as lattices or gels. In addition, although these variations sometimes are presented interchangeably, each has

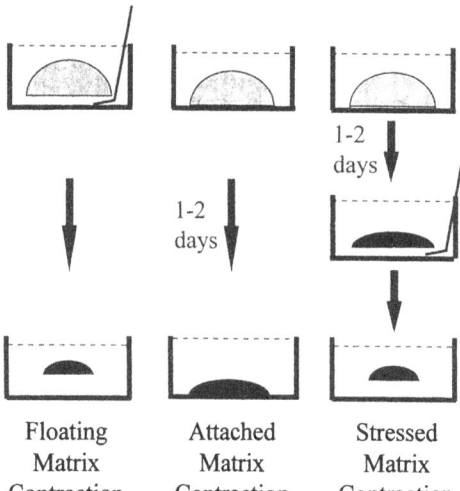

**Fig. 1.** In vitro models of wound contraction

Floating Matrix Contraction

Attached Matrix Contraction

Stressed Matrix Contraction

**Table 1.** Features of in vitro wound contraction

|  | Floating-matrix contraction | Attached-matrix contraction | Stressed-matrix contraction |
|---|---|---|---|
| Starting conditions | Trypsinized cells in a newly polymerized matrix floating in medium | Trypsinized cells in a newly polymerized matrix attached to a culture dish | Cells in an attached-collagen matrix 1–2 days, mechanical stress |
| After contraction | No mechanical stress develops, stellate cell morphology, cell quiescence and apoptosis | Mechanical stress develops, bipolar cell morphology, cell proliferation | Mechanical stress dissipated, stellate cell morphology, cell quiescence and apoptosis |
| In vivo correlate | Initial wound contraction as a consequence of cell migration | Granulation tissue formation, appearance of myofibroblasts | Myofibroblast contraction, cell regression at the end of wound contraction |

its own unique features and relationship to the in vivo situation, as summarized in Table 1 and discussed below in greater detail.

## 4 Floating-Matrix Contraction

Floating-matrix contraction was originally introduced by BELL et al. [2] as the "dermal equivalent" component of an in vitro skin graft [3]. The matrices are released from the culture dish immediately after polymerization. During contraction, the size of the matrix decreases in three dimensions. The floating matrix offers no external resistance to fibroblasts and, under these conditions, the cells do not differentiate into myofibroblasts [23]. Instead, the cells develop stellate morphology with long processes and a cytoskeletal meshwork [2, 4], similar to fibroblasts in dermis. The floating-matrix contraction model has been useful for comparing different cell populations, and cells harvested from granulation tissue [27, 32, 70, 77] or hypertrophic scar [31, 99] generally show an increased ability to contract the matrices compared with control cells.

## 5 Attached-Matrix Contraction

Unlike the situation during floating-matrix contraction, the collagen matrix remains attached on the culture dish (or other support) during contraction. As a result, although contraction begins in a similar manner as during floating-matrix contraction, the fibroblasts eventually encounter mechanical resistance to the forces that they exert. As a result, mechanical stress develops. The cells become bipolar, orient along lines of tension [5, 94] and develop prominent actin stress fibers and fibronexus junctions [43, 58, 67, 98].

If floating-matrix contraction results in formation of a "dermal equivalent", then attached-collagen-matrix contraction results in formation of a "granulation-tissue equivalent", containing cells with overall morphological features that resemble myofibroblasts. The force exerted on collagen by cells under these conditions is comparable with that generated in skin wounds undergoing contraction [13, 19, 53].

## 6 Role of Cell Motility in Contraction of Floating and Attached Collagen Matrices

Fibroblast contraction of floating collagen matrices and the early phase of contraction of attached collagen matrices (before the matrices begin to resist the pull of the cells) occur as a byproduct of cell spreading and motility [20, 23, 34, 44, 87], but the collagen fibrils, rather than the cells, translocate. The forces exerted by the cells are propagated throughout the interconnected collagen fibril network (40), and fibril reorganization occurs in a proximal to distal manner [34, 105]. Reorganized collagen fibrils can be stabilized by non-covalent interactions [39], but covalent crosslinking may also be important [102]. Fibroblast attachment to collagen necessary for contraction depends on $\alpha2\beta1$ integrins [42, 51, 90, 91]. Despite the fact that contraction of collagen matrices does not require fibronectin [38, 42] or the fibronectin receptor $\alpha5\beta1$ [97], monoclonal antibodies against a unique fibronectin domain have been shown to inhibit contraction [1, 76].

## 7 Cell Proliferation in Floating versus Mechanically Stressed Collagen Matrices

One of the major differences between fibroblasts in floating versus mechanically stressed matrices concerns cell growth. That is, fibroblasts cultured in mechanically stressed collagen matrices proliferate [71, 73, 74], whereas cells cultured in floating collagen matrices become quiescent [89, 100]. Under the latter conditions, platelet-derived growth factor (PDGF) and epidermal growth factor (EGF) receptors become desensitized, i. e., lose their normal signaling capacity [59, 64, 96] (see below), essentially subjecting the cells to growth-factor withdrawal, even in the continued presence of growth factors in the cells' environment [35, 81].

## 8 Stressed-Matrix Contraction

Stressed-matrix contraction, in a sense, combines the attached- and floating-matrix contraction variations (Fig. 1). That is, during an initial period (>1 day) of attached-matrix contraction, mechanical stress develops. Then, when the mechanically stressed matrices are released and allowed to float in culture medium, the cells rapidly contract the matrix further, as mechanical stress is dissipated. In this case, cell contraction is accompanied by release of ectocytotic vesicles, collapse of actin filament bundles, and disruption of fibronexus junctions [58, 67, 98], and the cells acquire morphological features similar to those observed after floating matrix contraction.

## 9 Collagen-Matrix Contraction and Cell Signaling

Signal-transduction pathways become activated during collagen matrix contraction for diverse reasons. For instance, during floating-matrix contraction, the initial adhesive interactions between fibroblasts and collagen result in activation of focal adhesion kinase [84], extracellular signal-regulated protein kinase (ERK) 1/2 [57] and phospholipase C-$\zeta$ [104]. Moreover, placing cells in collagen matrices results in increased expression of $\alpha 2$ integrin [51, 103] and collagenase [55, 65]. Occupancy of integrin $\alpha 2 \beta 1$, activation of protein tyrosine kinase, and phospholipase C-$\zeta$ have been implicated in the changes in collagenase expression [6, 56, 104].

In the case of stressed-matrix contraction, the adhesive interactions of the cell population reach the steady state before contraction is initiated. Moreover, the entire cell population contracts rapidly in a relatively synchronized fashion. Therefore, stressed-matrix contraction provides a model in which to study contraction-stimulated signal-transduction processes and their downstream consequences, independent of initial cell-matrix adhesion.

Upon releasing mechanically stressed matrices from their attachment sites, basal contraction (in the absence of serum or growth factors) (Fig. 2) activates a $Ca^{2+}$-dependent signaling pathway, resulting within minutes in increases in cellular phosphatidic acid, diacylglycerol and cAMP [45, 46]. $Ca^{2+}$ enters the

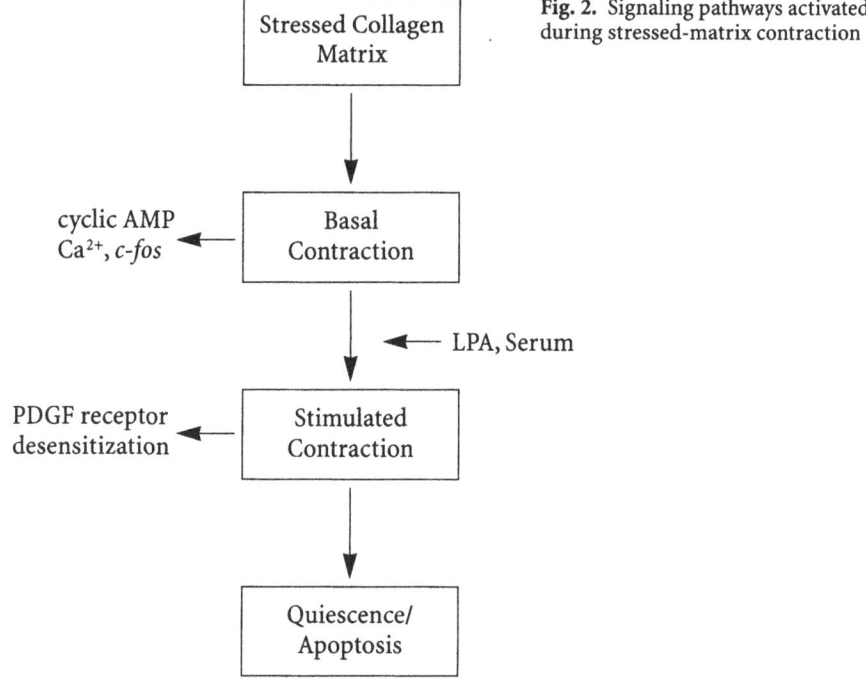

**Fig. 2.** Signaling pathways activated during stressed-matrix contraction

cells through ~3- to 5-nm plasma-membrane passages with openings that can be detected by fluorescein isothiocyanate (FITC)-dextran added to the culture medium (Fig. 3) [61]. These passages reseal in less than 5 s in the presence of divalent cations. Similar plasma-membrane passages have been detected in vivo in diverse cells types within mechanically active tissues [7, 11, 48, 66]. Contraction also results in activation of the MAP kinases, ERK 1, 2 [86], p38, and c-Jun amino terminal kinase (JNK) (Lee and Grinnell, unpublished observations).

$Ca^{2+}$ influx and other as yet unidentified factors lead to markedly increased c-fos transcription, which peaks 50–60 min after initiating contraction. Two other immediate early genes, fosb and c-jun, also increase transiently after fibroblast contraction, but fra-1, fra-2, and c-myc, and the transcription factor NF-$\kappa$B do not appear to change. Therefore, contraction appears to activate a select group of genes [86].

In the presence of serum or lysophosphatidic acid (LPA), which stimulate stressed matrix contraction (see below), PDGF receptors rapidly become desensitized. The mechanism of desensitization depends on decreased PDGF-receptor kinase activity rather than increased protein tyrosine phosphatase activity [62]. Subsequently, DNA synthesis declines rapidly [67] and the cells undergo marked regression [72], probably as a consequence of apoptosis [28] (M. Carlson, M. Zhu, and F. Grinnell, unpublished observations).

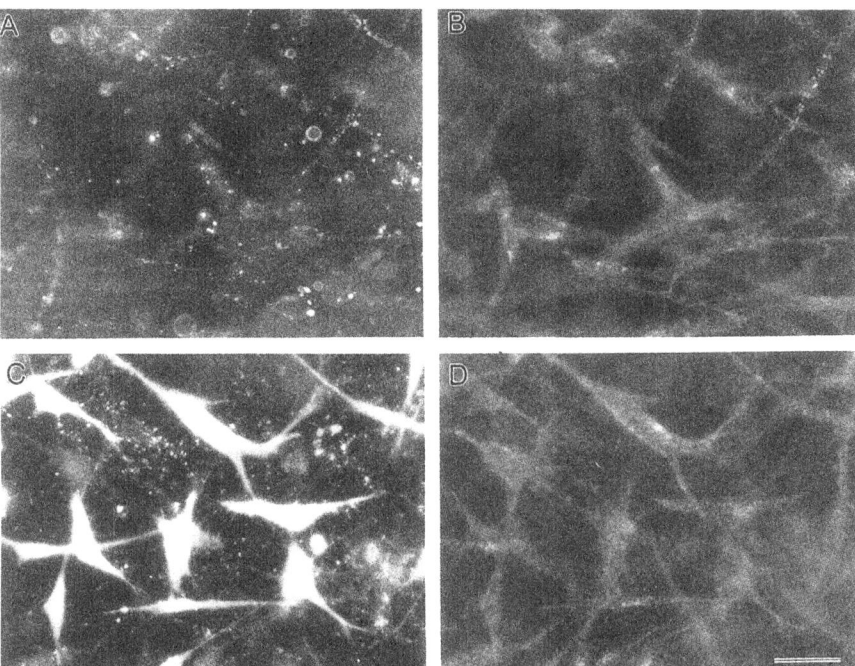

**Fig. 3 A – D.** Fluorescein isothiocyanate (FITC)-dextran uptake during fibroblast contraction of stressed-collagen matrices. Fibroblasts in stressed collagen matrices were incubated for 10 min with 10 mg/ml 4 kDa FITC-dextran after which half the matrices were released to initiate contraction. After 10 min, the samples were washed and counterstained with rhodamine isothiocyante (RITC)-wheat germ agglutinin (WGA). **A, B** Cells in stressed matrices; **C, D** cells undergoing contraction; **A, C** FITC-dextran; **B, D** RITC-WGA. **C** and **D** show that essentially all of the cells in the matrix become fluorescently labeled during contraction, whereas little FITC-dextran can be detected in cells in stressed matrices (A/B). Bar = 50 μm. See [61] for details

## 10 Regulation of Matrix Contraction by Growth Factors

In addition to serum [38, 93], a variety of specific growth factors have been shown to promote collagen matrix contraction. Interestingly, LPA, a bioreactive lipid released from activated platelets [69], can stimulate floating or stressed matrix contraction [52, 60, 80]; whereas PDGF stimulates floating matrix contraction [9, 42, 96], but not stressed matrix contraction [60]. Also, increasing cellular cAMP levels inhibits floating-matrix contraction [22, 100], but not stressed-matrix contraction [45, 46].

Overall, the above data suggest that different signaling pathways regulate floating- and stressed-matrix contraction. The linkage between these pathways and downstream contractile mechanisms have yet to be determined, however. Based on pharmacological studies, a variety of factors have been implicated in contraction, including the actin cytoskeleton [2, 5, 38], myosin light-chain kinase [24], myosin light-chain phosphorylation [52], protein kinase C [37], protein tyrosine kinase [6, 56] and protein tyrosine phosphatase [60].

Also, it should be noted that a variety of other growth factors in addition to PDGF and LPA stimulate collagen-matrix contraction under some conditions. These include TGF-$\beta$ [27, 68], endothelin [41] and thrombin [78]. The mechanism of stimulation by TGF-$\beta$ probably depends on increased expression of integrin $\alpha2\beta1$ [82] and differentiation of cells to the myofibroblast phenotype [16, 85, 106].

## 11  Future Studies

Future studies are required to identify the mechanisms by which growth factors stimulate collagen-matrix contraction. As indicated above, PDGF and LPA probably stimulate myosin light-chain phosphorylation and matrix contraction by different signal-transduction pathways [8, 54, 95]. Why the PDGF regulatory mechanism no longer functions once fibroblasts are in mechanically stressed collagen matrices remains an unsolved puzzle. The possibility of regulating wound contraction in vivo by manipulating growth factors depends on our understanding of how the growth factors function in contraction. In addition, it would be worthwhile to identify upstream factors that lead from contraction to activation of the MAP kinase signal-transduction pathways. Preliminary evidence suggests that ERK activation may be biphasic and involve a contraction-stimulated autocrine mechanism (D. Lee and F. Grinnell, unpublished observation). The linkage between activation of the MAP kinase and transcription of immediate early genes requires analysis as well. Finally, it will be important to identify the factors that contribute to apoptosis of cells after stressed-matrix contraction, especially the possibility that apoptosis in this model system results from inhibition of the PI3-kinase-AKT/protein kinase B signaling pathway [49, 50] through a combination of growth factor desensitization (growth factor withdrawal) and disruption of fibronexus junctions (loss of fibronectin receptor occupancy).

**Acknowledgements.** These studies were supported by NIH Grant #GM31321 and by the NIH Skin Diseases Research Center Grant #AR4194.

## References

1. Asaga H, Kikuchi S, Yoshizato K (1991) Collagen gel contraction by fibroblasts requires cellular fibronectin but not plasma fibronectin. Exp Cell Res 193:167–174
2. Bell E, Ivarsson B, Merrill C (1979) Production of a tissue-like structure by contraction of collagen lattices by human fibroblasts of different proliferative potential in vitro. Proc Nat Acad Sci U S A 76:1274–1278
3. Bell E, Sher S, Hull B, Merrill C, Rosen S, Chamson A, Asselineau D, Dubertret L, Coulomb B, Lapiere C, Nusgens B, Neveux Y (1983) The reconstitution of living skin. J Invest Dermatol 81:2s–10s
4. Bellows CG, Melcher AH, Aubin JE (1981) Contraction and organization of collagen gels by cells cultured from periodontal ligament, gingiva, and bond suggest functional differences between cell types. J Cell Sci 50:299–314
5. Bellows CG, Melcher AH, Aubin JE (1982) Association between tension and orientation of periodontal ligament fibroblasts and exogenous collagen fibers in collagen gels in vitro. J Cell Sci 58:125–138

6. Broberg A, Heino J (1996) Integrin alpha2beta1-dependent contraction of floating collagen gels and induction of collagenase are inhibited by tyrosine kinase inhibitors. Exp Cell Res 228:29–35
7. Cheng GC, Libby P, Grodzinsky AJ, Lee RT (1996) Induction of DNA synthesis by a single transient mechanical stimulus of human vascular smooth muscle cells. Circulation 93:99–105
8. Chrzanowska-Wodnicka M, Burridge K (1996) Rho-stimulated contractility drives the formation of stress fibers and focal adhesions. J Cell Biol 133:1403–1415
9. Clark RA, Folkvord JM, Hart CE, Murray MJ, McPherson (1989) Platelet isoforms of platelet-derived growth factor stimulate fibroblasts to contract collagen matrices. J Clin Invest 84:1036–1040
10. Clark RAF (1996) Wound repair: overview and general considerations. In: Clark RAF (ed) The molecular and cellular basis of wound repair, Plenum Press, New York, pp 3–50
11. Clarke MS, Caldwell RW, Chiao H, Miyake K, McNeil PL (1995) Contraction-induced cell wounding and release of fibroblast growth factor in heart. Circ Res 76:927–934
12. Darby I, Skalli O, Gabbiani G (1990) Alpha-smooth muscle actin is transiently expressed by myofibroblasts during experimental wound healing. Lab Invest 63:21–29
13. Delvoye P, Wiliquet P, Leveque JL, Nusgens BV, Lapiere CM (1991) Measurement of mechanical forces generated by skin fibroblasts embedded in a three-dimensional collagen gel. J Invest Dermatol 97:898–902
14. Desmoulière A, Gabbiani G (1994) Modulation of fibroblastic cytoskeletal features during pathological situations: the role of extracellular matrix and cytokines. W Cell Motil Cytoskeleton 29:195–203
15. Desmoulière A, Gabbiani G (1996) The role of the myofibroblast in wound healing and fibrocontractive disease. In: Clark RAF (ed) The molecular and cellular basis of wound repair. Plenum Press, New York, pp 391–423
16. Desmoulière A, Geinoz A, Gabbiani F, Gabbiani G (1993) Transforming growth factor-beta 1 induces alpha-smooth muscle actin expression in quiescent and growing cultured fibroblasts. J Cell Biol 122:103–111
17. Desmoulière A, Redard M, Darby I, Gabbiani G (1995) Apoptosis mediates the decrease in cellularity during the transition between granulation tissue and scar. Am J Pathol 146:56–66
18. Desmoulière A, Rubbia-Brandt L, Abdiu A, Walz T, Macieira-Coelho A, Gabbiani G (1992) Alpha-smooth muscle actin is expressed in a subpopulation subpopulation of cultured and cloned fibroblasts and is modulated by γ-interferon. Exp Cell Res 201:64–73
19. Eastwood M, McGrouther DA, Brown RA (1994) A culture force monitor for measurement of contraction forces generated in human dermal fibroblast cultures: evidence for cell-matrix mechanical signalling. Biochim Biophys Acta 1201:186–192
20. Eastwood M, Porter R, Khan U, McGrouther G, Brown R (1996) Quantitative analysis of collagen gel contractile forces generated by dermal fibroblasts and the relationship to cell morphology. J Cell Phys 166:33–42
21. Eddy RJ, Petro JA, Tomasek JJ (1988) Evidence for the nonmuscle nature of the "myofibroblast" of granulation tissue and hypertrophic scar. Am J Pathol 130:252–260
22. Ehrlich HP, Griswold TR (1984) Epidermolysis bullosa dystrophica recessive fibroblasts produce increased concentrations of cAMP within a collagen matrix. J Invest Dermatol 83:230–233
23. Ehrlich HP, Rajaratnam JB (1990) Cell locomotion forces versus cell contraction forces for for collagen lattice contraction: an in vitro model of wound contraction. Tissue Cell 22:407–417
24. Ehrlich HP, Rockwell WB, Cornwell TL, Rajaratnam JBM (1991) Demonstration of a direct role for myosin light chain kinase in fibroblast-populated collagen lattice contraction. J Cell Physiol 146:1–7
25. Elsdale T, Bard J (1972) Collagen substrata for studies on cell behavior. J Cell Biol 54:626–637
26. Estes JM, Vande Berg JS, Adzick NS, MacGillivray TE, Desmoulière A, Gabbiani G (1994) Phenotypic and functional features of myofibroblasts in sheep fetal wounds. Differentiation 56:173–181

27. Finesmith TH, Broadley KN, Davidson JM (1990) Fibroblasts from wounds of different stages of repair vary in their ability to contract a collagen gel in response to growth factors. J Cell Physiol 144:99-107
28. Fluck J, Querfeld C, Cremer A, Niland S, Krieg T, Sollberg S (1998) Normal human primary fibroblasts undergo apoptosis in three-dimensional contractile collagen gels. J Invest Dermatol 110:153-157
29. Gabbiani G, Hirschel BJ, Ryan GB, Statkov PR, Majno G (1972) Granulation tissue as a contractile organ. A study of structure and function. J Exp Med 135:719-734
30. Garbin S, Pittet B, Montandon D, Gabbiani G, Desmoulière A (1996) Covering by a flap induces apoptosis of granulation tissue myofibroblasts and vascular cells. Wound Rep Regen 4:244-251
31. Garner WL, Rittenberg T, Ehrlich HP, Karmiol S, Rodriques JL, Smith DJ, Phan SH (1995) Hypertrophic scar fibroblasts accelerate collagen gel contraction. Wound Rep Regen 3:185-191
32. Germain L, Jean A, Auger FA, Garrel DR (1994) Human wound healing fibroblasts have greater contractile properties than dermal fibroblasts. J Surg Res 57:268-273
33. Grinnell F (1994) Fibroblasts, myofibroblasts, and wound contraction. J Cell Biol 124:401-404
34. Grinnell F, Lamke CR (1984) Reorganization of hydrated collagen lattices by human skin fibroblasts. J Cell Sci 66:51-63
35. Grinnell F, Nakagawa S (1991) Spatial regulation of fibroblast proliferation: an explanation for cell regression at the end of wound repair. Prog Clin Biol Res 365:155-166
36. Gross J, Farinelli W, Sadow P, Anderson R, Bruns R (1995) On the mechanism of skin wound "contraction": a granulation tissue "knockout" with a normal phenotype. Proc Natl Acad Sci U S A 92:5982-5986
37. Guidry C (1992) Extracellular matrix contraction by fibroblasts: peptide promoters and second messengers. Cancer Metastasis Rev 11:45-54
38. Guidry C, Grinnell F (1985) Studies on the mechanism of hydrated collagen gel reorganization by human skin fibroblasts. J Cell Sci 79:67-81
39. Guidry C, Grinnell F (1986) Contraction of hydrated collagen gels by fibroblasts: evidence for two mechanisms by which collagen fibrils are stabilized. Coll Rel Res 6:515-529
40. Guidry C, Grinnell F (1987) Heparin modulates the organization of hydrated collagen gels and inhibits gel contraction by fibroblasts. J Cell Biol 104:1097-1103
41. Guidry C, Hook M (1991) Endothelins produced by endothelial cells promote collagen gel contraction by fibroblasts. J Cell Biol 115:873-880
42. Gullberg D, Tingström A, Thuresson AC, Olsson L, Terracio L, Borg TK, Rubin K (1990) Beta 1 integrin-mediated collagen gel contraction is stimulated by PDGF. Exp Cell Res 186:264-272
43. Halliday NL, Tomasek JJ (1995) Mechanical properties of the extracellular matrix influence fibronectin fibril assembly in vitro. Exp Cell Res 217:109-117
44. Harris AK, Stopak D, Wild P (1981) Fibroblast traction as a mechanism for collagen morphogenesis. Nature 290:249-251
45. He Y, Grinnell F (1994) Stress relaxation of fibroblasts activates a cyclic AMP signaling pathway. J Cell Biol 126:457-464
46. He Y, Grinnell F (1995) Role of phospholipase D in the cAMP signal transduction pathway activated during fibroblast contraction of collagen matrices. J Cell Biol 130:1197-1205
47. Hunt TK, Dunphy JE (1979) Fundamentals of wound management. Appleton-Century-Crofts, New York
48. Kaye D, Pimental D, Prasad S, Maki T, Berger HJ, McNeil PL, Kelly RA (1996) Role of transiently altered sarcolemmal membrane permeability and basic fibroblast growth factor release in the hypertrophic response of adult rat ventricular myocytes to increased mechanical activity in vitro. J Clin Invest 97:281-291
49. Kennedy SG, Wagner AJ, Conzen SD, Jordan J, Bellacosa A, Tsichlis PN, Hay N (1997) The PI 3-kinase/Akt signaling pathway delivers an anti-apoptotic signal. Genes Dev 11:701-713
50. Khwaja A, Rodriguez-Viciana P, Wennström S, Warne PH, Downward J (1997) Matrix adhesion and Ras transformation both activate a phosphoinositide 3-OH kinase and protein kinase B/Akt cellular survival pathway. Embo J 16:2783-2793

51. Klein CE, Dressel D, Steinmayer T, Mauch C, Eckes B, Krieg T, Bankert RB, Weber L (1991) Integrin alpha 2 beta 1 is upregulated in fibroblasts and highly aggressive melanoma cells in three-dimensional collagen lattices and mediates the reorganization of collagen I fibrils. J Cell Biol 115:1427–1436
52. Kolodney MS, Elson EL (1993) Correlation of myosin light chain phosphorylation with isometric contraction of fibroblasts. J Biol Chem 268:23850–23855
53. Kolodney MS, Wysolmerski RB (1992) Isometric contraction by fibroblasts and endothelial cells in tissue culture. J Cell Biol 117:73–82
54. Kureishi Y, Kobayashi S, Amano M, Kimura K, Kanaides H, Nakano T, Kaibuchi K, Ito M (1997) Rho-associated kinase directly induces smooth muscle contraction through myosin light chain phosphorylation. J Biol Chem 272:12257–12260
55. Lambert CA, Soudant EP, Nusgens BV, Lapiere CM (1992) Pretranslational regulation of extracellular matrix macromolecules and collagenase expression in fibroblasts by mechanical forces. Lab Invest 66:444–451
56. Langholz O, Rockel D, Mauch C, Kozlowska E, Bank I, Krieg T, Eckes B (1995) Collagen and collagenase gene expression in three-dimensional collagen lattices are differentially regulated by alpha 1 beta 1 and alpha 2 beta 1 integrins. J Cell Biol 131:1903–1915
57. Langholz O, Roeckel D, Petersohn D, Broermann E, Eckes B, Krieg T (1997) Cell-matrix interactions induce tyrosine phosphorylation of MAP kinases ERK1 and ERK2 and PLCgamma-1 in two-dimensional and three-dimensional cultures of human fibroblasts. Exp Cell Res 235:22–27
58. Lee TL, Lin YC, Mochitate K, Grinnell F (1993) Stress-relaxation of fibroblasts in collagen matrices triggers ectocytosis of plasma membrane vesicles containing actin, annexins II and VI, and $\beta1$ integrin receptors. J Cell Sci 105:167–177
59. Lin YC, Grinnell F (1993) Decreased level of PDGF-stimulated receptor autophosphorylation by fibroblasts in mechanically relaxed collagen matrices. J Cell Biol 122:663–672
60. Lin YC, Grinnell F (1995) Treatment of human fibroblasts with vanadate and platelet-derived growth factor in the presence of serum inhibits collagen matrix contraction. Exp Cell Res 221:73–82
61. Lin YC, Ho CH, Grinnell F (1997) Fibroblasts contracting collagen matrices form transient plasma membrane passages through which the cells take up fluorescein isothiocyanate-dextran and $Ca^{2+}$. Mol Biol Cell 8:59–71
62. Lin YC, Ho C-H, Grinnell F (1998) Decreased PDGF receptor kinase activity in fibroblasts contracting stressed collagen matrices. Exp Cell Res 240:377–387
63. Martin P (1997) Wound healing – aiming for perfect skin regeneration. Science 276:75–81
64. Marx M, Daniel TO, Kashgarian M, Madri JA (1993) Spatial organization of the extracellular matrix modulates the expression of PDGF-receptor subunits in mesangial cells. Kidney Intl 43:1027–1041
65. Mauch C, Adelmann-Grill B, Hatamochi A, Krieg T (1989) Collagenase gene expression in fibroblasts is regulated by a three-dimensional contact with collagen. FEBS Lett 250: 301–305
66. McNeil PL, Steinhardt RA (1997) Loss, restoration, and maintenance of plasma membrane integrity. J Cell Biol 137:1–4
67. Mochitate K, Pawelek P, Grinnell F (1991) Stress relaxation of contracted collagen gels: disruption of actin filament bundles, release of cell surface fibronectin, and down regulation of DNA and protein synthesis. Exp Cell Res 193:198–207
68. Montesano R, Orci L (1988) Transforming growth factor beta stimulates collagen-matrix contraction by fibroblasts: implications for wound healing. Proc Nat Acad Sci USA 85:4894–4897
69. Moolenaar WH (1995) Lysophosphatidic acid signalling. Curr Opin Cell Biol 7:203–210
70. Moulin V, Castilloux G, Jean A, Garrel DR, Auger FA, Germain L (1996) In vitro models to study wound healing fibroblasts. Burns 22:359–362
71. Nakagawa S, Pawelek P, Grinnell F (1989) Extracellular matrix organization modulates fibroblast growth and growth factor responsiveness. Exp Cell Res 182:572–582
72. Nakagawa S, Pawelek P, Grinnell F (1989) Long-term culture of fibroblasts in contracted collagen gels: effects on cell growth and biosynthetic activity. J Invest Dermatol 93:792–798

73. Nishiyama T, Akutsu N, Horii I, Nakayama Y, Ozawa T, Hayashi T (1991) Response to growth factors of human dermal fibroblasts in a quiescent state owing to cell-matrix contact inhibition. Matrix 11:71–75
74. Nishiyama T, Horii I, Nakayama Y, Ozawa T, Hayashi T (1990) A distinct characteristic of the quiescent state of human dermal fibroblasts in contracted collagen gel as revealed by no response to epidermal growth factor alone, but a positive growth response to a combination of the factor and saikosaponin b. Matrix 10:412–419
75. Nodder S, Martin P (1997) Wound healing in embryos: a review. Anat Embryol (Berl) 195:215–228
76. Obara M, Yoshizato K (1997) A novel domain of fibronectin revealed by epitope mapping of a monoclonal antibody which inhibits fibroblasts-mediated collagen gel contraction. FEBS Lett 412:48–52
77. Petri JB, Saalbach A, Haupt B, Pierer M, Hausten U-F, Herrmann K (1997) In vitro analysis of adhesion molecule expression and gel contraction of human granulation tissue fibroblasts. Wound Rep Regen 5:69–76
78. Pilcher BK, Kim DW, Carney DH, Tomasek JJ (1994) Thrombin stimulates fibroblast-mediated collagen lattice contraction by its proteolytically activated receptor. Exp Cell Res 211:368–373
79. Pittet B, Rubbia-Brandt L, Desmouliere A, Sappino AP, Roggero P, Guerret S, Grimaud JA, Lacher R, Montandon D, Gabbiani G (1994) Effect of gamma-interferon on the clinical and biologic evolution of hypertrophic scars and Dupuytren's disease: an open pilot study. Plast Reconst Surg 93:1224–1235
80. Rayan GM, Parizi M, Tomasek JJ (1996) Pharmacologic regulation of Dupuytren's fibroblast contraction in vitro. J Hand Surg [Br] 21:1065–1070
81. Rhudy RW, McPherson JM (1988) Influence of the extracellular matrix on the proliferative response of human skin fibroblasts to serum and purified platelet-derived growth factor. J Cell Phys 137:185–191
82. Riikonen T, Koivisto L, Vihinen P, Heino J (1995) Transforming growth factor-beta regulates collagen gel contraction by increasing alpha 2 beta 1 integrin expression in osteogenic cells. J Biol Chem 270:376–382
83. Roberts AB, Sporn MB (1996) Transforming growth factor $\beta$. In: Clark RAF (ed) The molecular and cellular basis of wound repair. Plenum Press, New York, pp 275–308
84. Roeckel D, Krieg T (1994) Three-dimensional contact with type I collagen mediates tyrosine phosphorylation in primary human fibroblasts. Exp Cell Res 211:42–48
85. Rønnov-Jessen L, Petersen OW (1993) Induction of alpha-smooth muscle actin by transforming growth factor-$\beta$1 in quiescent human breast gland fibroblasts. Lab Invest 68:696–707
86. Rosenfeldt H, Lee DJ, Grinnell F (1998) Increased c-fos mRNA expression by human fibroblasts contracting stressed collagen matrices. Mol Cell Biol 18:2659–2667
87. Roy P, Petroll WM, Cavanagh HD, Chuong CJ, Jester JV (1997) An in vitro force measurement assay to study the early mechanical interaction between corneal fibroblasts and collagen matrix. Exp Cell Res 232:106–117
88. Rudolph R, Berg JV, Ehrlich HP (1992) Wound contraction and scar contracture. In: Cohen IK, Diegelmann RF, Lindblad WJ (eds) Wound healing: biochemical and clinical aspects. Saunders, Philadelphia, pp 96–114
89. Sarber R, Hull B, Merrill C, Soranno T, Bell E (1981) Regulation of proliferation of fibroblasts of low and high population doubling levels grown in collagen lattices. Mech Ageing Dev 17:107–117
90. Schiro JA, Chan BM, Roswit WT, Kassner PD, Pentland AP, Hemler ME, Eisen AZ, Kupper TS (1991) Integrin alpha 2 beta 1 (VLA-2) mediates reorganization and contraction of collagen matrices by human cells. Cell 67:403–410
91. Schon M, Schon MP, Kuhrober A, Schirmbeck R, Kaufmann R, Klein CE (1996) Expression of the human alpha2 integrin subunit in mouse melanoma cells confers the ability to undergo collagen-directed adhesion, migration, and matrix reorganization. J Invest Dermatol 106:1175–1181
92. Skalli O, Gabbiani G (1988) The biology of the myofibroblast in relationship to wound contraction and fibrocontractive disease. In: Clark RAF, Henson PM (eds) The molecular and cellular basis of wound repair. Plenum Press, New York, pp 373–402

93. Steinberg BM, Smith K, Colozzo M, Pollack R (1980) Establishment and transformation diminish the ability of fibroblasts to contract a native collagen gel. J Cell Biol 87:304–308
94. Stopak D, Harris AK (1982) Connective tissue morphogenesis by fibroblast traction. I. Tissue culture observations. Dev Biol 90:383–398
95. Tapon N, Hall A (1997) Rho, Rac and Cdc42 GTPases regulate the organization of the actin cytoskeleton. Curr Opin Cell Biol 9:86–92
96. Tingström A, Heldin C-H, Rubin K (1992) Regulation of fibroblast-mediated collagen gel contraction by platelet-derived growth factor, interleukin-1a and transforming growth factor-$\beta$1. J Cell Sci 102:315–322
97. Tomasek JJ, Akiyama SK (1992) Fibroblast-mediated collagen gel contraction does not require fibronectin-alpha 5 beta 1 integrin interaction. Anat Rec 234:153–160
98. Tomasek JJ, Haaksma CJ, Eddy RJ, Vaughan MB (1992) Fibroblast contraction occurs on release of tension in attached collagen lattices: Dependency on an organized actin cytoskeleton and serum. Anat Rec 232:359–368
99. Tsai C, Hata K, Torii S, Matsuyama M, Ueda M (1995) Contraction potency of hypertrophic scar-derived fibroblasts in a connective tissue model: In vitro analysis of wound contraction. Ann Plast Surg 35:638–646
100. van Bockxmeer FM, Martin CE, Constable IJ (1984) Effect of cyclic AMP on cellular contractility and DNA synthesis in chorioretinal fibroblasts maintained in collagen matrices. Exp Cell Res 155:413–421
101. Welch MP, Odland GF, Clark RA (1990) Temporal relationships of F-actin bundle formation, collagen and fibronectin matrix assembly, and fibronectin receptor expression to wound contraction. J Cell Biol 110:133–145
102. Woodley DT, Yamauchi M, Wynn KC, Mechanic G, Briggaman RA (1991) Collagen telopeptides (cross-linking sites) play a role in collagen gel lattice contraction. J Invest Dermatol 97:580–585
103. Xu J, Clark RA (1996) Extracellular matrix alters PDGF regulation of fibroblast integrins. J Cell Biol 132:239–249
104. Xu J, Clark RA (1997) A three-dimensional collagen lattice induces protein kinase C-zeta activity: role in alpha2 integrin and collagenase mRNA expression. J Cell Biol 136:473–483
105. Yamato M, Adachi E, Yamamoto K, Hayashi T (1995) Condensation of collagen fibrils to the direct vicinity of fibroblasts as a cause of gel contraction. J Biochem 117:940–946
106. Yokozeki M, Moriyama K, Shimokawa H, Kuroda T (1997) Transforming growth factor-beta 1 modulates myofibroblastic phenotype of rat palatal fibroblasts in vitro. Exp Cell Res 231:328–336

# Extracellular Matrix, Integrins and Focal Adhesions

D. Dogic, B. Eckes, M. Aumailley

## 1 Introduction

Focal adhesions are defined as cell adhesion-related events in vitro, such as the strip-like structures formed within cells during their attachment [12, 17, 33]. Focal adhesions were first identified by transmission electron microscopy [1] followed by their characterisation using interference reflection as well as immunofluorescence microscopy [2]. In vivo, focal adhesion-like assemblies that are structurally and functionally similar to focal adhesions formed in vitro are found in certain cell types. These include the dense plaques of smooth-muscle cells, and the myotendinous and neuromuscular junctions of skeletal muscles [8, 52, 53]. A large number of cultivated normal or transformed cells are capable of forming focal adhesions in vitro; the prerequisite for classical focal-adhesion assembly being the presence of an extracellular-matrix substrate.

In this substrate-induced cell adhesion, the integrins, which are cellular receptors specifically mediating the interactions with extracellular-matrix proteins, self-aggregate and initiate the assembly of focal adhesions [14, 30, 56]. This process results in the recruitment and clustering of additional cytoplasmic as well as membrane-linked proteins, such as paxillin, vinculin, talin and $\alpha$-actinin (Fig. 1). A large number of cytoplasmic proteins participating in focal-adhesion formation is known, but the selectivity of their recruitment by integrins, although highly possible, needs to be investigated further. These different events lead to maturation of the adhesion organelles and to the presence in the final structure of an essential component, polymerised actin, that possibly gives the "strip-like" shape to focal adhesions [29]. Actually, focal adhesions could be considered as prolongations of actin filaments as they form only along the outer-most extremities of individual microfilaments. Indeed, the actin polymer barbed ends, characterised by high growth, are present and anchored in focal adhesions [34] where actin polymerisation takes place, in agreement with microfilament orientation [33, 39]. Therefore,

Current Topics in Pathology, Volume 93
A. Desmoulière, B. Tuchweber (Eds.)
© Springer-Verlag Berlin Heidelberg 1999

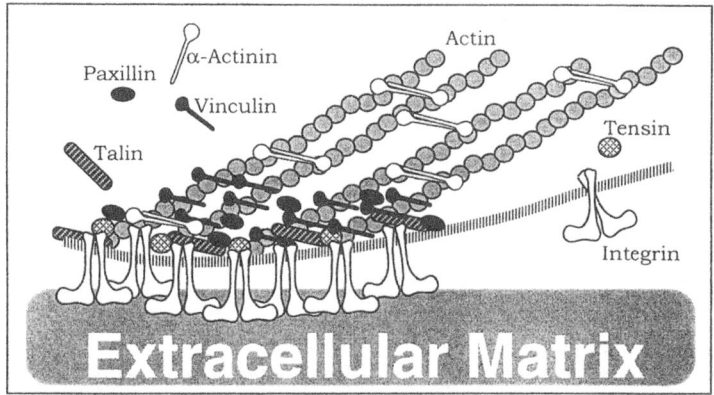

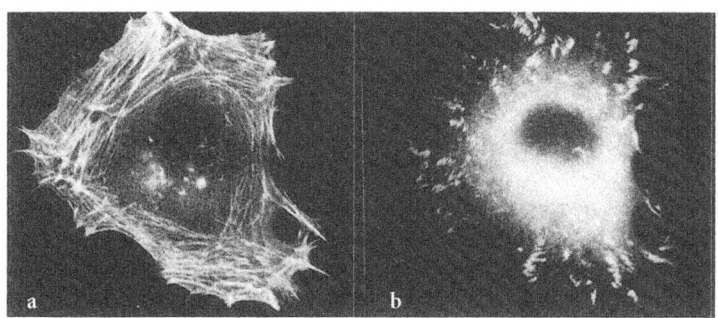

**Fig. 1 A, B.** Schematic representation and immunofluorescence staining of focal adhesion complexes. **A** Clustering of integrins and recruitment of diverse focal-contact proteins including actin microfilaments are schematically presented. **B** After 60 min of adhesion to fibronectin, cells were processed for double-staining of fibrillar actin with fluorescein-conjugated phalloidin (*a*) and vinculin with anti-vinculin antibody followed by Cy3-conjugated secondary antibody (*b*)

mature adhesion organelles, or focal contacts, serve to anchor the actin microfilament system and, in this way, contribute to the determination of cell shape during cell adhesion, spreading, migration and related events [29, 37]. Changes in cell shape are assured by the dynamics of actin filaments in terms of polymerisation and depolymerisation, and of reorganisation of preexisting microfilaments [41]. Two focal-adhesion proteins, vasodilator-stimulated phosphoprotein (VASP) and profilin, may control the rate of actin polymerisation and, consequently and in concert with other focal adhesion-associated components and the extracellular matrix, may impinge on cell shape, spreading and mobility [24].

The central players in the formation, the role and the regulation of the adhesion organelles are the integrins, which provide the physical link between the extracellular matrix and intracellular components [30]. Integrins are a large family of transmembrane proteins formed by heterodimerisation of two polypeptides, the $\alpha$ and $\beta$ subunits. To date, 16 $\alpha$ and 8 $\beta$ subunits have been identified and shown to combine into 22 distinct heterodimers [30]. Considering the fact that integrin cytoplasmic domains are devoid of enzymatic activity together with their potential role in signal transduction, it is expected that an individual receptor has high specificity for extracellular as well as intracellular ligands. As mentioned above, information is rather scarce concerning specific recruitment of cytoplasmic proteins and only a few players have been proposed for this task [28, 46, 50]. More is known about the interactions and the specificity of integrins for extracellular-matrix proteins and a rather exhaustive list of ligands present in the extracellular space has been reported [26, 30, 51]. This includes a large spectre of molecules as different as extra-cellular-matrix components, circulating factors and members of the complement system, bacterial and viral proteins, or cellular-counter receptors. Connective-tissue macromolecules, such as laminins, collagens, and fibronectins are mostly recognised by integrins of the $\beta 1$ subfamily [3, 30].

Specific recognition of extracellular-matrix proteins by integrin receptors occurs by a molecular mechanism, not yet completely understood, that certainly involves integrin conformational change [44]. This leads to integrin activation that is critical for induction of intracellular-signalling pathways and initiation of focal-contact formation. Signalling events taking place after integrin ligation, in parti-cular after cell adhesion, include activation of protein kinases such as pp125FAK (focal adhesion kinase), p59ILK (integrin linked kinase) and PKC (protein kinase C), changes in phospholipid metabolism, elevation of intracellular pH and $Ca^{2+}$ levels and specific down- or upregulation of certain genes [14, 20, 27]. Several focal-contact proteins, such as tensin and paxillin, are susceptible to phosphorylation on tyrosine (possibly by pp125FAK) upon cell adhesion and integrin ligation [9, 48]. Protein phosphorylation on tyrosine residues creates binding sites for Src homo-logy 2 (SH2) domain-containing proteins, such as tensin, several kinases and adapter proteins [14]. In this way, the Ras-MAP kinase pathway may be activated, leading to the induction of specific genes [42, 49].

## 2 Extracellular-Matrix Proteins in Focal Adhesion Formation: The Model of Laminins

"Outside-in" signalling, signalling from the extracellular matrix to the cell's interior, is mediated by direct interaction of integrins with the extracellular matrix and results in focal-adhesion assembly along the cell surface, followed by a variety of different cellular responses, such as proliferation, migration, differentiation or apoptosis. In this context, the morphology, distribution and composition of focal-adhesion complexes is of special interest, as it reflects changes in cellular activities due to cell interactions with extracellular-matrix proteins.

The laminin family is a group of prominent basement-membrane adhesive glycoproteins constituted by the assembly of three chains, the $\alpha$, $\beta$ and $\gamma$ chains [4, 10]. To date, 11 isoforms are identified, 10 of them resulting from the combination between one of the five known $\alpha$ ($\alpha 1 - 5$) chains with the $\gamma 1$ chain and either the $\beta 1$ or $\beta 2$ chains, and one resulting from the association of the $\alpha 3$, $\beta 3$ and $\gamma 2$ chains. Further isoforms are likely to be identified soon, given the intense and fruitful search for new chains. By means of several approaches, including affinity chroma-tography on laminin or proteolytic or recombinant fragments, in vitro ligand–

receptor binding assays, and inhibition of the interactions with peptides or receptor- or substrate-specific antibodies, different cell-binding sites have been mapped on laminin 1 or identified on other isoforms and the integrins involved in their recognition were characterised. Two cell-binding sites of laminin 1, one localised on the long arm and another contributed by the short arms, corresponding to, respectively, the proteolytic fragments E8 and E1–4, have been shown to interact with $\alpha 6\beta 1/\alpha 7\beta 1$ and $\alpha 1\beta 1/\alpha 2\beta 1$ integrins, respectively [3]. On other laminin isoforms, the cell adhesion-promoting activity is associated with the long-arm region of the molecules, which interacts with a different set of receptors, including $\alpha 3\beta 1$ and $\alpha 6\beta 1$ integrins [13, 18, 19, 47]. The functional importance of these interactions has recently been confirmed by the deleterious phenotypes observed·after gene targeting in mice or by the discovery that mutations in the genes coding for laminin or integrin chains are associated with very severe human diseases, such as epidermolysis bullosa junctionalis or progressive muscular dystrophy [6, 11].

In vitro, laminins promote cell attachment and spreading accompanied by focal-adhesion formation in, however, a laminin-specific manner [25]. Interference reflection microscopy observation revealed that focal adhesions formed by cells on laminin were smaller and more dispersed than those formed on fibronectin [25], although they contain the same structural proteins (vinculin, paxillin, talin) as shown by indirect immunofluorescence microscopy. Nevertheless, semi-quantitative biochemical analysis of isolated focal adhesions showed that, on laminin 1, the relative amounts of structural cytoskeletal-associated proteins are lower than on fibronectin (H. Sondermann et al., unpublished results). It indicates that, on fibronectin, either more focal contacts are formed or that individual focal contacts are more compact and contain a higher concentration of proteins than on laminin 1. The fact that similar numbers of isolated focal adhesions are observed on both substrates favours the second possibility. Interestingly, adhesion structures formed on laminin 1 have a higher content in $\alpha$-actinin, a molecule usually associated with the entire length of actin microfilaments, which may indicate a more dispersed configuration of focal contacts. Consequently, the cytoskeleton and associated adhesion forces could be differentially distributed in cells adhering to fibronectin or laminin 1, and enable the induction of different substrate-specific signalling events.

Further differences in focal adhesions are observed when cells are in contact with different laminin isoforms [21]. Laminin 1 induces the formation of filopodia-like processes and of compact and well-individualised focal-adhesion complexes, while laminin 5 and other isoforms trigger the development of lamellipodia containing tiny focal contacts arranged into long and parallel arrays (Fig. 2). Analysis of these focal adhesions by indirect immunofluorescence revealed the presence of several structural proteins as well as the $\alpha 6$ and $\beta 1$ integrin subunits in both cases. By contrast, while the $\alpha 3$ integrin subunit was detected in complexes formed on laminin 5 or on other laminin isoforms, such as those found in the kidney and having affinity for the $\alpha 3\beta 1$ integrins, it was not present in focal adhesions formed on laminin 1 [21] (D. Dogic et al., unpublished results). Similarly, under conditions where the $\alpha 3\beta 1$ integrin was occupied by a monoclonal antibody, assembly of focal adhesions closely resembled that observed when the integrin was occupied by its natural ligands [21]. These observations allow several important conclusions. First, ligation-induced recruitment of the $\alpha 3\beta 1$ integrins in focal adhesions is crucial for

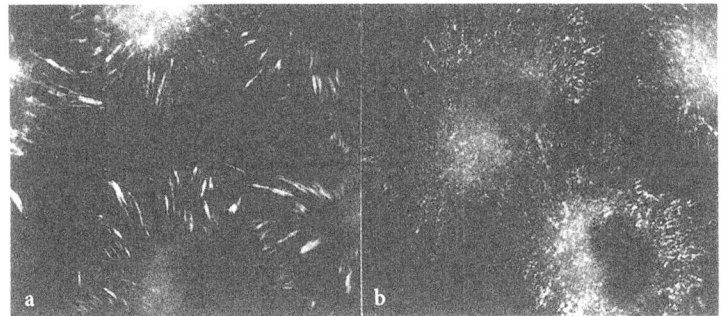

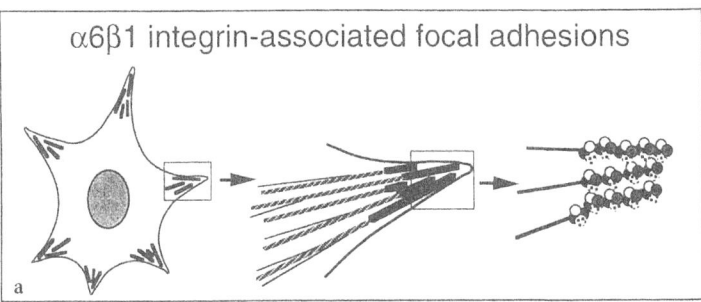

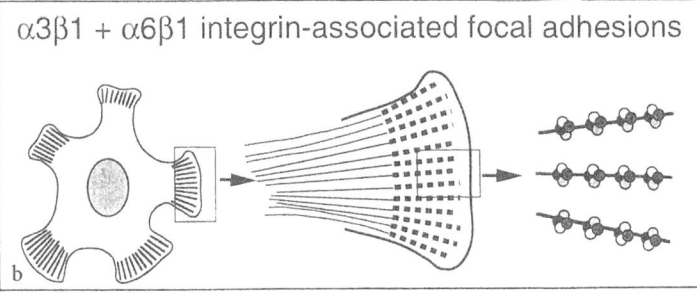

**Fig. 2 A, B.** Focal adhesions complexes formed on laminins. **A** Glass cover slips were coated with laminin 1 (*a*) or kidney laminins (*b*). After 60 min of adhesion, cells were incubated with monoclonal antibody for vinculin followed by Cy3-conjugated second antibody. Note the characteristic patterns induced by binding of either the $\alpha6\beta1$ integrin alone to laminin 1 (*a*) or both the $\alpha6\beta1$ and $\alpha3\beta1$ integrins to kidney laminins (*b*). **B** Schematic representation of the focal adhesions observed in **A** and drawing of their hypothetical organisation

the development of a specific morphology of cell spreading and of cell-adhesion structures. Second, the $\alpha3\beta1$ integrins trans-dominantly regulate the clustering of $\alpha6\beta1$ integrins and of cytoskeletal linker proteins, such as vinculin, paxillin, or talin. Third, when cells are exposed to a population of different laminin isoforms, such as in the kidney preparations and, as is most often the case, in vivo, they integrate a complex signal rather than adding single individual signals.

The striking difference in cell- and focal-adhesion morphology, depending on integrin involvement, suggests the induction of different signalling mechanisms leading to the regulation of specific cell activities. The induction of distinct signalling pathways triggered by $\alpha3\,\beta1$ or $\alpha6\,\beta1$ integrins alone or by $\alpha3\,\beta1$ and $\alpha6\,\beta1$ integrins together is further suggested by approaches involving direct interaction cloning of protein partners for the intracellular portions of integrin subunits with the two-hybrid system in yeast. Using this technique, new proteins have been found that specifically interact with either the $\alpha3$ alone or with both the $\alpha3$- and $\alpha6$-integrin subunits (V. WIXLER and M. AUMAILLEY, unpublished results).

## 3  The Influence of the Supramolecular Organisation of the Extracellular Matrix: Collagen Monomers and Polymers

In tissue, cells are surrounded by a variety of different extracellular-matrix proteins organised in complex supramolecular assemblies [5]. In vitro, it has been shown that cellular activities differ when cells are exposed to two- vs three-dimensional extracellular matrices. In particular, fibroblasts cultivated as a monolayer express much more collagen and much less collagenase than fibroblasts embedded in collagen lattices [35]. Although the signalling intermediates are qualitatively the same [36], collagen and collagenase expression are under the control of different integrins, namely $\alpha1\,\beta1$ and $\alpha2\,\beta1$ integrins, respectively [35]. With respect to focal-adhesion formation, cellular interactions with the extracellular matrix have, however, been mostly characterised by the use of extracted, purified and usually individual extracellular-matrix components. Although very instrumental in dissecting single molecular mechanisms, this may not reflect the in vivo complexity.

Indeed, adhesion of fibroblasts to collagen monomers induces a homogeneous layer of very well spread cells, whereas on fibrillar collagens, cells are aligned among themselves by adopting an elongated bipolar morphology, with numerous thin filopodia-like processes [40]. Furthermore, focal contacts and microfilament networks are structurally different. On monomeric collagen, the actin cytoskeleton is well developed across the entire cell body and focal adhesions are present at the microfilament extremities. In contrast, on fibrillar collagen, the actin filament network is formed only by longitudinal fibres, reflecting the alignment of cells, and the focal adhesions appear as faint granular structures [40]. Distinct biological activities, depending on whether polymerisation takes place, have also been described for fibronectin [43]. Altogether, these observations show that cell morphology and architecture depend on the polymerisation state of the extracellular-matrix molecule. This may be due to the different cell-binding sites' accessibility to cells on monomeric or polymerised-matrix proteins. The cell-binding sites could be the same, but exposed to cells in a different way, or new cell-binding sites could be created by the process of polymerisation (Fig. 3). Moreover, the spatial organisation of extracellular-matrix macromolecules could change the forces applied at focal adhesions and directly influence the cytoskeletal organisation, cell orientation and morphology.

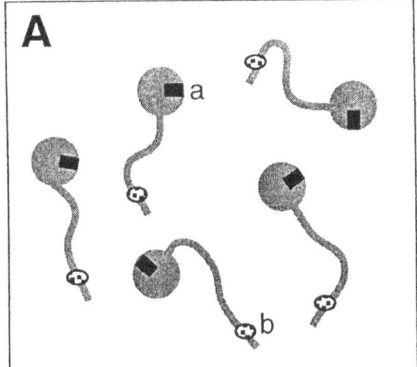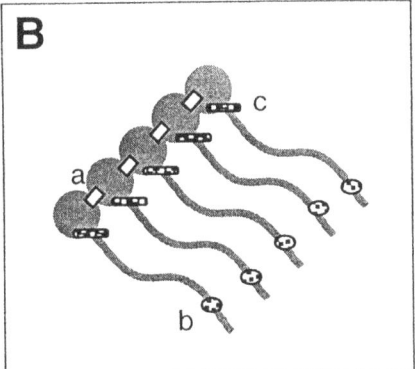

Fig. 3 A, B. Cell binding sites of extracellular matrix molecules and quaternary structure. Hypothetical cell binding sites present on extracellular matrix monomers (A) or polymers (B). In monomers (A), two cell-binding sites, *a* and *b*, are exposed while on polymers (B) one cell-binding site (*a*) is now masked and another is newly created (*c*) due to polymerisation or consequent conformational changes

## 4  The Intracellular Architecture in Focal-Adhesion Formation: The Role of its Integrity

Most focal-adhesion components are multifunctional, containing binding sites for other molecules, thereby participating in the network of interactions in focal adhesions that are necessary for signalling events taking place at these sites. It is logical to assume that all focal-contact proteins are necessary for proper function of these adhesive structures in terms of adhesion, signalling and overall cytoskeletal organisation. Cells, however, that are deficient in one or more focal-adhesion protein or that have functionally inactive proteins do not necessarily lose the ability to form focal adhesions, which nevertheless present subtle alterations [15, 38, 45, 54]. Surprisingly, cells deficient in pp125FAK are still capable of forming focal adhesions, in an even larger number than wild-type cells, suggesting that the kinase is required for the turnover, rather than for the initiation of focal-adhesion assembly [31].

How other components of the cytoskeleton that are not directly present in focal adhesions are involved in their regulation is unknown. To address this issue, we have analysed focal-adhesion formation in vimentin-deficient fibroblasts [22]. Vimentin belongs to the group of intermediate filaments and, in the fibroblast cytoskeleton, it is the most abundant protein of this class [23]. Vimentin-deficient mice created by homologous recombination and that are homozygous for the mutation are, however, viable and breed [16]. Nevertheless, cultivated fibroblasts isolated from vimentin-null mice present several alterations in their phenotype, including perturbations of focal-adhesion formation and of the re-organisation of actin-based cytoskeleton. In wild-type fibroblasts, focal adhesions form at the anchoring points of actin microfilaments, keep the same length and adopt a characteristic radial orientation (Fig. 4). The actin microfilaments are organised into circular filaments crossing with longitudinal stress fibres, thereby forming a polygonal network. This typical geometrical pattern of fibrillar actin and focal-

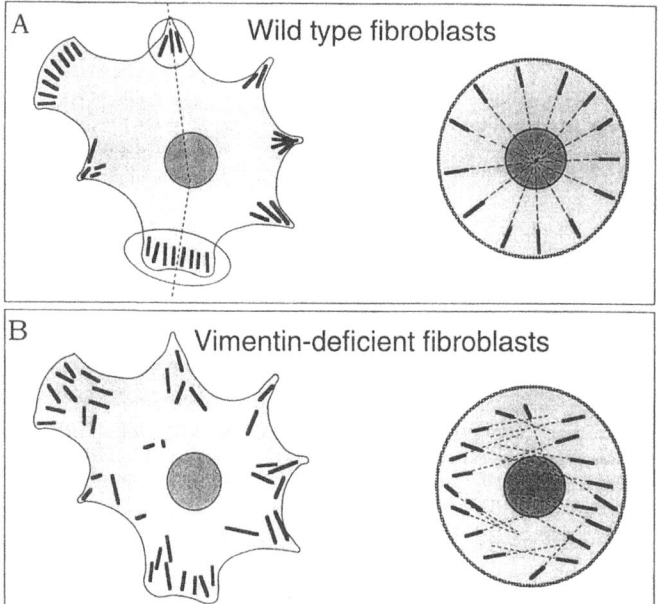

**Fig. 4 A, B.** Schematic representation of focal adhesion organisation in normal (A) and vimentin-deficient fibroblasts (B). In wild-type fibroblasts, the focal adhesions are distributed in an orderly pattern and the prolongations of individual focal adhesions or groups of focal adhesions fall in a single point in the centre of the cell. By contrast, in vimentin-deficient fibroblasts, the adhesion structures are not geometrically distributed and their longitudinal axis are randomly orientated [22]

adhesion organisation is absent in vimentin-negative fibroblasts. Here, focal adhesions assemble randomly throughout the ventral-cell surface. Their length, orientation, number and position are largely variable within the same cell and the cell population (Fig. 4). This is associated with a modification of fibrillar-actin assembly and the total absence of the circular network. At present, we do not know whether vimentin intermediate filaments participate directly or indirectly to the organisation of focal adhesions. Co-localisation of vimentin and vinculin has been observed in fibroblasts [7], making possible a direct effect of vimentin. Alternatively, the absence of vimentin is deleterious to the actin cytoskeleton, which in turn leads to malformations of focal adhesions. The actin-based cytoskeleton is likely responsible for coordination of focal-adhesion formation and necessary for their remodelling and maintenance. Interactions between the actin and the intermediate filament networks could be mediated by cytoskeletal linker proteins [57]. Moreover, physical properties of the cytoskeleton suggest interconnection of all three classes of the cytoskeleton elements [32, 55]. In this model, all elements of the cytoskeleton are under tension, which is essential for transfer of mechanical stimuli via integrins to the cytoskeleton. Intermediate filaments participate in integration of different cytoskeletal elements, including microfilaments along with focal adhesions and microtubules into a unique structural unit, assuring mechanical stability of the cells and participating in different cell activities.

In conclusion, the outcome of interactions between cells and the extracellular matrix is specifically and directly dictated by both the extracellular-matrix proteins and the receptors involved. It is, however, modulated by the three-dimensional structure of the extracellular matrix and it strictly requires the integrity of the cytoskeletal architecture. Although, at the molecular level, distinct and unique signals may be elicited, at the cellular or tissue levels, the signals do not seem to be additive, but rather result from the integration as a whole of an array of information.

**Acknowledgements.** The authors gratefully acknowledge the support of the Centre National de la Recherche Scientifique, the Association pour la Recherche sur le Cancer, the University of Cologne, and the Deutsche Forschungsgemeinschaft.

# References

1. Abercrombie M, Heaysman JE, Pegrum SM (1971) The locomotion of fibroblasts in culture. IV. Electron microscopy of the leading lamella. Exp Cell Res 67:359–367
2. Abercrombie M, Dunn GA (1975) Adhesions of fibroblasts to substratum during contact inhibition observed by interference reflection microscopy. Exp Cell Res 92:57–62
3. Aumailley M, Gimond C, Rousselle P (1996) Integrin-mediated cellular interactions with laminins. In: "The Laminins", Ekblom P, Timpl R (eds) Harwood Academic Publishers, pp 127–158
4. Aumailley M, Krieg T (1996) Laminins: a family of diverse multifunctional molecules of basement membrane. J Invest Dermatol 106:209–214
5. Aumailley M, Gayraud B (1998) Structure and biological activity of the extracellular matrix. J Mol Med 76:253–265
6. Aumailley M, Smyth N (1998) The role of laminins in basement membrane function. J Anat 193:1–21
7. Bershadsky AD, Tint IS, Svitkina TM (1987) Association of intermediate filaments with vinculin-containing adhesion plaques of fibroblasts. Cell Motil Cytoskel 8:274–283
8. Bloch RJ, Hall ZW (1983) Cytoskeleton components of the vertebrate neuromuscular junction: vinculin, a-actinin and filamin. J Cell Biol 97:217–223
9. Bockholt SM, Burridge K (1993) Cell spreading on extracellular matrix proteins induces tyrosine phosphorylation of tensin. J Biol Chem 269:14565–14567
10. Burgeson RE, Chiquet M, Deutzmann R, Ekblom P, Engel J, Kleinman H, Martin GR, Meneguzzi G, Paulsson M, Sanes J, Timpl R, Tryggvason K, Yamada Y, Yurchenco P (1994) A new nomenclature for laminins. Matrix Biol 14:209–211
11. Burgeson RE, Christiano AM (1997) The dermal-epidermal junction. Curr Opin Cell Biol 9:651–658
12. Burridge K, Fath K, Kelly T, Nuckolls G, Turner C (1988) Focal adhesions: transmembrane junctions between the extracellular matrix and the cytoskeleton. Ann Rev Cell Biol 4:487–525
13. Carter WG, Ryan MC, Gahr PJ (1991) Epiligrin, a new cell adhesion ligand for integrin $\alpha3\beta1$ in epithelial basement membranes. Cell 65:599–610
14. Clark EA, Brugge JS (1995) Integrins and signal transduction pathways: the road taken. Science 268:233–238
15. Coll JL, Ben-Ze'ev A, Ezzell RM, Rodriguez Fernandez JL, Beribault H, Oshima RG, Adamson ED (1995) Targeted disruption of vinculin genes in F9 and embryonic stem cells changes cell morphology, adhesion, and locomotion. Proc Natl Acad Sci U S A 92:9161–9165
16. Colucci-Guyon E, Portier MM, Dunia I, Paulin D, Pournin S, Babinet C (1994) Mice lacking vimentin develop and reproduce without an obvious phenotype. Cell 79:679–694
17. Craig WC, Johnson RP (1996) Assembly of focal adhesions: progress, paradigms, and portents. Curr Opin Cell Biol 8:74–85

84 D. Dogic et al.

18. Delwel GO, Hogervorst F, Kuikman I, Paulsson M, Timpl R, Sonnenberg A (1993) Expression and function of the cytoplasmic variants of the integrin $\alpha$ subunit in transfected K562 cells. J Biol Chem 268:25865–25875
19. Delwel GO, de Melker AA, Hogerworst F, Jaspers LH, Fles DLA, Kuikman I, Lindblom A, Paulsson M, Timpl R, Sonnenberg A (1994) Distinct and overlapping ligand specificities of the $\alpha$3A $\beta$1 and $\alpha$6A $\beta$1 integrins: recognition of laminin isoforms. Mol Biol Cell 6:151–160
20. De Nichilo MO, Yamada KM (1996) Integrin $\alpha$v$\beta$5-dependent serine phosphorylation of paxillin in cultured human macrophages adherent to vitronectin. J Biol Chem 271:11016–11022
21. Dogic D, Rousselle P, Aumailley M (1998) Cell adhesion to laminin 1 or 5 induces isoform-specific clustering of integrins and other focal adhesion components. J Cell Sci 111:793–802
22. Eckes B, Dogic D, Colucci-Gugon E, Wang N, Maniotis A, Ingber D, Merkling A, Aumailley M, Delouvée A, Koteliansky V, Babinet C, Krieg T (1998) Impaired mechanical stability, migration, and contractile capacity in vimentin-deficient fibroblasts. J Cell Sci 111:1897–1907
23. Fuchs E, Weber K (1994) Intermediate filaments: structure, dynamics, function, and disease. Annu Rev Biochem 63:345–382
24. Gilmore AP, Burridge K (1996) Molecular mechanisms for focal adhesion assembly through regulation of protein-protein interactions. Structure 4:647–651
25. Gimond C, Mercier I, Weber I, Aumailley M (1996) Adhesion complexes formed by OVCAR-4 cells on laminin 1 differ from those observed on fibronectin. Cell Adh Commun 3:527–539
26. Haas TA, Plow E (1994) Integrin-ligand interaction: a year in review. Curr Opin Cell Biol 6:656–662
27. Hannigan GE, Leung-Hagesteijn C, Fitz-Gibbon L, Coppolino MG, Radeva G, Filmus J, Bell JC, Dedhar S (1996) Regulation of cell adhesion and anchorage-dependent growth by a new $\beta$1-integrin-linked protein kinase. Nature 379:91–96
28. Hotchin NA, Gandarillas A, Watt PM (1995) Regulation of cell surface $\beta$1 integrin levels during keratinocyte terminal differentiation. J Cell Biol 128:1209–1219
29. Huttenlocher A, Sandborg RR, Horwitz AF (1995) Adhesion in cell migration. Curr Opin Cell Biol 7:697–706
30. Hynes RO (1992) Integrins: versatility, modulation, and signaling in cell adhesion. Cell 69:11–25
31. Ilic D, Furuta Y, Kanazawa S, Takeda N, Sobue K, Nakatsuji N, Nomura S, Fujimoto J, Okada M, Yamamoto T, Aizawa S (1995) Reduced cell motility and enhanced focal contact formation in cells from FAK-deficient mice. Nature 377:539–543
32. Ingber DE, Dike L, Hansen L, Kerp S, Liley H, Maniotis A, McName H, Mooney D, Plopper G, Sims J, Wang N (1994) Cellular tensegrity: exploring how mechanical changes in the cytoskeleton regulate cell growth, migration, and tissue pattern during morphogenesis. Int Rev Cytol 150:173–224
33. Jockusch BM, Bubeck P, Giehl K, Kroemker M, Moschner J, Rothkegel M, Rüdiger M, Schlüter K, Stanke G, Winkler J (1995) The molecular architecture of focal adhesions. Annu Rev Cell Dev Biol 11:379–416
34. Kreis TE, Geiger D, Schlessinger J (1982) Mobility of microinjected rhodamin actin within living chicken gizzard cells determined by fluorescence photobleaching recovery. Cell 29:835–845
35. Langholz O, Rockel D, Mauch C, Kozlowska E, Bank I, Krieg T, Eckes B (1995) Collagen and collagenase gene expression in three-dimensional collagen lattices are differentially regulated by $\alpha$1 $\beta$1 and $\alpha$2 $\beta$1 integrins. J Cell Biol 131:1903–1915
36. Langholz O, Roeckel D, Petersohn D, Broermann E, Eckes B, Krieg T (1997) Cell-matrix interactions induce tyrosine phosphorylation of MAP kinases ERK1 and ERK2 and PLC$\gamma$-1 in two-dimensional and three-dimensional cultures of human fibroblasts. Exp Cell Res 235:22–27
37. Lauffenburger DA, Horwitz AF (1996) Cell migration: a physically integrated molecular process. Cell 84:359–369
38. Lo SH, Yu QC, Degenstein L, Chen LB, Fuchs E (1997) Progressive kidney degeneration in mice lacking tensin. J Cell Biol 136:1349–1361
39. Luna EJ, Hitt AL (1992) Cytoskeleton-plasma membrane interactions. Science 256:955–964

40. Mercier I, Lechaire JP, Desmouliere A, Gaill F, Aumailley M (1996) Interactions of human skin fibroblasts with monomeric or fibrillar collagens induce different organization of the cytoskeleton. Exp Cell Res 225:245–256
41. Mitchison TJ, Cramer LP (1996) Actin-based cell motility and cell locomotion. Cell 84: 371–379
42. Morino N, Mimura T, Hamasaki K, Tobe K, Ueki K, Kikuci K, Takehara K, Kadowaki T, Yazaki Y, Nojima Y (1995) Matrix/Integrin interaction activates the mitogen-activated protein kinase, p44erk-1 and p42erk-2. J Biol Chem 270:269–273
43. Morla A, Zhang Z, Ruoslahti E (1994) Superfibronectin is a functionally distinct form of fibronectin. Nature 367:193–196
44. Mould PA (1996) Getting integrins into shape: recent insights into how integrin activity is regulated by conformational changes. J Cell Sci 109:2613–2618
45. Nuckolls GH, Romer LH, Burridge K (1992) Microinjection of antibodies against talin inhibits the spreading and migration of fibroblasts. J Cell Sci 102:753–762
46. Rojiani MV, Finlay BB, Gray V, Dedhar S (1991) In vitro interaction of a polypeptide homologous to human Ro/SS-A antigen (calreticulin) with a highly conserved amino acid sequence in the cytoplasmic domain of integrin $\alpha$ subunit. Biochemistry 30:9859–9866
47. Rousselle P, Aumailley M (1994) Kalinin is more efficient than laminin in promoting adhesion of primary keratinocytes and some other cells and has a different requirement for integrin receptors. J Cell Biol 125:205–214
48. Schaller MD Parsons JT (1995) pp125FAK-dependent tyrosine phosphorylation of paxillin creates a high-affinity binding site for crk. Mol Cell Biol 15:2635–2645
49. Schlaepfer DD, Hanks SK, Hunter T, van der Geer P (1994) Integrin-mediated signal transduction linked to Ras pathway by GRB2 binding to focal adhesion kinase. Nature 372: 786–791
50. Shattil SJ, O'Toole T, Eigenthaler M, Thon V, Williams M, Babior BM, Ginsberg MH (1995) b3-endonexine, a novel polypeptide that interacts specificaly with the cytoplasmic tail of the integrin $\beta$3 subunit. J Cell Biol 131:807–816
51. Stewart M, Thiel M, Hogg N (1995) Leukocyte integrins. Curr Opin Cell Biol 7:690–696
52. Tidball JG, O'Halloran T, Burridge K (1986) Talin at the myotendinous junction. J Cell Biol 103:1465–1472
53. Turner CE, Kramarcy N, Sealock R, Burridge K (1991) Localisation of paxillin, a focal adhesion protein, to smooth muscle dense plaques, and the myotendinous and neuromuscular junctions of skeletal muscle. Exp Cell Res 192:651–655
54. Volberg T, Geiger B, Kam Z, Pankov R, Simcha I, Sabanay H, Coll JL, Adamson E, Ben-Ze'ev A (1995) Focal adhesion formation by F9 embryonal carcinoma cells after vinculin gene disruption. J Cell Sci 108:2253–2260
55. Wang N, Butler JP, Ingber DE (1993) Mechanotransduction across the cell surface and through the cytoskeleton. Science 260:1124–1127
56. Yamada KM, Geiger B (1997) Molecular interactions in cell adhesion complexes. Curr Opin Cell Biol 9:76–85
57. Yang Y, Dowling J, Yu QC, Kouklis P, Cleveland DW, Fuchs E (1996) An essential cytoskeletal linker protein connecting actin microfilaments to intermediate filaments. Cell 86:655–665

# What Is New in Mechanical Properties of Tissue-Engineered Organs

F. A. Auger, F. Berthod, F. Goulet, L. Germain

## 1 Introduction

Tissue engineering is a promising new field based on expertise in cell biology, medicine and mechanical engineering. It raises exciting hopes of producing autologous tissue substitutes to replace altered organs. This challenge involves highly specialized technology in order to provide the proper shape to the tissue and promote the maintenance of its native physiological properties. Primary cell populations may lose some of their functional and morphological properties in vitro in the absence of a proper environment. In order to maintain cell integrity, a three-dimensional matrix that mimics the in vivo environment as closely as possible was developed, according to the type of tissue produced [1, 5, 18, 26, 27, 29, 34, 35].

Mechanical strength is a critical feature of most bioengineered organs, allowing them to be handled and transplanted, and to withstand their functional role. But how can we succeed in reproducing mechanical properties of a tissue in vitro? A universal set of building rules called "tensegrity" has been developed to explain body, organ, tissue and cell architecture [21, 22, 38]. Tensegrity describes an architectural system in which structures stabilize themselves by balancing the counteracting forces of compression and tension along a network of rigid and flexible elements. The rigid components of the framework can be compared with struts that bear compression, and the flexible components with cables that induce tension. The stability of the whole structure is guaranteed by pre-stress forces that submit struts to continuous compression induced by tension generated by the cables. This architecture remains stiff if cables and struts are inert elements, but can be highly adaptable to external stress when flexible and rigid components modify their length, subsequently modifying both tension, locally, and compression induced in the whole construct. The human body is made of struts and cables, corresponding, respectively, to bones and muscles. This internal skeleton based

Current Topics in Pathology, Volume 93
A. Desmoulière, B. Tuchweber (Eds.)
© Springer-Verlag Berlin Heidelberg 1999

upon the tensegrity concept is markedly lighter than a crustacean shell, which is so heavy that it greatly limits the extension of the species to a few centimetres.

Internal architecture of cells is also based on the tensegrity concept. Struts correspond to microtubules, and cables to microfilaments and intermediate filaments. Microtubules form the compression-bearing skeleton on which actin filaments attach. The cytoskeleton is pre-stressed by tension induced by actin on microtubules. In addition, cell architecture can be modified by changing tension forces induced by actin, and adjusting microtubule length. This process leads to variations in cell shape, but more importantly may promote cell migration. Cell movement is enabled by the adhesion of the cytoskeleton through integrin receptors to the extracellular matrix, by microtubules elongation and by increase in actin-induced tension. When cells are firmly attached at both ends to their surrounding substrate, the same phenomenon leads to the remodelling of extracellular matrix instead of migration [22, 38].

The extracellular matrix follows the rules of tensegrity; struts correspond to collagen fibrils, and cables to cells. Thus, the tensegrity concept is a continuum of molecules, fibrils and tissues interconnected to promote a mechanical coherence of the whole body. Of course, organization of these structural components is orchestrated by numerous endocrine, paracrine and autocrine factors modulated in response to external stress, central control and, at least in part, by human will [22].

Finally, in vitro reconstruction of tissues involves isolation and maintenance of the correct cell types integrated in the proper extracellular matrix. Then, cells must be stimulated by the right hormones, growth factors and specific culture conditions to recreate a structure as similar as possible to their tissue of origin.

Tensegrity is at the basis of contractile tissue properties. Our group has been involved since 1985 with in vitro skin, blood vessel, bronchi and ligament bioengineering. These different types of tissues share a common feature; they can modulate their strength in response to physiological or mechanical stimuli.

## 2 Mechanical Properties of Reconstructed Skin

Skin exhibits mechanical characteristics in physiological situations to withstand mechanical stress. The epidermis demonstrates mechanical strength, while the dermis displays strength and elasticity [24, 25]. Skin can adapt itself to specific stress. Indeed, skin reacts to friction forces by epidermis thickening, while dermis increases its collagen content. This last observation was elegantly demonstrated by LAMBERT and coworkers, who showed that fibroblasts embedded in a collagen gel were induced by a pre-translational activation to markedly increase their collagen synthesis following gel stretching [28]. In addition to a whole augmentation of collagen content, a special increase of specific types of collagen was observed. Collagen XII synthesis was increased in stressed collagen gels compared with floating ones [7, 23]. Indeed, collagen XII could modulate biomechanical properties of tissues by encouraging a compaction of collagen bundles [33]. This adaptive behavior is explained by tensegrity, since tissue equilibrium is broken by stretching and reacts by reinforcing its rigid network. Tissue-engineered skin in vitro was demonstrated to promote the re-expression of collagen XII and XIV, while these molecules were irreversibly lost in conventional culture systems [4].

In contrast, the dermis needs to contract itself to fill in a skin defect in the case of deep wounds. This contraction process is promoted by a reinforcement of the flexible component of tissue architecture, i.e., the fibroblast and its differentiation into myofibroblasts [11, 15, 32].

Fibroblasts are known to contract collagen fibrils until a specific collagen density is reached [1, 2, 14, 19, 20, 35]. This process is a physiological response, leading to an extracellular-matrix remodelling that mimics the in vivo environment. In the case of a wound, tissue contraction aims to draw wound edges together, thus accelerating healing. This process could be explained by an increase in fibroblast locomotion or a change in cell phenotype [3, 15, 32]. In wound tissue, fibroblasts switch their phenotype to myofibroblasts, which share common properties with smooth-muscle (SM) cells [9, 12, 13, 30, 32]. Myofibroblasts express an actin isoform usually produced by SM cells, the $\alpha$-SM actin, in much larger amounts than fibroblasts. This phenotype change can be partially induced by growth factors, such as transforming growth factor beta (TGF$\beta$), produced in inflammatory conditions [10]. As discussed above, in the tensegrity model, an increase in $\alpha$-SM actin content with greater contractile properties than actin will promote cell contraction, which will transmit tension forces to collagen bundles, inducing the tissue to contract.

# 3 Mechanical Properties of Reconstructed Blood Vessels

Our group is also involved in the in vitro reconstruction of small-diameter blood vessels, and recently performed a breakthrough in the field of tissue-engineered blood-vessel production [26, 27].

A dual mechanical property is observed in the case of blood vessels. The mechanical challenge faced by blood vessels is to withstand blood pressure in addition to adjusting it by contraction or dilatation of their internal diameter. The blood-vessel mechanical strength depends on adventitia made of fibroblasts, while contractile properties are promoted by media made of SM cells. In addition, blood vessels need to be elastic to bear the pulsating blood pressure.

Our group produced the first completely biological tissue-engineered blood vessel featuring a high-burst strength, a positive-surgical handling and a functional endothelium. The complete vessel had a burst strength (measured by internal hydrostatic pressurization) of more than 2500 mmHg compared with 1680 mmHg for human saphenous veins [27]. This strength was promoted by fibroblasts cultured for 5 weeks in monolayer culture condition. This long culture period enabled them to produce their own extracellular matrix, made mostly of collagen. Collagen fibrils were arranged in a network of closely packed bundles, which gave a high resistance to the graft [6, 27].

Furthermore, the media reconstruction made of SM cells cultured in similar conditions promoted the reconstruction of a tubular tissue in which SM cells recovered their native state of differentiation. This was demonstrated by the expression of desmin [27], a marker of highly differentiated SM cells [37]. This specific marker was considered irreversibly lost in SM cells cultured on plastic [37].

Finally, as discussed in the Introduction, the right cells cultured in the right conditions promote the in vitro reconstruction of tissues that display nearly the same mechanical properties as their in vivo counterpart [27].

## 4 Mechanical Properties of Reconstructed Bronchi

We previously reported that collagen and fibroblast concentrations in culture can greatly influence the kinetics of contraction of collagen gels [15, 29, 35]. When these parameters are kept constant in all the experiments, human bronchial fibroblastic cells can exert extracellular-matrix remodelling by their capacity to contract, reorganize and orient collagen fibers vertically within floating-collagen gels [18]. When the cells are seeded in an anchored collagen gel, they remodel the surrounding matrix to reproduce the horizontal alignment of collagen fibers observed in the bronchial mesenchyme, which supports the pseudo-stratified epithelium [34]. These data agree with previous observations demonstrating the effect of the constraints induced by external anchorages on the resulting orientation of the cells and the collagen fibers in vitro [1, 14 – 17, 26, 29, 34, 35].

## 5 Mechanical Properties of Reconstructed Ligaments

Ligament function in vivo maintains joint stability by tensile resistance and compliance. Ligaments contain a high ratio of collagen fibers organized in a wavy pattern oriented in a direction parallel to their long axis. The challenge of ligament reconstruction in vitro is to produce a compliant tissue with high mechanical resistance [16]. The strategy developed by our group to reach this goal was to produce a ligament made of fibroblasts in vitro, extracted from human anterior cruciate ligament, seeded within a collagen matrix anchored at both ends with bone pieces. Bones can greatly facilitate ligament transplantation in humans [16, 17].

These tissues are constantly remodelled in response to mechanical forces, and this greatly contributes to the reinforcement of their structures. Indeed, traction forces are known to induce tissues to produce more collagen in order to increase their tensile strength [28]. Our group demonstrated that in vitro-reconstructed ligaments maintained under static elongation contained cells and collagen bundles oriented in a direction parallel to the constraint applied [17]. We are currently testing the effects of cyclic stretching on the resulting strength of the tissue to mimic ligament behavior in vivo. We hope that such mechanical stimuli will strengthen the bioengineered ligament scaffold through cellular metabolic responses.

# 6 Conclusion

At least minimal strength is necessary for most tissue-engineered organs to be transplanted in humans. Synthetic biopolymers can be used to reinforce tissues [8], but artificial compounds usually need to be removed or replaced. In addition, biopolymer merely bears mechanical stress, but cannot react to it. Living tissues react to stress and adapt themselves, e.g., by increasing their collagen production. In addition, they are able to repair themselves by self-renewal pathways and, thus, resist continuous mechanical stress more efficiently than inert compounds. We demonstrated that the tissue engineering approach allows biological tissues to remodel extracellular matrix in order to bear mechanical stresses. This was observed in reconstructed skin in which collagen XII and XIV expressions were induced [4] and also elegantly demonstrated in reconstructed blood vessels in which physiological strength of adventitia was recovered [27]. Similarly, human ligament cells seeded in the matrix of a bioengineered ligament subjected to continuous static tension, secrete and contract the collagen network, leading to an aligned matricial structure [16, 17]. In addition, extracellular-matrix remodelling has been observed in bronchial equivalents [18, 34].

Finally, the correct choice of cells cultured under proper conditions seems to be the key for success in tissue engineering. Specialized cells seem to have the receptors and structural elements essential for tissue-integrity restoration. Furthermore, if this reconstruction is not totally achieved in vitro, it will be completed after transplantation in the human body, which is the best bioreactor a cellular biologist could ever imagine.

**Acknowledgements.** The authors acknowledge Drs Vincent Bernier, Louis-Philippe Boulet, Michel Boutet, Jamila Chakir, Réjean Cloutier, Odile Damour, Dominique Garrel, Robert Garrone, Michel Guillot, Georges Hébert, Normand Houle, Andréa Jean, Raymond Labbé, Jean Lamontagne, Michel Laviolette, Claire Lethias, Carlos Lòpez Valle, Véronique Moulin, Albert Normand, Denis Rancourt, Alphonse Roy, Félix-André Têtu, Michel van der Rest and Wen Xu for their close collaboration in our tissue-engineering programs. They are also grateful to Geneviève Bordeleau, Stéphane Bouchard, Charlotte Caron, Gilbert Castilloux, Christine Demers, Jean Dubé, Marie-Josée Godbout, Rina Guignard, Hugues Lafrance, Eve Langelier, Nicolas L'Heureux, Annie Marier, Martine Michel, Bernard Nöel, Stéphanie Pâquet, Jean-Sébastien Paquette, Pierre Rompré, Louis-Mathieu Stevens, Pierre-Philippe Stevens, and Maxime Talbot for the work done in relation to this review. This study was supported by the Medical Research Council of Canada, Réseau des Grands Brûlés du Fonds de la Recherche en Santé du Québec (FRSQ), Fondation des Pompiers du Québec pour les Grands Brûlés, Fondation de l'Hôpital du Saint-Sacrement, Fondation des Maladies du Coeur, Club Richelieu, Canadian Orthopaedics Association and France-Québec exchange program. L. Germain and F. A. Auger were recipients of scholarships from FRSQ.

# References

1. Auger FA, Lòpez Valle CA, Guignard R, Tremblay N, Nöel B, Goulet F, Germain L (1995) Skin equivalents produced using human collagens. In Vitro Cell Dev Biol 31: 432–439
2. Bell E, Ivarsson B, Merril C (1979) Production of a tissue-like structure by contraction of collagen lattices by human fibroblasts of different proliferative potential in vitro. Proc Natl Acad Sci U S A 76:1274–1278

3. Berthod F, Auger FA (1997) Experimental application of skin substitutes for dermatological purposes. In: Rouabhia M (ed) Skin substitute production by tissue engineering: clinical and fundamental applications. Landes Bioscience, Austin, pp 211–237

4. Berthod F, Germain L, Guignard R, Lethias C, Garrone R, Damour O, van der Rest M, Auger FA (1997) Differential expression of collagen XII and XIV in human skin and in human reconstructed skin. J Invest Dermatol 108:737–742

5. Berthod F, Sahuc F, Hayek D, Damour O, Collombel C (1996) Deposition of collagen fibril bundles by long-term culture of fibroblasts in a collagen sponge. J Biomed Mater Res 32: 87–94

6. Birk DE, Lisenmayer TF (1994) Collagen fibril assembly, deposition, and organization into tissue-specific matrices. In: Yurchenko PD, Birk DE, Mecham PR (eds) Extracellular matrix assembly and structure. Academic Press, San Diego, pp 91–128

7. Chiquet-Ehrismann R, Tannheimer H, Koch M, Brunner A, Spring J, Martin D, Baumgartner S, Chiquet M (1994) Tenascin-C expression by fibroblasts is elevated in stressed collagen gels. J Cell Biol 127:2093–2101

8. Cloutier R, Lacasse D, Normand A (1993) ACL reconstruction with LAD: a five-year follow-up. J Bone Joint Surg Br 74 [Suppl III]:273–274

9. Darby I, Skally O, Gabbiani G (1990) α-smooth muscle actin is transiently expressed by myofibroblasts during experimental wound healing. Lab Invest 63:21–29

10. Desmoulière A, Geinoz A, Gabbiani F, Gabbiani G (1993) TGFβ1 induces α-smooth muscle actin expression in granulation tissue myofibroblasts and in quiescent and growing cultured fibroblasts. J Cell Biol 122:103–111

11. Desmoulière A, Rubbia-Brandt L, Abdiu A, Walz T, Macieira-Coelho A, Gabbiani G (1992) α-smooth muscle actin is expressed in a subpopulation of cultured and cloned fibroblasts and is modulated by γ-interferon. Exp Cell Res 201:64–73

12. Gabbiani G., Ryan GB, Majno G (1971) Presence of modified fibroblasts in granulation tissue and their possible role in wound contraction. Experientia 27:549–550

13. Gabbiani G, Hirschel BJ, Ryan GB, Statkov PR, Majno G (1972) Granulation tissue as a contractile organ. A study of structure and function. J Exp Med 135:719–734

14. Germain L, Auger FA (1995) Tissue engineered biomaterials: biological and mechanical characteristics. In: Wise DL, Trantolo DJ, Altobelli DE, Yaszemski MJ, Gresser JD, Schwartz ER (eds) Encyclopedic handbook of biomaterials and bioengineering vol 1. Marcel Dekker Inc., New York, pp 699–734

15. Germain L, Jean A, Auger FA, Garrel DR (1994) Human wound healing fibroblasts have greater contractile properties than dermal fibroblasts. J Surg Res 57:267–273

16. Goulet F, Germain L, Caron C, Rancourt D, Normand A, Auger FA (1997) Tissue engineered ligament. In: Yahia LH (ed) Ligaments and ligamentoplasties. Springer-Verlag, Berlin Heidelberg New York, pp 367–377

17. Goulet F, Germain L, Rancourt D, Caron C, Normand A, Auger FA (1997) Tendons and ligaments. In: Lanza R, Langer R, Chick WL (eds) Textbook of tissue engineering. Landes Bioscience, Austin, pp 633–644

18. Goulet F, Boulet L-P, Chakir J, Tremblay N, Dubé J, Laviolette M, Auger FA (1996) Morphological and functional properties of bronchial cells isolated from normal and asthmatic subjects. Am J Respir Cell Mol Biol 15:312–318

19. Grinnell F, Lamke R (1984) Reorganization of hydrated collagen lattices by human skin fibroblasts. J Cell Sci 66:51–53

20. Guidry C, Grinnel F (1985) Studies on the mechanism of hydrated collagen gel reorganization by human fibroblasts. J Cell Sci 79:67–81

21. Ingber DE (1993) Cellular tensigrity: defining new rules of biological design that govern the cytoskeleton. J Cell Sci 104:613–627

22. Ingber DE (1998) The architecture of life. Scientific American Jan:48–57

23. Koch M, Bernasconi C, Chiquet M (1992) A major oligomeric fibroblast proteoglycan identified as a novel form of type-XII collagen. Eur J Biochem 207:847–856

24. Lafrance H, Guillot M, Germain L, Auger FA (1995) Method for the evaluation of tensile properties of skin equivalents. Med Eng Phys 17:537–543

25. Lafrance H, Yahia L'H, Germain L, Guillot M, Auger FA (1995) Study of the tensile properties of living skin equivalents. Biomed Mater Eng 5:195–208

26. L'Heureux N, Germain L, Labbé R, Auger FA (1993) In vitro construction of a human blood vessel from cultured vascular cells: a morphologic study. J Vasc Surg 17:499–509
27. L'Heureux N, Pâquet S, Labbé R, Germain L, Auger FA (1998) A completely biological tissue-engineered human blood vessel. FASEB J 12:47–56
28. Lambert CA, Soudant EP, Nusgens BV, Lapière CM (1992) Pretranslational regulation of extracellular matrix macromolecules and collagenase expression in fibroblasts by mechanical forces. Lab Invest 66:444–451
29. López Valle CA, Auger FA, Rompré P, Bouvard V, Germain L (1992) Peripheral anchorage of dermal equivalents. Br J Dermatol 127:365–371
30. Majno G, Gabbiani G, Hirschel BJ, Ryan GB, Statkov PR (1971) Contraction of granulation tissue in vitro: similarity to smooth muscle. Science 173:548–550
31. Moulin V, Auger FA, O'Connor-McCourt M, Germain L (1997) Fetal and postnatal sera differentially modulate human dermal fibroblast phenotypic and functional features in vitro. J Cell Phys 171:1–10
32. Moulin V, Castilloux G, Jean A, Garrel DR, Auger FA, Germain L (1996) In vitro models to study wound healing fibroblasts. Burns 22:359–362
33. Nishiyama T, McDonough AM, Bruns RR, Burgeson RE (1994) Type XII and XIV collagens mediate interactions between banded collagen fibers in vitro and may modulate extracellular matrix deformability. J Biol Chem 269:28193–28199
34. Paquette JS, Goulet F, Boulet L-P, Tremblay N, Chakir J, Germain L, Auger FA (1998) Three-dimensional production of bronchi in vitro, Can Respir J 5:1
35. Rompré P, Auger FA, Germain L, Bouvard V, Lòpez Valle CA, Thibault J, LeDuy A (1990) The influence of initial collagen and cellular concentrations on the final surface area of dermal and skin equivalents: a Box-Behnken analysis. In Vitro Cell Dev Biol 26:983–990
36. Schürch W, Seemayer TA, Gabbiani G (1992) Myofibroblast. In: Sternberg SS (ed) Histology for pathologists 5. Raven Press, New York, pp 109–114
37. Thyberg J, Hedin U, Sjolund M, Palmberg L, Bottger BA (1990) Regulation of differentiated properties and proliferation of arterial smooth muscle cells. Arteriosclerosis 10:966–990
38. Wang N, Butler JP, Ingber DE (1993) Mechanotransduction across the cell surface and through the cytoskeleton. Science 260:1124–1127

# Fibroblast – Cytokine – Extracellular Matrix Interactions in Wound Repair

A. Siméon, F. Monier, H. Emonard, Y. Wegrowski, G. Bellon,
J. C. Monboisse, P. Gillery, W. Hornebeck, F. X. Maquart

## 1 Introduction

The activity of connective tissue cells is controlled by numerous factors in their environment. Soluble molecules, such as hormones, growth factors and cytokines, may interact with specific receptors at the cell surface. This interaction may activate the various intracellular transduction pathways and finally modulate the expression of some specific genes. Other extracellular signals are provided by the insoluble extracellular matrix macromolecules, e.g., collagens, elastin, proteoglycans and connective tissue glycoproteins. These insoluble molecules, when interacting with specific membrane receptors of the integrin family, are able to activate similar intracellular transduction pathways to their soluble counterparts.

Among the various outcomes of these effectors are modulation of cell proliferation and the expression of some specific proteins, including new extracellular matrix macromolecules which may provide signals for connective tissue cells. However, specific proteinases, such as matrix metalloproteinases (MMPs), may also be secreted and/or activated. This may lead to extracellular matrix degradation and liberation of peptides which may, by themselves, constitute new signals for connective tissue cells. Consequently, loops of regulation exist inside the connective tissues, which depend on the interactions between connective tissue cells and extracellular matrix macromolecules or their degradation fragments (Fig. 1). Such loops might be implicated in the wound repair process.

The term "matrikine" is proposed to designate extracellular matrix-derived peptides that regulate connective tissue cell activity. Several examples of such peptides have been described recently; for instance, for peptides derived from elastin [2, 13], laminin and fibronectin [5], and the glycoprotein SPARC/osteonectin/BM-40 [3]. In this review, we will focus on a tripeptide, glycyl-histidyl-lysine (GHK) which may originate in several extracellular matrix proteins and possesses many activating effects on mesenchymal cells.

Current Topics in Pathology, Volume 93
A. Desmoulière, B. Tuchweber (Eds.)
© Springer-Verlag Berlin Heidelberg 1999

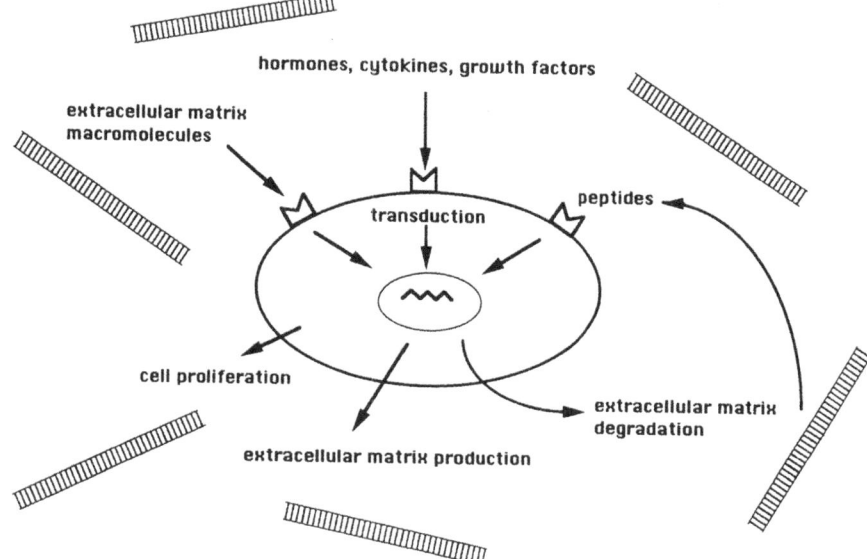

**Fig. 1.** Schematic representation of the interactions between connective tissue cells, extracellular matrix macromolecules and their degradation fragments

## 2 Glycyl-Histidyl-Lysine (GHK): A Typical Matrikine

GHK is a matrix-derived tripeptide that modulates new connective tissue formation. It was initially isolated from human plasma [9] and described as a growth factor for differentiated cells [10]. GHK spontaneously forms a high affinity complex with copper (II) ions: GHK–Cu. Further experiments from our laboratory and others demonstrated that GHK–Cu is a potent activator of the wound healing process.

The structure of GHK–Cu is shown in Fig. 2. Copper is bound to the N-terminal end of the peptide – the amide bond between glycine and histidine – and the imidazole ring of histidine [4]. In biological solutions, however, it is likely that the complex contains two peptides for one copper ion.

Particular interest was devoted to GHK when it appeared that this sequence was present in several extracellular matrix proteins, mainly collagen $\alpha 2$(I), $\alpha 2$(V) and $\alpha 2$(IX) chains, the glycoprotein SPARC/osteonectin/BM40, thrombospondin-1, and fibrin $\alpha$ chain (Fig. 3). We suggested that partial proteolysis of such extracellular matrix proteins in the wound might activate connective tissue repair [7].

## 3 GHK–Cu Activates Connective Tissue Cells

The first evidence of a positive effect of GHK–Cu on wound healing was demonstrated by Downey et al. more than 10 years ago [1]. In these experiments, full-thick-

**Fig. 2.** Structure of the glycyl-histidyl-lysine (GHK)–Cu complex

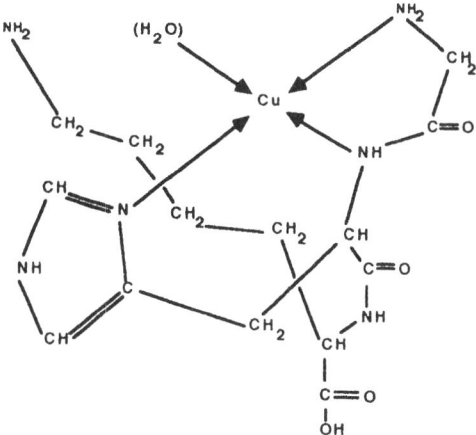

**Fig. 3.** Glycyl-histidyl-lysine (GHK)-containing sequences in extracellular matrix proteins. The number of amino acid residues preceding the GHK tripeptide is indicated for each protein

1025
Collagen α2(I) : DGPPGRDGQP<u>GHK</u>GERGYPGNIG

313
Collagen α2(V) : PGLPGLKGHR<u>GHK</u>GLEGPKGEVG

4
Collagen α2(IX) : GLK<u>GHK</u>GEKGEDGFPG

136
SPARC/osteonectin/BM-40 : TKCTLEGTKK<u>GHK</u>LHLDYIGPCK

260
Thrombospondin-1 : SSPAIRTNYI<u>GHK</u>TKDLQAICGI

474
Fibrin α chain : TVTKTVIGPD<u>GHK</u>ETVKEVVTSE

ness excision wounds were made on the backs of rats. Groups of rats received serial applications of GHK–Cu solution inside the wound, whereas control rats received application of the same volume of normal saline. Measurements of the wound circumference at various times after excision demonstrated a significant acceleration of the wound closure in the GHK–Cu treated rats compared with the controls.

In vivo and in vitro experiments [11] demonstrated that GHK – Cu was chemotactic for endothelial cells, with significant effects for concentrations as low as $10^{-12}$ M. It was also chemotactic for fibroblasts, but at higher concentrations ($10^{-6}$ M). In monolayer cultures of fibroblasts, we demonstrated that GHK–Cu induced a dose-dependent stimulation of collagen synthesis, with a maximal effect at the $10^{-9}$ M concentration [6]. It is important to note that copper ions alone were highly toxic for fibroblasts; addition of $CuCl_2$ to fibroblast cultures at the same molar concentration as GHK–Cu induced the death of more than 90% of the cells present in the culture. This result suggests that the binding of copper ions by GHK–Cu permits the delivery of this metal to the cells without inducing toxicity.

## 3.1 GHK–Cu Increases New Connective Tissue Formation in Wounds

To investigate the effects of the copper–peptide complex in vivo, we decided to use the wound chamber model described by Schilling [12]. In this model, a stainless steel wire-mesh cylinder is surgically inserted under the skin of rats. The void volume of the cylinder is then the site of an inflammatory reaction that reproduces all the steps of the normal wound-healing process. In groups of rats, we injected directly into the cylinder, increasing concentrations of GHK–Cu solution. Control rats received an injection of the same volume of normal saline. Rats were sacrificed at various times after chamber insertion and the chamber content was collected for analysis [8].

Simple macroscopical observation of the cylinders showed an increased amount of newly deposited connective tissue in the chambers injected with GHK–Cu, compared with the controls. Histological studies at day 3 showed an increased number of inflammatory cells in the treated chambers, with several new capillaries already visible. At day 14, control cylinders were filled by fibroblasts infiltrating the fibrinous material deposited in the chambers. In contrast, a well-organized fibrosis was already visible in the GHK–Cu-injected cylinders, showing an acceleration of the healing process.

Biochemical analysis of the wound chamber content demonstrated that GHK–Cu increased the dry weight of material deposited in the chambers and also total proteins, uronic acid (an index of the glycosaminoglycan/proteoglycan content), and collagen content of the chambers. DNA content, an index of cellularity, was also increased, but to a lesser degree. Interestingly, hydroxyproline-containing peptides were significantly increased in the treated chambers, showing that not only collagen synthesis but also collagen degradation were stimulated, indicating an intense wound tissue remodeling in GHK–Cu-injected chambers.

A typical dose-effect curve, showing the GHK–Cu stimulation of collagen accumulation in the chambers is shown in Fig. 4. A significant increase was observed for doses of GHK–Cu of as low as 0.4 mg per injection. Maximal stimulation was obtained for the concentration of 2.0 mg per injection.

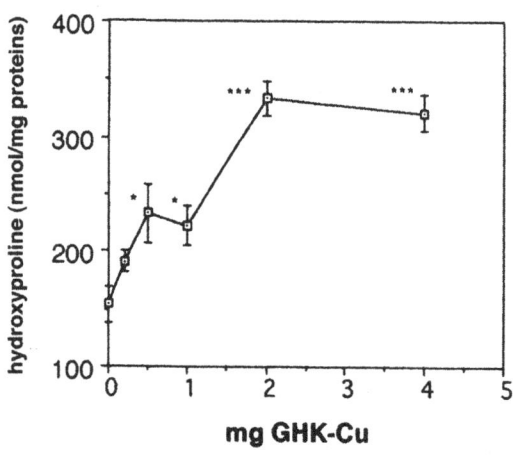

**Fig. 4.** Dose-dependent accumulation of collagen in glycyl-histidyl-lysine (GHK)–Cu-injected chambers. Groups of rats received the injection of the desired amount of *GHK–Cu* directly into the wound chamber every 3 days for 3 weeks. Chambers were collected at day 29 for analysis. Results show the mean ± SD of six rats (one wound chamber per rat). $* p < 0.05$, $*** p < 0.001$

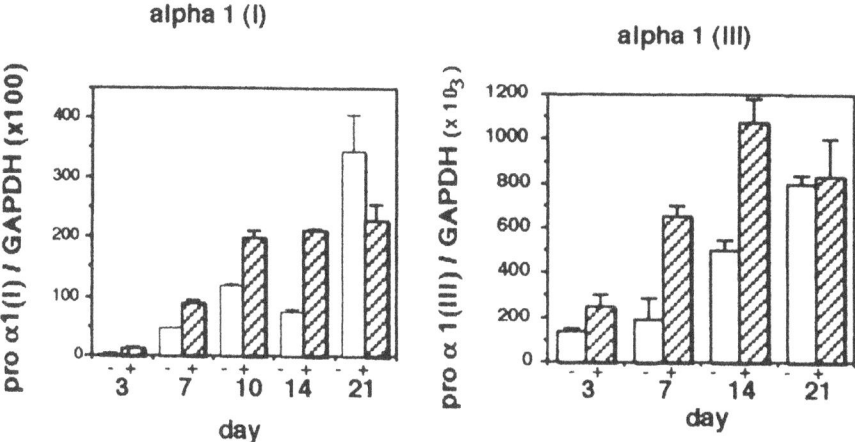

**Fig. 5.** Measurement of $\alpha 1$ (I) and $\alpha 1$ (III) collagen chain mRNAs in wound chambers serially injected with 2.0 mg glycyl-histidyl-lysine (GHK)–Cu (*hatched bars*) and control wound chambers (*open bars*). Results are mean of four wound chambers (one chamber per rat) ± SD

Northern-blot and dot-blot analysis of collagen mRNAs (Fig. 5) showed that $\alpha 1$ (I) chain mRNA was significantly increased as soon as day 3 after the first GHK–Cu injection. A significant increase was also found at days 7, 10 and 14, with a maximal increase at day 14. Similar results were observed for collagen $\alpha 1$ (III) chain mRNA, with a maximal increase at day 7 after the first GHK–Cu injection.

## 3.2 GHK–Cu Increases Extracellular Matrix Remodeling in Wounds

The increased number of hydroxyproline-containing peptides in the wound chambers injected with GHK–Cu suggested that extracellular matrix remodeling might be modulated by the copper–tripeptide complex, and prompted us to investigate the effects of GHK–Cu on MMPs expression and activation in the wound chamber model. Digestion of [$^{3}$H]-labeled acid-soluble collagen from rat skin demonstrated that the wound fluid of the chambers contained a high level of collagenase (MMP-1) activity, which increased progressively from day 3 to day 18. There was, however, no difference between the GHK–Cu-injected chambers and the controls.

Gelatin zymography of the wound fluid from the chambers demonstrated that MMP-2 (gelatinase A) and MMP-9 (gelatinase B) were the two major MMPs expressed in the experimental wounds during the early phases of the healing process (day 3). At this time, both enzymes were present in the "pro", inactive form, only. Pro-MMP-9 concentrations decreased rapidly in the wound fluid and disappeared completely after day 12. There was no difference in pro-MMP-9 expression between control and GHK–Cu-injected chambers. However, pro-MMP-2 expression increased progressively during the wound-healing process, reaching a maximum at day 12, then decreasing until day 22. GHK–Cu injections stimulated the expression of pro-MMP-2 at days 12 and 18.

Activated MMP-2 appeared in the wound fluid at day 7. In the control wound chambers, it remained present at a low level for the duration of the healing process, whereas it was strongly increased in GHK–Cu-injected chambers at days 18 and 22 after insertion. Western-blot experiments demonstrated that the MMP-2 protein was actually increased in the wound chambers injected with GHK–Cu. We verified, in separate experiments, that copper ions alone did not stimulate the activation of MMP-2. These results show that, in addition to the stimulation of extracellular-matrix accumulation, GHK–Cu is also able to modulate the expression and activation of some specific MMPs in wounds and might contribute to wound remodeling.

# 4 Conclusion

Not only cytokines and growth factors are involved in the regulation of connective tissue cells, but also a number of other factors present in their environment. The tripeptide GHK is a typical example of a short fragment from extracellular-matrix macromolecules that modulates the activity of connective tissue cells. Other examples of such short peptides have been described; for instance, VGVAPG, an elastin-derived peptide [2]. We suggest that this kind of regulation may play a significant role in the wound healing process.

# References

1. Downey D, Larrabee WF, Voci V, Pickart L (1985) Acceleration of wound healing using glycyl-histidyl-lysine-Cu$^{(II)}$. Surg Forum 48:573–575
2. Kamoun A, Landeau JM, Godeau G, Wallach J, Duchesnay A, Pellat B, Hornebeck W (1995) Growth stimulation of human skin fibroblasts by elastin-derived peptides. Cell Adhes Commun 3:273–281
3. Lane TF, Sage EH (1994) The biology of SPARC, a protein that modulates cell-matrix interactions. FASEB J 8:163–173
4. Lau S, Sarkar B (1981) The interaction of copper (II) and glycyl-L-histidyl-L-lysine, a growth-modulating tripeptide from plasma. Biochem J 199:649–656
5. Lopes-Moratalla N, Del Mar Calouge M, Lopez-Zabalza MJ, Perez-Mediavilla LA, Subira ML, Santiago E (1995) Activation of human lymphomononuclear cells by peptides derived from extracellular matrix proteins. Biochim Biophys Acta 1265:181–188
6. Maquart FX, Pickart L, Laurent M, Gillery P, Monboisse JC, Borel JP (1988) Stimulation of collagen synthesis in fibroblast cultures by the tripeptide-copper complex glycyl-L-histidyl-L-lysine-Cu$^{++}$. FEBS Lett 238:343–346
7. Maquart FX, Gillery P, Monboisse JC, Pickart L, Laurent M, Borel JP (1990) Glycyl-L-histidyl-L-lysine, a triplet from the $\alpha$2(I) chain of human type I collagen, stimulates collagen synthesis by fibroblast cultures. Ann NY Acad Sci 580:573–574
8. Maquart FX, Bellon G, Chaqour B, Wegrowski J, Patt LM, Trachy RE, Monboisse JC, Chastang F, Birembaut P, Gillery P, Borel JP (1993) In vivo stimulation of connective tissue accumulation by the tripeptide–copper complex glycyl-L-histidyl-L-lysine-Cu$^{2+}$ in rat experimental wounds. J Clin Invest 92:2368–2376
9. Pickart L, Thaler M (1973) Tripeptide in human serum which prolongs survival of normal liver cells and stimulates the growth of hepatoma cells. Nat New Biol 243:85–87

10. Pickart L (1981) The use of glycyl-histidyl-lysine in culture systems. In Vitro Cell Mol Biol 17:459–466
11. Raju KS, Alessandri J, Ziche M, Gullino PM (1982) Ceruloplasmin, copper ions and angiogenesis. J Natl Cancer Inst 69:1182–1188
12. Schilling TA, Joel W, Shurley MT (1959) Wound healing: a comparative study of the histochemical changes in granulation tissue contained in stainless steel wire mesh and polyvinyl sponge cylinders. Surgery 46:702–710
13. Tajima S, Wachi H, Seyama H (1996) Tropoelastin-derived degradation products downregulate elastin expression in vascular smooth muscle cell in cultures. Connect Tissue 28:231–235

# Myofibroblastic Differentiation and Extracellular Matrix Deposition in Early Stages of Cholestatic Fibrosis in Rat Liver

B. Tuchweber, A. Desmoulière, A. M. A. Costa, I. M. Yousef, G. Gabbiani

## 1 Introduction

Many studies have described changes in the hepatic extracellular matrix (ECM) and the cells involved in its production during liver injury [1, 2]. In acute liver damage, there may be complete parenchymal regeneration, scar formation, or a combination of both, and fibrogenesis seems to be transient [3]. Several cells of the liver can produce various ECM components. However, the hepatic stellate cell (HSC, also known as Ito or fat-storing cell) is the main source of ECM [24, 25] and has been shown to play a role in fibrogenesis for wound repair in acute injury of the liver [2, 18]. The HSCs can proliferate and rapidly express $\alpha$ smooth muscle (SM) actin, which is indicative of the cell's involvement in matrix deposition [2, 25–27].

In chronic liver injury, fibrogenesis leads to excessive deposition of ECM, which progresses to fibrosis and cirrhosis [2, 6, 10, 16]. As in acute injury, it has been established that the HSC participates in fibrogenesis. However, work from this [11, 30] and other [1, 3, 17, 23] laboratories has provided evidence that, in various models of fibrosis, cells other than the HSC may participate in the accumulation of ECM components.

In this paper, we will discuss the very early changes of portal fibroblasts and expression of ECM components in the rat model of fibrosis induced by bile duct ligation (BDL), which simulates the features of human biliary fibrosis and cirrhosis. Detailed descriptions of some of the findings were published previously [11, 30].

## 2 Proliferation and Differentiation of Portal Fibroblasts

The kinetics of the proliferation of different liver cell subpopulations was studied at 6 h, and 1, 2, 3, and 7 days after BDL. The proliferative response was evaluated by proliferating cell nuclear antigen (PCNA) immunohistochemistry [30]. As early as

Current Topics in Pathology, Volume 93
A. Desmoulière, B. Tuchweber (Eds.)
© Springer-Verlag Berlin Heidelberg 1999

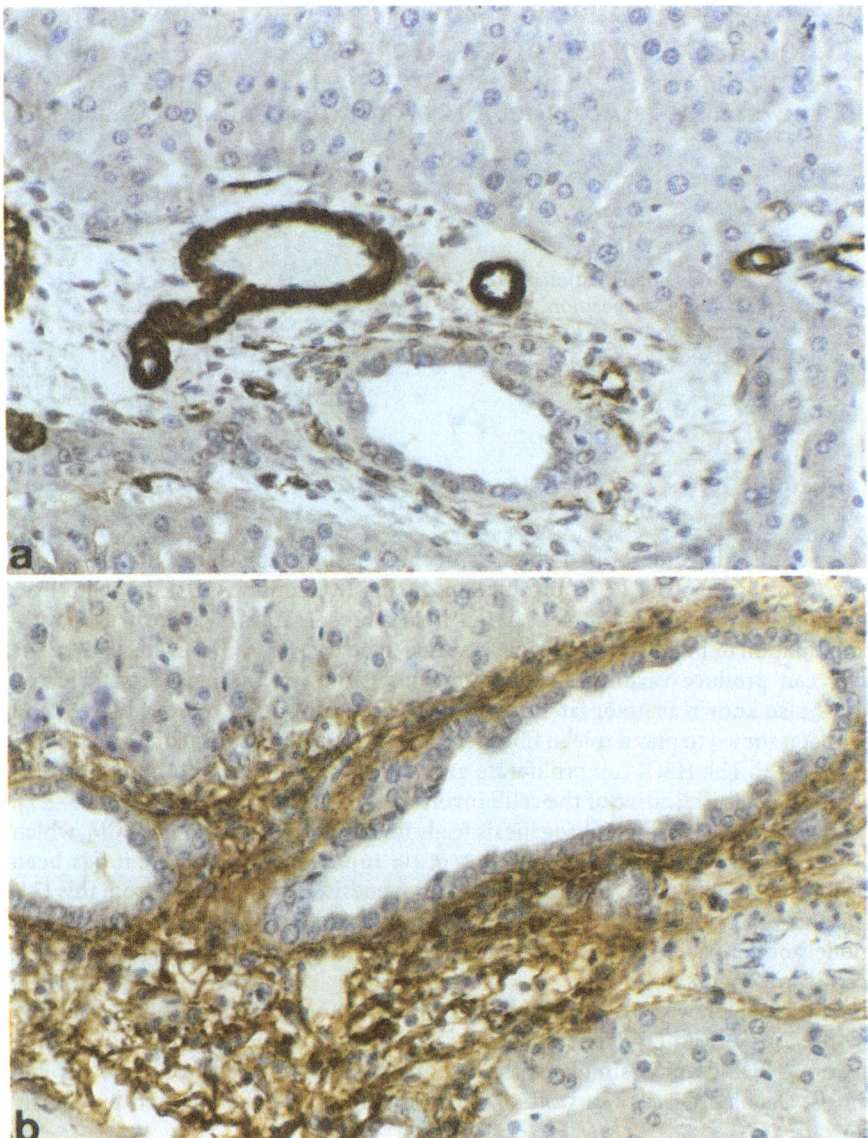

**Fig. 1a, b.** Immunoperoxidase staining for $\alpha$-smooth muscle actin (**a**) or lysyl oxidase (**b**) 24 h after bile-duct ligation. In the portal zone, $\alpha$-smooth muscle actin is restricted as in controls to vascular smooth muscle cells, whereas, at the same time, a strong reactivity for lysyl oxidase appears. × 300

6 h after BDL, there was proliferation of the bile duct epithelial cells, a well-docu-mented finding in biliary obstruction research in both animals and humans [2, 10, 17, 29]. This was followed by a marked expansion of fibroblastic cells in the stroma adjacent to proliferating ductules. The labeling index of portal fibroblasts reached a peak at 48 h after BDL, and gradually decreased until the day 7.

Similarly, there was a transient proliferation of hepatocytes and a significant expansion of HSCs in zones 1 and 3 of the acinus. Differentiation of periductular portal fibroblasts was examined by measuring expression of $\alpha$-SM actin and desmin [30]. Immunohistochemistry, immunoelectron microscopy with the immunogold technique, and immunofluorescence evaluation showed, in the fibroblastic cells surrounding the proliferating ductules, no $\alpha$-SM actin expression in controls and at 24 h after BDL (Fig. 1a), a slight $\alpha$-SM actin expression at 48 h after BDL and a significant $\alpha$-SM actin expression at 72 h after BDL. The propor-tion of cells expressing $\alpha$-SM actin in this area increased until day 7. However, $\alpha$-SM actin was not expressed in HSCs of the liver lobule. This observation contrasts with the sequence observed following damage to the parenchyma by chemical agents, such as carbon tetrachloride [20, 21, 24, 25, 27]. Here, fibrogenesis was associated with phenotypic modulation (expression of $\alpha$-SM actin) of HSCs and parenchymal cell necrosis and inflammation. It seems likely then that different potentially fibrogenic cells and mechanisms participate in fibrosis induced by various agents.

To further characterize the myofibroblastic phenotypic features of portal fibro-blasts, desmin expression was evaluated along with $\alpha$-SM actin. Until 72 h after BDL, desmin expression increased in fibroblastic cells in the stroma surrounding proliferating ductules, as it did in HSCs, particularly in zone 1 of the liver lobule. However, double immunofluorescence staining by confocal microscopy showed that, at that time, most of the periductular fibroblasts expressing $\alpha$-SM actin were desmin negative, pointing to heterogeneous cytoskeletal protein expression in fibroblasts during liver fibrogenesis.

## 3 Extracellular Matrix Deposition

Since rapid modulation of expression of $\alpha$-SM actin occurred in portal fibroblasts after BDL, we examined whether these cells could produce deposition of ECM com-ponents in portal areas [11]. By immunofluorescence, it was shown that laminin expression occurred in the stroma surrounding proliferating ductules, and was increased by BDL from 48 h until day 7 after ligation. Fibronectin EIIIA, which, under normal conditions, is only observed in blood vessels, was strongly expressed in portal areas as well as in sinusoids as early as 24 h after BDL (Fig. 2). The level of expression of fibronectin EIIIA was higher at 48 h, and, at this time, collagen IV, collagen I, procollagen III and elastin were also highly expressed in the portal zone. In the early stages after BDL (24 – 48 h), tenascin was increased in the areas adjacent to proliferating ductules, but at later times, (3 – 7 days), expression of the protein was localized to the periphery of the lesion. Of interest was the observation that lysyl oxidase (Fig. 1 b) was markedly expressed as early as 24 h after BDL and was restricted to the periductular area. Similarly, tissue inhibitor of metalloproteinase-1

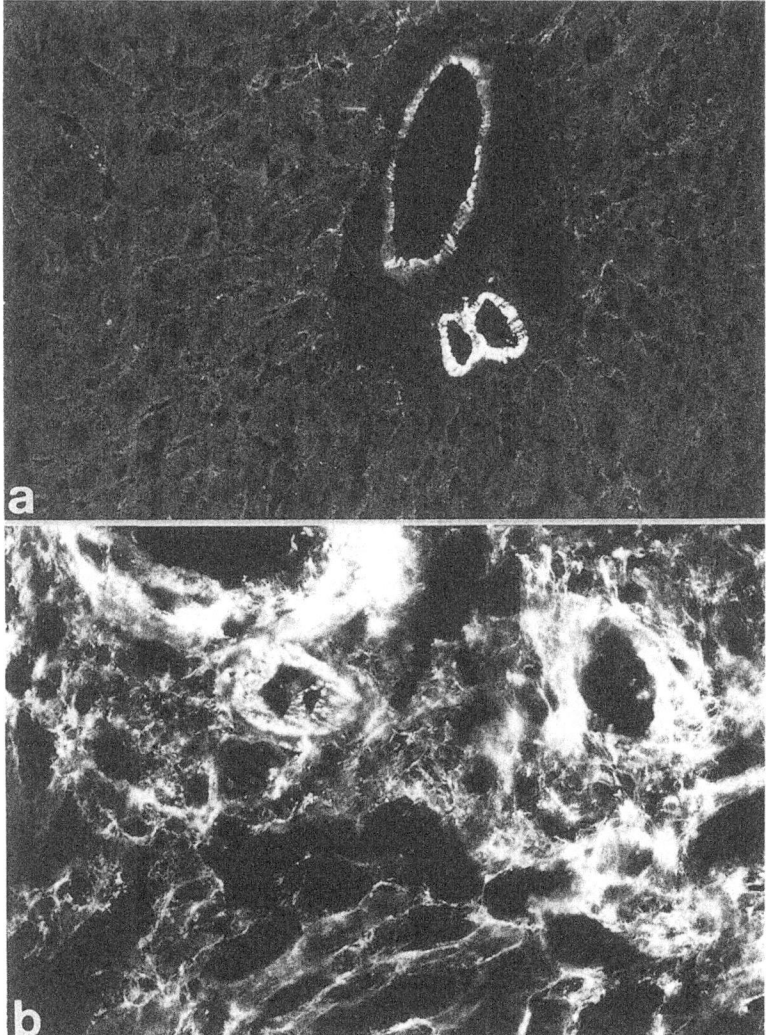

**Fig. 2a, b.** Fibronectin EIIIA immunofluorescence staining in control (**a**) and 24 h (**b**) after bile-duct ligation. In sham-operated controls, fibronectin EIIIA expression is restricted to vessel wall. By 24 h, fibronectin EIIIA is expressed both in portal zones and along sinusoids. **a** × 240; **b** × 280

(TIMP-1) mRNA expression was greatly increased in periductular areas 24 h after BDL. From these observations it is clear that changes in ECM deposition and degradation occur very early in the development of fibrosis after BDL, and seem to precede myofibroblastic differentiation. The acquisition of $\alpha$-SM actin by portal fibroblasts may represent an adaptive response of this cell to altered ECM, providing further support for the importance of the ECM as a modulator of cell phenotype and behavior.

## 4 Possible Factors Involved in ECM Changes and Portal Fibroblast Proliferation and Differentiation

Recently, there has been much interest in elucidating the mechanism(s) through which changes in matrix composition and in expression of matrix-degrading enzymes and their inhibitors modulate structure and function of liver cells [4, 9, 13, 14, 19, 28]. The early changes in ECM after BDL are likely the result of increased intraductular pressure and activation of portal fibroblasts and mononuclear phagocytes [1, 6, 7, 11, 17]. In addition, the participation of bile duct epithelial cells and hepatocytes, particularly from periportal areas, in the ECM deposition cannot be excluded.

Our studies [11] showed a very early expression of lysyl oxidase, which may play a role in the stabilization and maturation of collagen and elastin. Similarly, in cutaneous wound healing [15] and lung fibrosis induced by cadmium [8], lysyl oxidase was expressed in very early phases of fibrogenesis. Since studies with cultured fibroblasts indicated that transforming growth factor $\beta1$ (TGF$\beta1$) increases accumulation of lysyl oxidase [5], it is likely that this cytokine is involved in the response after BDL. TGF$\beta1$ could also be responsible for the secretion and maturation of other matrix proteins. Many studies have demonstrated that TGF$\beta1$ can alter the modulation of fibroblasts into myofibroblasts [12]; thus, this cytokine could also participate alone or with others, e. g., tumor necrosis factor (TNF), platelet-derived growth factor (PDGF), or interleukin 1 (IL-1), in the differentiation of the fibroblasts of the periductular stroma.

In the model of cholestatic injury, there is fibrosis without significant parenchymal cell injury or inflammation. However, we have observed very early expansion of EDI-positive cells in portal and periductular areas, indicating that, in addition to hepatic cells, monocytes may contribute to cytokine release [30]. Recently [22], it was reported that neutrophils are also present in periductular areas from 2–10 days after BDL, and are increased in the circulation. In addition, treatment with anti-neutrophil serum was shown to reduce the severity of fibrosis, and the expression of collagen mRNA in total liver tissue.

In summary, in the experimental model of fibrosis induced by BDL, fibroblasts within the portal tracts are mainly involved in the fibrogenesis process. ECM deposition and the expression of lysyl oxidase occur very soon after BDL, and seem to precede the expression of $\alpha$-SM actin in periductular fibroblasts. The rapid induction of TIMP-1 in cholestasis also indicates that, not only is there an increase in ECM deposition, but there may be a decrease in matrix degradation. The myofibroblastic differentiation may reflect an adaptive response of the fibroblast to the altered ECM environment. The specific signals from the changed ECM associated with cholestasis which modify the phenotypic characteristics of periductular fibroblasts need to be defined.

**Acknowledgements.** This work was supported in part by the Association pour la Recherche sur le Cancer (France), the Medical Research Council of Canada, the Swiss National Science Foundation (Grant no. 31–50568.97), and the Centre Jacques Cartier (Lyon, France).

# References

1. Abdel-Aziz G, Rescan PY, Clément B, Lebeau G, Rissel M, Grimaud JA, Campion JP, Guillouzo A (1991) Cellular sources of matrix proteins in experimentally induced cholestatic rat liver. J Pathol 164:167–174
2. Aronson DC, De Haan J, James J, Bosch KS, Ketel AG, Houtkooper JM, Heijmans HS (1988) Quantitative aspects of the parenchyma-stroma relationship in experimentally induced cholestasis. Liver 8:116–126
3. Bhunchet E, Wake K (1992) Role of mesenchymal cell populations in porcine-serum induced rat liver fibrosis. Hepatol 6:1452–1473
4. Bissell DM (1992) Effects of extracellular matrix on hepatic behavior. In: Clément B, Guillouzo A (eds) Cellular and molecular aspects of cirrhosis. ISERM/J Libbey Eurotext Ltd, Montrouge, France, pp 189–197
5. Boak AM, Roy R, Berk J, Taylor L, Polgar P, Goldstein RH, Kagan HM (1994) Regulation of lysyl oxidase expression in lung fibroblasts by transforming growth factor-$\beta 1$ and prostaglandin E2. Am J Respir Cell Mol Biol 11:751–755
6. Burt AD (1993) Cellular and molecular aspects of hepatic fibrosis. J Pathol 170:105–114
7. Burt AD, MacSween RNM (1993) Bile-duct proliferation: its true significance? Histopathology 23:599–602
8. Chichester CO, Palmer KC, Hayes JA, Kagan HM (1981) Lung lysyl oxidase and prolyl hydroxylase: increases induced by cadmium chloride inhalation and the effect of $\beta$-aminopropionitrile in rats. Am Rev Respir Dis 124:709–713
9. Clément B, Loréal O, Rescan PY, Levavasseur F, Diakonova M, Rissel M, L'Helgoualch H, Guillouzo A (1992) Cellular origin of the hepatic extracellular matrix. In: Gressner AM, Ramadori G (eds) Molecular and cell biology of liver fibrogenesis. Kluwer, Dordrecht, The Netherlands, pp 85–98
10. Desmet VJ (1987) Cholestasis: extrahepatic obstruction and secondary biliary cirrhosis. In: MacSween RNM, Anthony PP, Scheuer PJ (eds) Pathology of the liver. Churchill Livingston, Edinburgh, pp 364–423
11. Desmoulière A, Darby I, Costa AMA, Raccurt M, Tuchweber B, Sommer P, Gabbiani G (1997) Extracellular matrix deposition, lysyl oxidase expression, and myofibroblastic differentiation during the initial stages of cholestatic fibrosis in the rat. Lab Invest 76:765–778
12. Desmoulière A, Geinoz A, Gabbiani F, Gabbiani, G (1993) Transforming growth factor-$\beta 1$ induces $\alpha$-smooth muscle actin expression in granulation tissue myofibroblasts and in quiescent and growing cultured fibroblasts. J Cell Biol 122:103–111
13. Emonard H, Guillouzo A, Lapiere CM, Grimaud JA (1990) Human liver fibroblast capacity for synthesizing intestinal collagenase in vitro. Cell Mol Biol 36:461–467
14. Friedman SL, Roll FJ, Boyles J, Arenson DM, Bissell DM (1989) Maintenance of differentiated phenotype of cultured rat hepatocytes by basement membrane matrix. J Biol Chem 264:10756–10762
15. Fushidatakemura H, Fukuda M, Maekawa N, Chanoki M, Kobayashi H, Yashiro H, Ishii M, Hamada T, Otani S, Ooshima A (1996) Detection of lysyl oxidase gene expression in rat skin during wound healing. Arch Dermatol Res 288:7–10
16. Gressner AM (1991) Liver fibrosis: perspectives in pathobiochemical research and clinical outlook. Eur J Clin Chem Clin Biochem 29:293–311
17. Hines JE, Johnson SJ, Burt AD (1993) In vivo responses of perisinusoidal cells (lipocytes) and macrophages to cholestatic liver injury. Am J Pathol 142:511–518
18. Inuzuka S, Veno T, Tanikawa K (1994) Fibrogensis in acute liver injuries. Pathol Res Pract 190:903–909
19. Iredale JP, Arthur MJP (1994) Hepatocyte-matrix interactions. Gut 35:729–732
20. Johnson SJ, Hillan KJ, Hines JE, Ferrier R, Burt AD (1992) Proliferation and phenotypic modulation of perisinusoidal (Ito) cells following acute liver injury: temporal relationship with TGF1 expression. In: Clément B, Guillouzo A (eds) Cellular and molecular aspects of cirrhosis. ISERM/J Libbey Eurotext Ltd, Montrouge, France, pp 219–222
21. Johnson SJ, Hines JE, Burt AD (1992) Macrophage and perisinusoidal cell kinetics in acute liver injury. J Pathol 166:351–358

22. Maher JJ, Lozier JS, Shi Z, Saito JM (1997) Neutrophil depletion attenuates hepatic fibro-genesis in bile duct-ligated rats. Hepatol 26:185A
23. Miyazaki H, Van Eyken P, Roskams T, De Vos R, Desmet VJ (1993) Transient expression of tenascin in experimentally induced cholestatic fibrosis in rat liver: an immunohistochemi-cal study. J Hepatol 19:353–366
24. Pinzani M (1995) Novel insight into the biology and physiology of the Ito cell. Pharmacol Ther 66:387–412
25. Ramadori G (1991) The stellate cell (Ito cell, fat-storing cell, lipocyte, perisinoisidal cell) of the liver. New insights into pathophysiology of an intriguing cell. Virchows Arch B Cell Pathol 61:147–158
26. Rockey DC, Boyles JK, Gabbiani G, Friedman SL (1992) Rat hepatic lipocytes express smooth muscle actin upon activation in vivo and in culture. J Submicrosc Cytol Pathol 24:193–203
27. Schmitt-Gräff A, Krüger S, Bochard F, Gabbiani G, Denk H (1991) Modulation of alpha smooth muscle actin and desmin expression in perisinusoidal cells of normal and diseased humans livers. Am J Pathol 138:1233–1242
28. Schuppan D, Milani S (1992) The extracellular matrix in cellular communications. In: Gressner AM, Ramadori G (eds) Molecular and cell biology of liver fibrogenesis. Kluwer, The Netherlands, pp 52–71
29. Slott PA, Liu MH, Tavoloni N (1990) Origin, pattern, and mechanism of bile duct prolifera-tion following biliary obstruction in rat. Gastroenterology 99:466–477
30. Tuchweber B, Desmoulière A, Bochaton-Piallat ML, Rubbia-Brandt L, Gabbiani G (1996) Proliferation and phenotypic modulation of portal fibroblasts in the early stages of chole-static fibrosis in the rat. Lab Invest 74:1–14

# Gene Therapy of Wounds with Growth Factors

J. M. DAVIDSON, J. S. WHITSITT, B. PENNINGTON, C. B. BALLAS, S. EMING, S. I. BENN

## 1 Introduction

The wound site is a miniature battleground, where the host tissue must stop the loss of blood and body fluid, fight off infection, restore tissue integrity and minimize loss of function to the damaged tissue. This is accomplished through a cascade of cellular and biochemical events. It is clear that part of the communication machinery that coordinates these events is the expression of soluble signaling molecules, the cytokines, which are synthesized and released by effector cells to act upon their targets. One of the most important groups of these molecules to be investigated during the last decade is cellular growth factors [11]. As their name implies, these molecules are able, at least in cell culture, to bring about dramatic changes in the rate of growth of cells or the production of cell products, such as extracellular matrix. Because of these special properties of growth factors, the hypothesis that they might accelerate the process of wound repair was tested and confirmed in a wide variety of experimental animal models [5, 6]. Subsequently, many of these purified growth factors, including transforming growth factor beta (TGF-$\beta$), platelet-derived growth factor (PDGF), epidermal growth factor (EGF) and basic fibroblast growth factor (bFGF), have gone on to clinical trials that have shown partial success [7, 14, 16, 20, 23, 25]. Often, these trials have used prodigious quantities of the growth factors, yet usually the outcome has not been impressive enough to warrant further pursuit of the compounds as clinical materials.

A very important aspect of the growth factor wound-healing paradigm is the effective delivery of these polypeptides to the wound site; however, the wound site is a relatively hostile environment. These molecules are all relatively small proteins that might be freely diffusible, but they are often bound to a carrier molecule that serves as both a protector and a delivery system. Thus, growth factors that are normally expressed by inflammatory or resident cells at sites of tissue repair act over

Current Topics in Pathology, Volume 93
A. Desmoulière, B. Tuchweber (Eds.)
© Springer-Verlag Berlin Heidelberg 1999

**Table 1.** DNA-Transfer Techniques

| |
|---|
| Chemical |
|     Calcium phosphate precipitation |
|     Diethyl-aminoethyl(DEAE)-dextran |
|     Polybrene/DMSO |
|     Liposomes |
|     Nanoparticles |
| Physical |
|     Irradiation |
|     Microinjection |
|     Muscle injection |
|     Electroporation |
|     Biolistics (particle bombardment, "gene gun") |
| Biological |
|     Retrovirus |
|     Adenovirus |
|     Adeno-associated virus |
|     Vaccinia virus |
|     Lentivirus |

very short distances. In contrast, when growth factors are added to wounds, either as topical formulations or injections into the interstitial space, this results in the haphazard delivery of some of the growth factor molecules to their targets. One can readily imagine that a great deal of the growth factor activity is either lost by binding to other kinds of molecules in the extracellular space or by being subjected to degradative action of the many enzymes that are released by inflammatory- and connective-tissue cells during the course of wound repair and remodeling.

At the wound site, the positive response to growth factors is counteracted by the inefficiency of these growth factors in the face of high levels of protein-degrading activity. Introduction of growth factor genes might be an ideal mechanism for drug delivery by local, autogenous expression. Gene therapy is now in widespread use as a laboratory technique for introducing new or modified genes into cells, tissues and organisms. There are numerous technologies for introduction of foreign DNA into organs such as skin (Table 1). While gene therapy is often employed as a last resort, it is an excellent means of drug delivery. Thus, we began, about 5 years ago, a line of experimentation to determine whether growth factor genes could be introduced into experimental wounds in animals, and whether they could produce significant biological effects. In this paper, we report on findings with several different cytokines in several different model systems, which indicate that using the appropriate delivery system, gene therapy with growth factors is certainly feasible, shows little immediate risk and is biologically effective.

## 2 Experimental Design

The underlying philosophy in these experiments is to obtain the transient expression of growth factors at the wound site. Persistent expression would be unphysiological and possibly harmful, since many of the growth factors are oncogenes. Although a number of transfection systems, particularly those using viruses, are highly efficient, they often lead to an undesirable host reaction to viral components. In the case of retroviruses, these vectors favor the permanent integration of the transgene into a host chromosome. Given the range of biological effects of growth factors and their association with malignant growth as well as normal wound healing, we wanted to make sure we had a system that could be predicted to express rapidly and then turn off the expression of these potent molecules. For this reason, all of our experimentation has used conventional DNA plasmids with no viral-insertional sequences. As the project has evolved, we have shifted promoter systems from early studies with the Rous sarcoma virus (RSV), later studies with the simian virus 40 (SV40), and finally with the cytomegalovirus (CMV) promoters. Each of these promoters increases the expression of transgenes in target cells and tissues by an order of magnitude.

Three types of model wound systems have been explored. The most frequently used model is the standard incisional wound in the laboratory rat. These longitudinal wounds are placed at four parallel sites on the backs of normal Sprague-Dawley rats. At intervals after the time of surgery, the biomechanical properties of the incisional site are measured with an Instron tensiometer. The second model, which provides more complete biochemical and histological data, is the implantation of a small polyvinyl alcohol (PVA) sponge disc under the skin of the rat. This creates a wound space into which cells progressively invade, providing an abundant wound bed of granulation tissue. The third model, which we have used in some studies, simply involves the exposure of the abdominal fascia of the rat to allow targeting of transgenes to a connective-tissue compartment.

Transfection methods have evolved during the course of our studies. The initial methods followed up on the observations that naked DNA in simple sucrose solutions could be injected into skeletal muscle with long-term expression of the transgene by a few cells. Following these protocols, we performed studies using the PVA-sponge model. Subsequently, injection of naked DNA was modified by the use of liposome carriers. This technology involves the encapsulation of DNA in a particle with a lipid bilayer, which facilitates the entry of DNA into cells. Liposome technology is now in wide use in both in vitro and in vivo experimental applications.

The third technology is based on the development of specialized transfection techniques that could be used to introduce DNA into plant cells that had thick cell walls. This technology, which goes under the various names of biolistic transfection, particle-mediated acceleration, or more simply the "gene gun", has been developed independently by several organizations. The basic principles for operation are the same in most versions (Fig. 1). Small, microscopic particles (0.9–2.6 µg) of dense material, either tungsten or gold, are coated with the DNA of interest. These particles are then loaded into a carrier system and placed in a device that, through use of either a shock wave generated by an electric spark or a gas discharge, propels the particles toward the target at sufficient velocities to allow some of the particles to penetrate cells and become lodged in the cytoplasm. With appropriate forces, this is not harmful to the cells or the tissue, and a portion of the DNA introduced into the cells is transiently expressed, much in the same fashion as if delivered by other means. With a low frequency, stable transfection may occur. The principle advantages of this technology are that it is relatively inexpensive, the

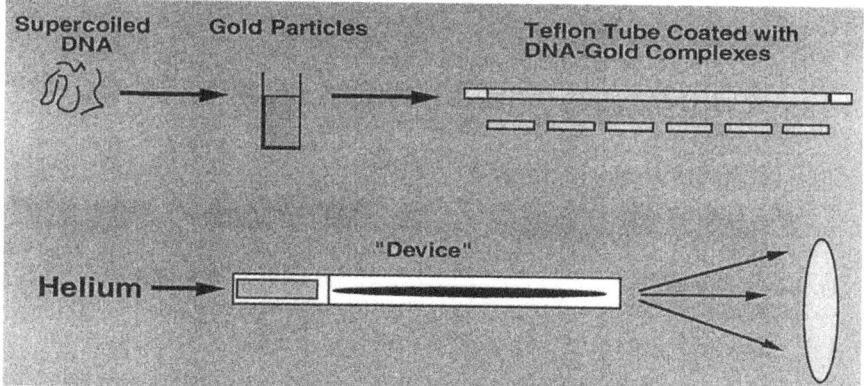

**Fig. 1.** Principles of particle-mediated gene transfer. Plasmid DNA is first precipitated onto gold particles which are then coated on the inside of PTFE tubing. Segments cut from the tubing are loaded into a helium-driven device that uses a rapid, high-pressure discharge (200–800 psi) to accelerate the particle into the cytoplasm of target cells/tissues (ACCELL gene delivery device; Agacetus, Geneva)

devices that have been developed are portable and not dangerous to the operator or the target, and the targeting is well confirmed on a given surface. The packaging of DNA onto the particles renders the transfection material stable under cool, dry conditions for many months. This latter aspect, the particle-mediated acceleration technology, differs widely from the use of either liposome- or virally-mediated systems in terms of the ease of application and shelf life. Obviously, the main attraction of the technology for our research has been the ease of use of such a device to target a surface wound.

Since many different growth factors and combinations have been shown to have an impact on wound repair, we have also produced plasmid constructs to perform in vivo studies with many different expression vectors. At this time, studies are being carried out with expression vectors encoding TGF-$\beta$, PDGF, bFGF, vascular endothelial growth factor (VEGF) and several other molecules. In most cases, these expression vectors encode the human forms of the proteins; however, our past experience using recombinant human growth factors in animal systems assures us that the species boundary is not an obstacle to the activity of these structurally conserved molecules.

## 3 Results

### 3.1 Direct DNA Transfer

Initial studies on wound transfection used a very simple system. We injected a $\beta$-galactosidase expression vector driven by the RSV promoter into sponge-granulation tissue using a sucrose vehicle. These early studies showed a positive out-

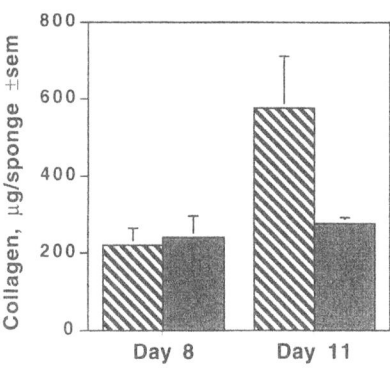

**Fig. 2.** Collagen content increases in sponge granulation tissue after direct transfection with a TGF-$\beta$1 expression vector. Polyvinyl alcohol sponges were implanted subcutaneously in 375-g rats and injected with 10 μg of an SV-40-driven plasmid vector expressing latent TGF-$\beta$1 (*hatched bars*). Controls (*solid bars*)were injected with an equal amount of $\beta$-galactosidase expression vector. Collagen content was measured at 8 days and 11 days after implantation by hydroxyproline determination

come, with a large number of the cells within granulation tissue expressing this transgene. Based on these findings, we moved on to the injection of TGF-$\beta$ expression vectors into the sponge granulation tissue. The vector was driven by the SV40 promoter and expressed the full-length latent form of porcine TGF-$\beta$1. In several experiments, we observed increased collagen content in sponges injected with expression vector, but not with other plasmid controls (Fig. 2). This suggested to us that the experiment could be expanded to treat other types of wounds. We also learned from these studies that the response was quite variable, suggesting that the transfection approach was not operating efficiently. Thus, we turned to more efficient transfection systems.

## 3.2 Liposome-Mediated Transfer

The use of liposomes as vehicles for cellular uptake of DNA is widespread. We have used a number of formulations, in particular a commercial formulation Transfectam (Promega) that was able to increase substantially the efficiency of transfection and of reporter-gene constructs, such as $\beta$-galactosidase or luciferase in the sponge granulation tissue model. At the same time, we began modification of our expression vectors, first switching to a constitutively active form of TGF-$\beta$1, in which two of the cysteines critical to latency had been converted to serine residues. This construct was clearly more active in a number of in vitro assays. There were marked differences in biological activity after transfection of various TGF-$\beta$ isoform vectors into HeLa cells. When latent murine TGF-$\beta$ is transfected into HeLa cells, the supernatants from these cells contain an activity that, upon acidification, is capable of increasing the elastin expression of target, smooth-muscle cells (Fig. 3). This is a characteristic feature of TGF-$\beta$. In contrast, experiments using the constitutively active form of porcine TGF-$\beta$ showed: (1) that supernatants from HeLa cells directly activated smooth-muscle cells without acidification, and (2) the construct could be directly transfected into smooth-muscle cells with the same result. Initially, this construct used the zinc-inducible metallothionein promoter, which allowed us to show that the elastin-inducing activity was only present in cul-

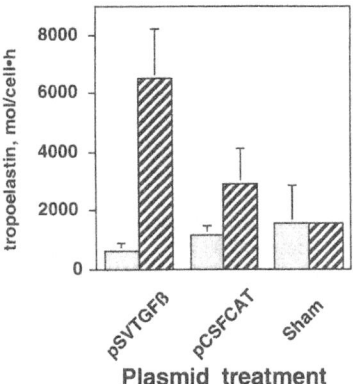

**Plasmid treatment**

**Fig. 3.** Production of biologically active, latent TGF-$\beta$1 by transfected cells. HeLa cells were transfected by the calcium phosphate procedure with vectors expressing latent TGF-$\beta$1 or chloramphenicol acetyl transferase. After 48 h culture, supernatants were removed, and a portion of each was transiently acidified by dialysis against 0.1 M HOAc to activate latent TGF-$\beta$. Untreated (*solid bars*) or acidified (*hatched bars*) supernatants were mixed with an equal volume of fresh medium and used to treat vocal fold fibroblasts. Tropoelastin production expressed as the mean was measured by enzyme-linked immunosorbent assay (ELISA) in fibroblast supernatants 48 h later. Only the acidified supernatants from TGF-$\beta$-transfected cells showed significant capacity to induce tropoelastin production in the target cell population

tures that had been treated with zinc. Since zinc alone is an accelerator of wound healing, only viral promoters have been used in vivo. A drawback of the liposome-mediated transfection system has been the expense of the reagent.

## 3.3 Biolistic Transfer

Having these preliminary results in hand, we turned to a new physical method for introducing DNA into cells: particle-mediated acceleration. This technology, which in our case has been developed by scientists at Agracetus (currently Powderject Vaccines, Inc.), involves the propulsion of micron-sized gold particles coated with DNA into the cytoplasm of cells using high-pressure helium as a propellant. Other investigators have shown, and we have confirmed, that optimal expression of reporter genes occurred in the system when the propellant pressure was set to embed most of the gold particles in the basal epidermal cell layer. Transfection of particles into the upper layer of the epidermis using lower pressures resulted in a more rapid sloughing of the gold-DNA and targeting into many nonviable cells in the superficial epidermis. Increasing pressure to target deeper connective-tissue cell layers resulted in many particles lodging in the extracellular matrix rather than in cell cytoplasm. The high cellularity of the basal epidermal cell layer seems to be the most efficient target site, at least in skin. Using this system, we calibrated reporter-gene expression (luciferase) for both pressure and site. We learned that the efficiency was very sensitive to the amount of stratum corneum left on the dermis. This variable was normalized by the use of commercial depilatory agents.

Expression in skin increased nearly two orders of magnitude by switching from the SV40 to the CMV promoter.

## 3.4 In Vivo Studies

Armed with this new device and high-level expression vectors, we proceeded to evaluate the effects of constitutively active TGF-$\beta$1 expression vectors on the mechanical strength of incisional wounds, from 7 days to 21 days after surgery. These studies showed positive results under many circumstances, at least in the rat [3]. We obtained, on average, 75–100 % increases in mechanical strength of incisions for periods up to 3 weeks after transfection, using a single administration of recombinant DNA to the skin up to 24 h before the time of surgery. Transfection with TGF-$\beta$ expression vectors has proved effective, not only in normal wound healing, but in diabetic wounds (Fig. 4) and, most recently, in wounds from aged animals. In the latter case, we have observed greater than 100 % increases in age-related wound tensile-strength deficits. Treatment after surgery has been somewhat complicated by the force of the helium discharge that, in our simple model system, tends to disrupt the integrity of the incision.

Recently, in collaboration with the group at the Shriner's Burns Hospital in Boston and the Department of Dermatology at the University of Cologne, we have shown that PDGF expression vectors are also capable of increasing wound tensile strength for days to weeks after transfection. Similar studies with more novel growth factor complementary DNA (cDNA) – activin A (provided by S. WERNER,

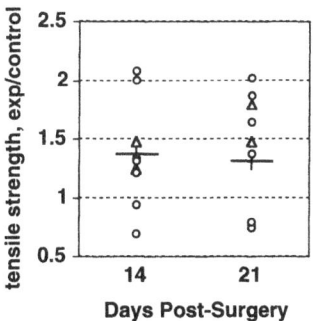

**Fig. 4.** Tensile strength of wounds in diabetic rats is increased by transfection with TGF-$\beta$1. An impaired healing model, the streptozotocin-diabetic rat incision, was tested for response to TGF-$\beta$1 transfection. In this experiment, constitutively active TGF-$\beta$1 was expressed in a plasmid vector driven by the cytomegalovirus promoter. Plasmid DNA (1 µg) was introduced into the epidermis at the wound site by particle-mediated bombardment with a device provided by Agracetus (Powderject Vaccines, Inc.). Control sites received 1 µg of a luciferase expression vector. Transfection sites were incised and closed with wound clips. Tensiometric evaluation of wound strength was performed at the indicated time points, and data are expressed as the ratio of experimental to control wound strengths in pairs of wounds on each animal. *Open triangles* represent animals that did not become hyperglycemic and may be considered normal. Relative responses were positive, similar and persistent in most animals. (Data are adapted from [3] with permission)

Max Planck Institut. Martinsreid) and connective-tissue growth factor (provided by G. GROTENDORST, University of Miami) – illustrate the fact that the wound-healing properties can be done without resorting to a large-scale production of the gene product. Both growth factors enhanced incisional-wound healing, and activin A has also shown activity in an excisional-wound model.

Another set of expression vectors we have evaluated encode the angiogenic and mitogenic cytokine bFGF. Because bFGF is not normally secreted by cells, we used fusion constructs that linked bFGF to the signal sequence of bovine immuno-globulin G (IgG) [22] or acidic FGF (aFGF) to the signal sequence of FGF-4 [13]. In other assays, this converts bFGF into a potent, secreted growth stimulus that induces cellular transformation. Interestingly, the transfection of these expression vectors produced no tissue response when introduced into intact skin, either alone or in combination with a TGF-$\beta$ expression vector. These results suggested that the vector product was not reaching the target cell efficiently. Therefore, we turned to an alternative transfection method by exposing the abdominal fascia and shooting the DNA directly into the abdominal wall. This produced a spectacular, angiogenic response with the expression vector in which bFGF was fused to the secretory signal peptide for bovine IgG [4].

## 4 Discussion

We have briefly described our findings using a number of vectors in different wound-repair systems, all of which strongly support the concept that gene therapy can be used to alter the course of wound repair much in the same way as has been accomplished by using the recombinant growth factors themselves. Our findings certainly echo the observations of ANDREE et al. [1], who showed previously that transfection of EGF into porcine skin produced increased rates of epithelialization. Recently, repeated application FGF vectors has also shown a positive effect on incisional wounds [26].

There are undoubtedly many other strategies for the gene therapy of skin, in particular, transfection of keratinocytes or fibroblasts in vitro and transplantation of those cells to target sites [2, 8, 10, 12, 15, 17–19, 21, 24]. Two overriding, philosophical issues have governed our line of experimentation: (1) we believe that potent molecules such as growth factors should only be expressed in a transient fashion; (2) effective remedies for wound healing should involve the local treatment of the problem. The successful form of gene therapy that we have described fulfills both of these criteria [9, 27]. The particle-mediated acceleration technology targets, in its present configuration, a circular area of about 3 cm$^2$. The propulsion of gold particles into the skin produces no permanent damage to the underlying tissue. A mild erythema may be noted for 1–2 h, but detailed histological evaluation of sections from targeted tissue shows no evidence of any persistent inflammatory response. Some individuals do exhibit an allergic reaction to gold; however, the bulk of the material is shed from the skin surface within several days of administration. The transient nature of the transfection is assured by two aspects of the methodology: first, targeting predominantly to the basal keratinocyte cell layer means that the target cells will, within several days, follow the normal course of keratinocyte development to be eventually sloughed off in the upper levels of the stratum corneum. This assures that the gold particles – and the DNA that they bear – is only temporarily present in the skin. When a deeper (higher pressure) transfection has been made, we have observed some accumulation of gold particles into mononuclear phagocytes. Second, the expression vectors that we currently use contain naked plasmid DNA lacking sequences or mechanisms to select for integration of the foreign DNA into the host-cell genome. Although it is certainly true, under laboratory conditions, that high numbers of cells exposed to high concentrations of naked plasmid DNA will incorporate this DNA into genomic material at some low frequency, the probabilities of this happening under the present transfection scheme are extremely low. The third safety factor is the fact that most foreign genes do not remain permanently active in such transgenic experiments; very often expression dies off within a matter of weeks or months unless the cell populations are maintained under constant, selective pressure. Therefore, we feel the safety margin of this method, were it ever to move into clinical practice, is quite high.

Another issue to be addressed with this methodology is the economics of gene therapy versus peptide therapy. As growth factors come to the market as recombinant proteins, it is likely that the cost of the therapy will remain high. Indeed, many clinical trials have not moved into the marketplace, at least in part, because of the cost associated with treating wounds with tens to hundreds of micrograms of highly purified recombinant protein. Gene therapy and DNA transfection obviate the need for specialized cell production and protein-purification facilities, as the only active reagent needed is quite standard in its chemistry: DNA. From our studies, it also appears that the effective doses needed to produce a biological response are quite low. We estimate that the administration of less than 1 µg of plasmid DNA results in the expression of 15 ng or more of recombinant protein. This is sufficient to produce a biological effect that lasts for at least 3 weeks and is equivalent to the administration of 1–10 µg of recombinant protein by topical or intradermal routes. There is no doubt that we have not yet perfected the methods in terms of efficiency.

The particle-mediated acceleration strategy offers therapeutic advantages to the clinician. The formulations we use – DNA coated onto gold particles – are remarkably stable. Their shelf life, in the laboratory at refrigerator temperatures, is at least 6 months. The delivery system is a surprisingly simple, mechanical device that requires little special training for its use. In the configuration we have employed, it is literally a revolver holding a 12-place cylinder. The delivery system is highly standardized. Another potential advantage of gene therapy as opposed to topical therapy is the ability to avoid issues of patient compliance and dosing variability. This form of treatment results in the expression of the therapeutic agent by the patient's own skin cells for a number of days. This could obviate a number of problems clinicians have, in an outpatient setting, in having patients apply medications to their own chronic wounds.

From an experimentalist's point of view, this system has remarkable advantages. First of all, we no longer need to deal with recombinant protein, but recombinant DNA. This means that manipulations of protein structure can be completed at the genetic level. It is remarkably easy to determine how minor modifications to the genetic structure of a cDNA will affect the biological outcome in an in vivo system.

It is also very straightforward to begin to build growth factor combinations, along the lines used with the bFGF constructs, either to facilitate diffusion of the molecules to their target sites, to protect them from degradation by proteinases, or even to incorporate into one, chimeric molecule more than one growth factor activity. Another distinct advantage of the particle-mediated bombardment technology is the ability to co-formulate several growth factor cDNAs into the same particle or to mix different populations of particles before loading them into the cartridge system. This enormous flexibility is going to allow us to explore much more rapidly the range and potential of applications of this novel DNA-mediated wound therapy.

In summary, particle-mediated bombardment is a simple, inexpensive and efficient method of introducing DNA into wound sites. Our studies have shown that we can efficiently express growth factors that have a positive impact on the rate of wound repair in normal, diabetic and aging animals. This technology is still evolving, but our early results suggest that gene therapy could develop into a genuine, practical method of drug delivery for an important clinical problem.

## References

1. Andree C, Swain WF, Page CP, Macklin MD, Slama J, Hatzis D, Eriksson E (1994) In vivo transfer and expression of a human epidermal growth factor gene accelerates wound repair. Proc Natl Acad Sci U S A 91:12188–12192
2. Badiavas E, Mehta PP, Falanga V (1996) Retrovirally mediated gene transfer in a skin equivalent model of chronic wounds. J Dermatol Sci 13:56–62
3. Benn SI, Whitsitt JS, Broadley KN, Nanney LB, Perkins D, He L, Patel M, Morgan JR, Swain WF, Davidson JM (1996) Particle-mediated gene transfer with transforming growth factor-beta1 cDNAs enhances wound repair in rat skin. J Clin Invest 98:2894–2902
4. Benn SI, Whitsitt JS, Davidson JM (1995) In vivo transfection of the rat with basic fibroblast growth factor fused to a secretory signal peptide is a potent inducer of angiogenesis. J Invest Dermatol 104:671
5. Bennett NT, Schultz GS (1993) Growth factors and wound healing: biochemical properties of growth factors and their receptors. Am J Surg 165:728–737
6. Bennett NT, Schultz GS (1993) Growth factors and wound healing: Part II. Role in normal and chronic wound healing. Am J Surg 166:74–81
7. Brown GL, Nanney LB, Griffen J, Cramer AB, Yancey JM, Curtsinger LJd, Holtzin L, Schultz GS, Jurkiewicz MJ, Lynch JB (1989) Enhancement of wound healing by topical treatment with epidermal growth factor (see comments). N Engl J Med 321:76–79
8. Carreau M, Quilliet X, Eveno E, Salvetti A, Danos O, Heard JM, Mezzina M, Sarasin A (1995) Functional retroviral vector for gene therapy of xeroderma pigmentosum group D patients. Hum Gene Ther 6:1307–1315
9. Cheng L, Ziegelhoffer PR, Yang N-S (1993) In vivo promoter activity and transgene expression in mammalian somatic tissues evaluated by using particle bombardment. Proc Natl Acad Sci U S A 90:4455–4459
10. Ciernik IF, Krayenbuhl BH, Carbone DP (1996) Puncture-mediated gene transfer to the skin. Hum Gene Ther 7:893–899
11. Davidson JM, Benn SI (1996) Regulation of angiogenesis and wound repair: interactive role of the matrix and growth factors. In: Sirica AE (ed) Cellular and molecular pathogenesis. Lippincott-Raven, New York, pp 79–107
12. Elder EM, Lotze MT, Whiteside TL (1996) Successful culture and selection of cytokine gene-modified human dermal fibroblasts for the biologic therapy of patients with cancer. Hum Gene Ther 7:479–487
13. Forough R, Xi Z, MacPhee M, Friedman S, Engleka KA, Sayers T, Wiltrout RH, Maciag T (1993) Differential transforming abilities of non-secreted and secreted forms of human fibroblast growth factor-1. J Biol Chem 268:2960–2968

14. Greenhalgh DG (1996) The role of growth factors in wound healing. J Trauma 41:159-167
15. Hengge UR, Walker PS, Vogel JC (1996) Expression of naked DNA in human, pig, and mouse skin. J Clin Invest 97:2911-2916
16. Knighton DR, Fiegel VD (1993) Growth factors and comprehensive surgical care of diabetic wounds. Curr Opin Gen Surg, pp 32-39
17. Krueger GG, Morgan JR, Jorgensen CM, Schmidt L, Li HL, Kwan MK, Boyce ST, Wiley HS, Kaplan J, Petersen MJ (1994) Genetically modified skin to treat disease: potential and limitations. J Invest Dermatol 103:76S-84S
18. Li L, Hoffman RM (1995) Model of selective gene therapy of hair growth: liposome targeting of the active Lac-Z gene to hair follicles of histocultured skin (letter). In Vitro Cell Dev Biol Anim 31:11-13
19. Lu B, Scott G, Goldsmith LA (1996) A model for keratinocyte gene therapy: preclinical and therapeutic considerations. Proc Assoc Am Physicians 108:165-172
20. Pierce GF, Tarpley JE, Allman RM, Goode PS, Serdar CM, Morris B, Mustoe TA, Vande Berg J (1994) Tissue repair processes in healing chronic pressure ulcers treated with recombinant platelet-derived growth factor BB. Am J Pathol 145:1399-1410
21. Rakhmilevich AL, Turner J, Ford MJ, McCabe D, Sun WH, Sondel PM, Grota K, Yang NS (1996) Gene gun-mediated skin transfection with interleukin 12 gene results in regression of established primary and metastatic murine tumors. Proc Natl Acad Sci U S A 93: 6291-6296
22. Rogelj S, Weinberg RA, Fanning P, Klagsbrun M (1988) Basic fibroblast growth factor fused to a signal peptide transforms cells. Nature 331:173-175
23. Rudkin GH, Miller TA (1996) Growth factors in surgery. Plast Reconstr Surg 97:469-476
24. Slama J, Andree C, Winkler T, Swain WF, Eriksson E (1995) Gene transfer. Ann Plast Surg 35:429-439
25. Steed D, Goslen B, Hambley R, Abell E, Hebda P, Webster M (1991) Clinical trials with purified platelet releasate, Prog Clin Biol Res 365:103-113
26. Sun L, Xu L, Chang H, Henry FA, Miller RM, Harmon JM, Nielsen TB (1997) Transfection with aFGF cDNA improves wound healing. J Invest Dermatol 108:313-318
27. Yang N-S, Burkholder J, Roberts B, Martinelli B, McCabe D (1990) In vivo and in vitro gene transfer to mammalian somatic cells by particle bombardment. Proc Natl Acad Sci U S A 87:9568-9572

# What's New in Human Wound-Healing Myofibroblasts?

V. Moulin, D. Garrel, F. A. Auger, M. O'Connor-McCourt,
G. Castilloux, L. Germain

## 1 Introduction

During wound healing and fibrocontractive diseases, clinical and experimental investigations have shown that fibroblastic cells acquire some morphological and biochemical features similar to those of smooth muscle cells [33]. These modified fibroblasts, called myofibroblasts, express de novo $\alpha$-SM actin temporarily during wound healing and permanently in fibrotic situations, such as hypertrophic scars or fibromatosis. Myofibroblasts are thought to be involved in contraction and have been observed in practically all fibrotic conditions involving retraction and re-organization of connective tissues [32].

Since their discovery 25 years ago by Gabbiani et al. [12], many studies have been performed on myofibroblasts, but some questions remain to be answered. Myofibroblasts that participate in wound repair are considered to be derived from local fibroblasts from surrounding dermal and subcutaneous tissues. The nature of the stimuli and the pathways of differentiation are still unknown, as well as factors regulating the disappearance of myofibroblasts at the end of normal wound healing. Furthermore, myofibroblast responses to cytokines or growth factors present in the wound are unknown. Another aspect of the healing process that is not understood is why, in contrast to the adult, fetal wounds heal without scarring [1]. Studies have shown that myofibroblasts are absent in fetal wounds [10]; however, a complete explanation for this empirical phenomenon is lacking.

## 2 Phenotypic Characteristics and Functional Properties of Human Wound-Healing Myofibroblasts

In order to understand the physiological events involved in wound healing, we have established human wound-healing myofibroblast (hWHM) cultures [16, 17] from

Current Topics in Pathology, Volume 93
A. Desmoulière, B. Tuchweber (Eds.)
© Springer-Verlag Berlin Heidelberg 1999

**Table 1.** Comparison of human dermal fibroblasts (hDF) cultured in fetal bovine serum (FBS), human wound-healing myofibroblasts (hWHM) and human dermal fibroblasts cultured in post-natal calf serum (PCS)

| Cell characteristics | hDF cultured in FBS | hWHM | hDF cultured in PCS |
|---|---|---|---|
| Diameter | + | +++ | ++ |
| Stress fibers | +/- | +++ | +++ |
| α-smooth muscle actin | + | +++ | +++ |
| Growth | +++ | + | ++ |
| Contractile capacity | + | +++ | ++ |
| Collagen synthesis | + | ++ | + |

+/-, slight; + to +++, low to significant increase.

experimental granulation tissues [9]. These cultures are stable for at least ten passages and never dedifferentiate to normal fibroblasts. They were compared with skin fibroblasts cultured from human dermis (Table 1) [30]. When cultured in monolayer, hWHM grew slowly, were large, star-shaped cells (Fig. 1A) and had cytoplasmic stress fibers (Fig. 2A), whereas fibroblasts had an elongated spindle shape with a small diameter (Fig. 1B) and a high growth rate [23]. All fibroblasts and hWHM contained vimentin. In contrast, α-smooth muscle (SM) actin, which was detected in 10% of dermal cells (Fig. 3A) [5], was present in 20%–80% of

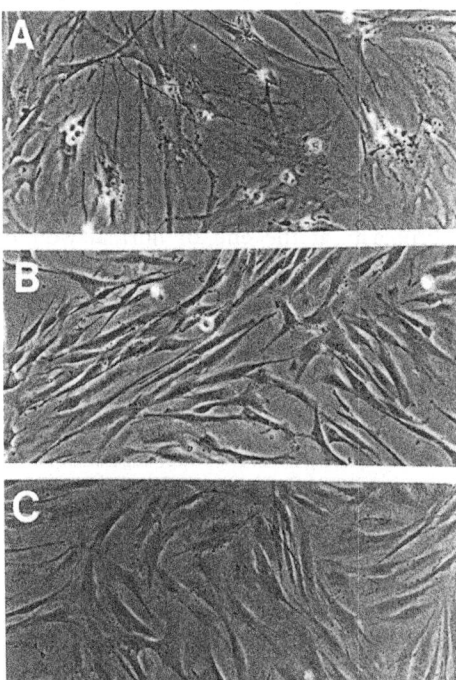

**Fig. 1A–C.** Morphological aspects of human wound-healing myofibroblasts (A) and normal human dermal fibroblasts cultured with fetal bovine serum (FBS) (B) or with post-natal calf serum (PCS) (C). Phase-contrast micrographs (bar: 80 μm)

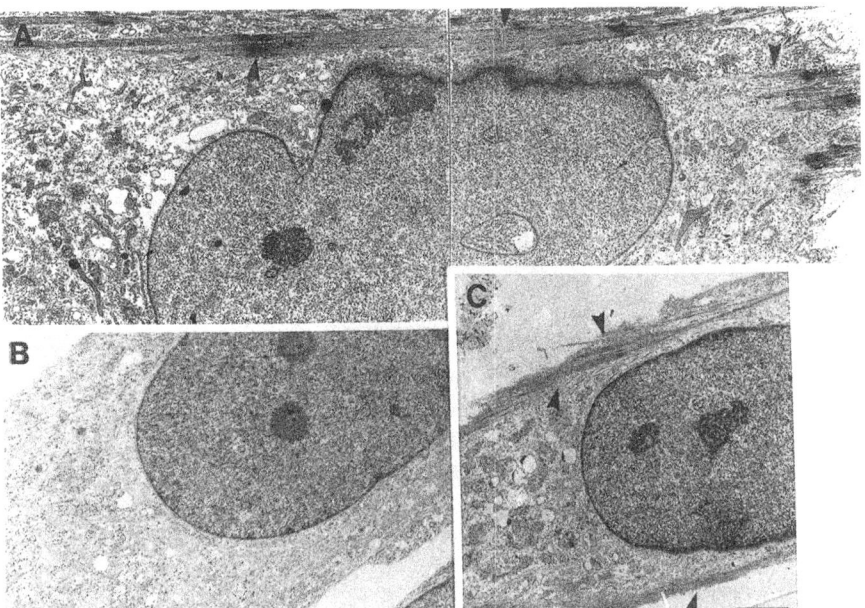

**Fig. 2 A–C.** Electron micrographs of wound-healing myofibroblasts (**A**) and of human dermal fibroblasts cultured in fetal bovine serum (FBS) (**B**) or cultured in post-natal calf serum (PCS) (**C**). *Arrowheads* show stress fibers, bar: 20 μm

hWHM cytoplasms (Fig. 3 D). The contractile property of the cells was evaluated using a three-dimensional tissue-engineered model [3, 30]. Our results show that, during the first few days, cells isolated from wound-healing tissues contracted the tissue-engineered equivalent more rapidly (reduction of 50%–75% of the initial surface area after 24 h) than dermal fibroblasts (reduction of 25% of the initial surface area after 24 h) (Fig. 4) [17]. The fact that a significant proportion of hWHM contains $\alpha$-SM actin suggests that the higher $\alpha$-SM-actin ratio may be responsible for the increased wound contraction. The assay of total and collagenous protein synthesis done by means of cell radiolabeling with [³H]-proline showed that hWHM produced significantly more proteins and collagen than fibroblasts. This correlates with the proposed role of these cells in the regeneration of the wound matrix.

## 3 Cytokine Effect on Fibroblasts and Human Wound-Healing Myofibroblasts

Many studies using normal dermal cells have been performed to understand the action of growth factors or other molecules on cell phenotype or function. Several growth factors have been shown to have an effect on $\alpha$-SM actin expression. Interferon $\gamma$ (IFN$\gamma$) decreases the amount of cytoplasmic $\alpha$-SM actin [5], whereas trans-

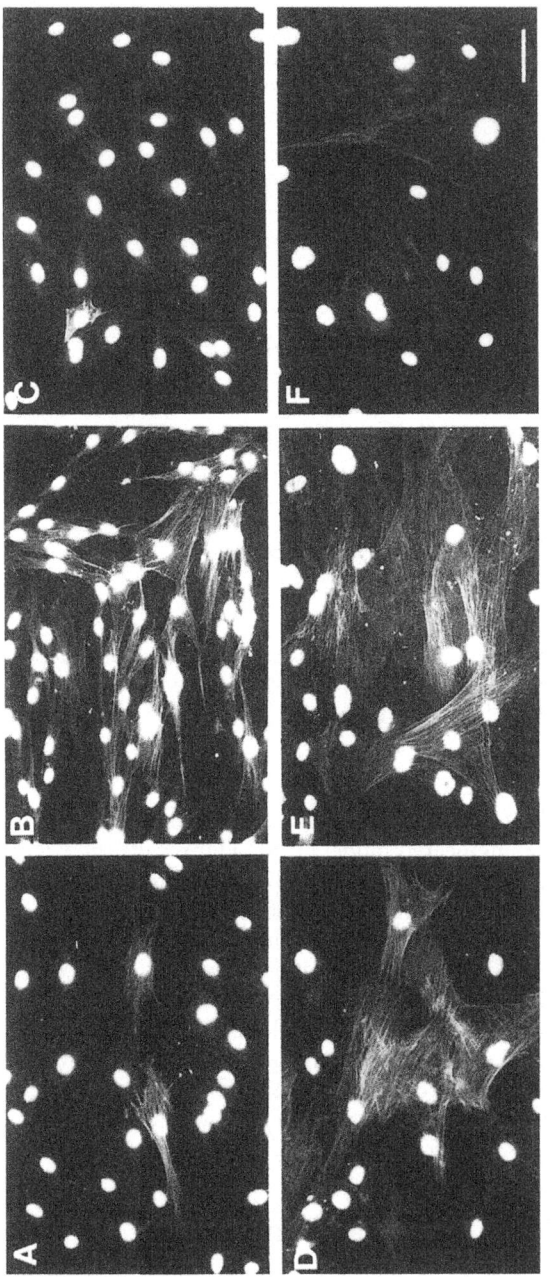

**Fig. 3 A – F.** Immunofluorescent staining of dermal fibroblasts (A, B, C) and wound-healing myofibroblasts (D, E, F) with anti-α-smooth muscle actin (α-SM actin) antibodies. Nucleus were stained using Hoechst dye. Cells were cultured for 7 days without treatment (A, D) or with transforming growth factor β1 (TGFβ1) (B, E) or interferon γ (IFNγ) (C, F) treatment. Bar: 40 μm. (From [25]; courtesy of Academic Press, Orlando, Fla.)

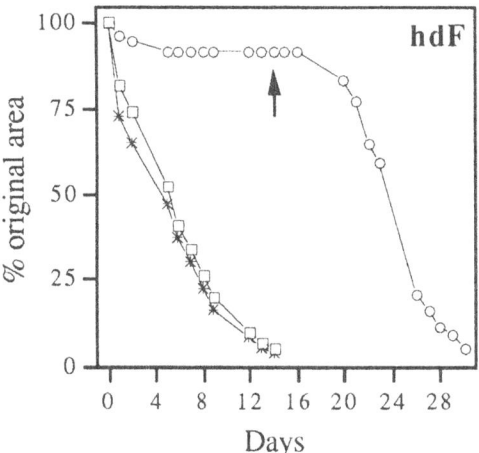

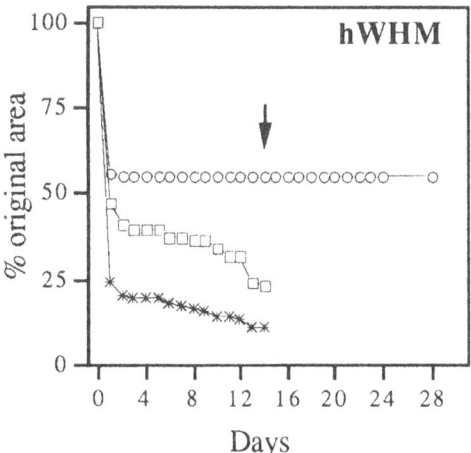

**Fig. 4.** Contraction of collagen gels by human dermal fibroblasts (*hdF*) or human wound-healing myofibroblasts (*hWHM*). Values are presented as the mean of three or more replicate gels ± SD. Absence of error bars signifies an error which was too small to illustrate. (-□-) untreated cells, (-*-) transforming growth factor $\beta 1$ (TGF$\beta 1$) treated cells, (-○-) interferon $\gamma$ (IFN$\gamma$) treated cells. *Arrows* indicate the day when IFN$\gamma$ treatment was stopped. (From [25]; courtesy of Academic Press, Orlando, Fla.)

forming growth factor $\beta 1$ (TGF$\beta 1$) seems to be the most important growth factor enhancing $\alpha$-SM-actin content in human dermal fibroblasts [7]. Other growth factors, such as platelet-derived growth factor (PDGF) or tumor necrosis factor $\alpha$ (TNF$\alpha$) have no activity upon differentiation of fibroblasts into myofibroblasts [6]. Studies of growth factor action on normal dermal fibroblast-populated collagen gels have shown that IFN$\gamma$ or interleukin-1 (IL-1) inhibit gel contraction, whereas TGF$\beta 1$ or PDGF enhance the contraction rate [29, 35]. Thus, several products present in the microenvironment of wounds are able to influence positively or negatively the expression of myofibroblastic features, and probably enhance or interfere with the evolution of wound healing. As myofibroblasts are derived from normal fibroblasts [5], their response to cytokines is assumed to be similar. The few studies that have reported the response of myofibroblasts to cytokines or growth factors have been performed using pathological myofibroblasts from Dupuytren's

**Table 2.** Summary of the effects of cytokines on human dermal fibroblasts (hDF) and human wound-healing myofibroblasts (hWHM)

| Cell characteristics | TGFβ1 effect (1 ng/ml) | | IFNγ effect (1000 U/ml) | |
|---|---|---|---|---|
| | hDF | hWHM | hDF | hWHM |
| Diameter | 0 | 0 | 0 | 0 |
| Morphology | 0 | 0 | 0 | 0 |
| Stress fibers | ++ | 0 | 0 | 0 |
| α-SM actin | +++ | + | ––– | – |
| Growth | + | 0 | – | 0 |
| Contractile capacity | + | ++ | – | –– |
| Reversibility of contractile capacity | n.d. | n.d. | +++ | +/– |
| Collagen synthesis | + | ++ | – | –– |
| Collagenase synthesis | 0 | 0 | 0 | 0 |

*TGF*, transforming growth factor; *IFN*, interferon; *SM*, smooth muscle.
0, similar; +/–, slight; + to +++, low to significant increase; – to –––, low to significant decrease; n.d., not determined.

disease, scleroderma or hypertrophic scars [14, 18]. However, since myofibroblasts from various origins differ in their phenotypic features [8] and growth rates [11], it is important to evaluate whether the cytokine response of hWHMs is distinct from that of fibroblasts and pathological myofibroblasts.

Accordingly, we compared hWHMs with fibroblasts from human dermal skin to determine whether they have the same response to cytokines (Table 2) [25]. Two cytokines, TGFβ1 (1 ng/ml) and IFNγ (1000 U/ml) were chosen because of their known effect on normal fibroblast α-SM actin content. In vitro, hWHMs and fibroblasts treated for 7 days with TGFβ1 or IFNγ did not show any change of their morphology or diameter. Following TGFβ1 treatment, the percentage of α-SM actin-positive cells increased in both fibroblastic cell types (Fig. 3B, E). However, TGFβ1 induced a greater increase (approximately sixfold) in the percentage of α-SM actin-positive cells in dermal fibroblasts than in hWHMs (1.1- to 2.5-fold). In the case of IFNγ treatment, the percentage of α-SM actin-positive cells decreased in both populations (Figs. 3C and 2F), but the decrease was greater for fibroblastic cells than hWHMs. In the same way, TGFβ1 and INFγ, significantly affected the growth rate of dermal fibroblasts (an increase and decrease, respectively), whereas the growth rate of hWHM was not significantly changed.

The presence of cytoplasmic microfilament bundles (stress fibers), the characteristic ultrastructural feature of myofibroblasts in situ, [33] was consistently observed in every hWHM strain (Fig. 2A). The hWHM cultures that were treated with TGFβ1 or IFNγ for 7 days did not show any ultrastructural modifications. In contrast, stress fibers were rare and small in cultured dermal fibroblasts (Fig. 2B). The number and organization of these stress fibers in the dermal fibroblasts were greatly increased in most of the cells following TGFβ1 treatment compared with untreated cells or cells treated with IFNγ.

Compared with dermal fibroblasts, hWHMs have a greater ability to contract collagen gels [17]. When cells were treated for 7 days with TGFβ1 before their inclusion in gels, an increase in contraction was observed during the first few days for both dermal fibroblasts and hWHMs. This augmentation was greater for hWHM strains than for fibroblasts (Fig. 4). Later on, the contraction rate was similar to that of untreated cells even though the TGF$\beta$1 treatment was continued. Treatment with IFN$\gamma$ reduced the contraction rate during the first day and, then, interrupted completely gel contraction in both fibroblasts and hWHMs. The reversibility of the inhibition induced by IFN$\gamma$ was evaluated by removing it from the culture medium after 14 days. For fibroblasts, contraction resumed after a 2-day lag period and, 2 weeks later, the extent of contraction was similar to that of untreated controls. By contrast, in hWHM-populated collagen gels, contraction resumed weakly or not at all when IFN$\gamma$ was removed. Similarly, TGF$\beta$1 treatment induced an increase and IFN$\gamma$ a decrease in collagen synthesis for both fibroblasts and hWHMs. However, the effect was less on dermal fibroblasts.

TGF$\beta$1 and IFN$\gamma$ do not greatly affect hWHM growth rate and morphology, compared with dermal fibroblasts. In contrast, cytokine treatment induced significant changes, sometimes irreversible, in the functional properties of hWHMs, such as collagen contraction and synthesis, whereas those of fibroblasts were only slightly changed [7, 25, 29]. Thus, we may conclude that the cytokine response of hWHMs is different from that of dermal fibroblasts and pathological myofibroblasts, since previous studies have shown less of an increase in collagen-gel contraction by hypertrophic scar myofibroblasts than with fibroblasts after TGF$\beta$1 treatment [15]. Also, myofibroblasts isolated from Dupuytren's nodules or hypertrophic scars had their growth rate greatly affected by IFN$\gamma$ [5, 19]. Together, these results indicate that hWHMs, dermal fibroblasts and myofibroblasts cultured from pathological tissues respond differently to TGF$\beta$1 and IFN$\gamma$.

Several lines of evidence suggest that TGF$\beta$1 is involved in the differentiation of fibroblasts into myofibroblasts [7, 25, 31, 34]. However, some properties of hWHMs observed in vitro do not seem to be induced by TGF$\beta$1: (1) their wide cell diameter, (2) their slow proliferation, and (3) their functional properties, such as collagen contraction and protein synthesis. Thus, our results suggest, as previously raised by DESMOULIÈRES ET AL. [7], that TGF$\beta$1 is insufficient to fully induce the myofibroblast phenotype.

## 4 Serum Effect on Fibroblasts

In contrast with the adult, the fetus has the remarkable ability to regenerate normal skin architecture without scarring after injury [1, 10, 22]. Numerous studies have been designed to determine which intrinsic properties of fetal cells or which fetal environmental factors are implicated in this remarkable phenomenon [2, 4, 20, 21, 26, 28]. It has been observed that myofibroblasts are present in adult wounds and absent from fetal healing tissues [10] and authors have suggested that amniotic fluid or intrinsic cell properties may be involved in the regeneration process leading to the absence of scarring. However, the exact mechanisms implicated in the control of cell growth, development and wound healing that result in scar-free tissue in the fetus remain unclear.

Since granulation tissue is highly vascularized, wound cells are exposed to multiple factors brought in situ by blood or by the surrounding cells. Serum carries several growth factors that enhance cell proliferation, migration and/or differentiation at wound sites. Consequently, we assessed the effects of fetal bovine serum (FBS) versus postnatal calf serum (PCS) on the behavior of normal dermal fibroblasts cultured in vitro (Table 1) [24]. Human dermal fibroblasts cultured with 10% FBS showed typical elongated spindle-shape morphology (Fig. 1 B). When cultured in 10% PCS, their morphological aspects changed with the appearance of large star-shaped cells exhibiting a high cytoplasmic to nuclear ratio under phase-contrast microscopy (Fig. 1 C) typical of hWHM morphology (Fig. 1 A). After treatment with PCS, electron microscopy showed the presence of cytoskeletal features that are characteristic of myofibroblasts, such as numerous cytoplasmic longitudinal bundles of microfilaments (stress fibers) arranged in a direction parallel to the long axis of the cells. Other features characteristic of myofibroblasts are a lower growth rate than normal fibroblasts and a high quantity of cytoplasmic $\alpha$-SM actin (Table 3). According to these two parameters, treatment of normal fibroblasts with PCS induced a change in the direction of cell differentiation into myofibroblasts [13, 14].

Functional aspects of fibroblasts cultured with PCS versus FBS were also studied. Contractile properties or protein synthesis and collagenase activity were chosen since a high capacity to contract a collagen gel and to synthesize proteins are other hallmarks of myofibroblasts. We demonstrated that fibroblasts cultured with PCS had a greater ability to contract gels than fibroblasts cultured with FBS. However, the collagen synthesis was not modulated by PCS, whereas the activity of some secreted gelatinases was decreased (Table 1). These data are consistent with in vivo observations that associate scarless fetal tissue repair with the fetal ability to efficiently organize collagen fibrils into a natural network rather than with a lack of collagen deposition [22].

Since TGF$\beta$ stimulates $\alpha$-SM actin expression in cultured fibroblastic cells [7, 25], TGF$\beta$ content in both sera was determined. Results from a radioreceptor and a biological assay showed that TGF$\beta$ was present in both sera at expected levels and that the majority of the TGF$\beta$ was in a latent form in both sera [27]. The data obtained using neutralizing antibodies against TGF$\beta$1 showed that active TGF$\beta$ is present when cells are cultured with medium containing PCS since the addition of anti-TGF$\beta$ antibodies to this medium can partially inhibit the $\alpha$-SM-actin increase

**Table 3.** Effect of sera and neutralizing antibodies to TGF$\beta$ on the proportion of fibroblasts expressing $\alpha$-smooth muscle actin ($\alpha$-SM actin). Cells were cultured in the presence of 10% post-natal calf serum (PCS) or fetal bovine serum (FBS) and/or neutralizing anti-transforming growth factor $\beta$ (TGF$\beta$) antibodies (Ab) (1/200) (mean of triplicates ± SD)

|  | $\alpha$-SM actin positive cells (%) | Student $t$ test |
| --- | --- | --- |
| hDF cultured in FBS | 11.11 ± 5.49 | – |
| hDF cultured in PCS | 43.36 ± 15.46 | $p < 0.05$ vs FBS |
| hDF cultured in PCS + anti-TGF$\beta$ | 26.67 ± 8.88 | $p < 0.05$ vs FBS; vs PCS |

hDF, human dermal fibroblast.

(Table 3). Thus, taken together, this indicates that the human dermal fibroblasts must activate or produce active TGF$\beta$ when they are cultured in medium containing PCS, but not in medium containing FBS. Selective activation could be attributed to the production of a specific TGF$\beta$-activating enzyme when cells are cultured in medium containing PCS. Alternatively, it could be due to the presence of a form of latent TGF$\beta$ in FBS that differs from that in PCS, the cellular enzymes being able to activate only the form in PCS. Thus, we conclude that TGF$\beta$1 is involved in human dermal fibroblast differentiation.

## 5 Conclusion

Knowledge of the molecular and cellular biology of human myofibroblasts is essential if we are to learn how to modulate the fundamental processes of wound healing, fibrosis and desmoplasia. Our results show that, in vitro, different factors such as TGF$\beta$1, IFN$\gamma$ and serum proteins induced changes in the differentiation status of fibroblasts. However, purified cytokines are not sufficient to induce stable and complete transformations and molecules allowing complete differentiation have not been found yet. Our data suggest that fibroblastic cells have a modulated response to cytokines according to their stage of differentiation and that hWHMs cannot be considered as pathological myofibroblasts with respect to their responses to cytokines. In the same way, our studies showed that serum components that affect fibroblast differentiation vary as a function of developmental stages.

Overall, these observations suggest that WHMs have to be studied as unique cells and not as normal fibroblasts. Their responses can be potently modulated by cytokines and this has critical consequences in the success of tissue repair.

**Acknowledgements.** The authors are grateful to Drs Georges Hébert, Normand Houle, Andréa Jean, Carlos López Valle, Martine Michel, Caroline Richard, Alphonse Roy, Félix André Têtu for their contributions to the work presented in this review, and Claude Marin for photographic assistance. This is NRCC publication number 41443. This study was supported by *Hydro-Québec, Fondation des Pompiers de Québec pour les Grands Brûlés, Fondation de l'Hôpital du Saint-Sacrement, Réseau des Grands Brûlés FRSQ-FPQGB* and a France–Quebec exchange Program in Biotechnology. L.G. and F.A.A. were recipients of scholarships from the *Fonds de la Recherche en Santé du Québec*.

## References

1. Adzick NS, Lorenz HP (1994) Cells, matrix, growth factors, and the surgeon: the biology of scarless fetal wound repair. Ann Surg 220:10–18
2. Alaish SM, Yager D, Diegelmann RF, Cohen IK (1994) Biology of fetal wound healing: hyaluronate receptor expression in fetal fibroblasts. J Pediatr Surg 29:1040–1043
3. Bell E, Ehrlich P, Sher S, Merrill C, Sarber R, Hull B, Nakatsuji T, Church D, Buttle DJ (1981) Development and use of a living skin equivalent. Plast Reconstr Surg 67:386–392
4. Bleacher JC, Adolph VR, Dillon PW, Krummel TM (1993) Fetal tissue repair and wound healing. Dermatol Clin 11:677–683

5. Desmoulière A, Rubbia-Brandt L, Abdiu A, Walz T, Macieira-Coelho A, Gabbiani G (1992) α-Smooth muscle actin is expressed in a subpopulation of cultured and cloned fibroblasts and is modulated by γ-interferon. Exp Cell Res 201:64–73

6. Desmoulière A, Rubbia-Brandt L, Grau G, Gabbiani G (1992) Heparin induces a-SM actin expression in cultured fibroblasts and in granulation tissue myofibroblasts. Lab Invest 67:716–726

7. Desmoulière A, Geinoz A, Gabbiani F, Gabbiani G (1993) Transforming growth factor-β1 induces α-smooth muscle actin expression in granulation tissue myofibroblasts and in quiescent and growing cultured fibroblasts. J Cell Biol 122:103–111

8. Desmoulière A, Gabbiani G (1994) Modulation of fibroblastic cytoskeletal features during pathological situations: the role of extracellular matrix and cytokines. Cell Motil Cytoskel 29:195–203

9. Diegelmann RF, Lindblad WJ, Cohen IK (1986) A subcutaneous implant for wound healing studies in humans. J Surg Res 40:229–235

10. Estes JM, Vande Berg JS, Adzick NS, MacGillivray TE, Desmoulière A, Gabbiani G (1994) Phenotypic and functional features of myofibroblasts in sheep fetal wound. Differentiation 56:173–181

11. Foo ITH, Naylor IL, Timmons MJ, Trejdosiewicz LK (1992) Intracellular actin as a marker for myofibroblasts in vitro. Lab Invest 67:727–733

12. Gabbiani G, Hirschel BJ, Ryan GB, Statkov PR, Majno G (1972) Granulation tissue as a contractile organ. A study of structure and function. J Exp Med 135:719–734

13. Gabbiani G, Chaponneier C, Huttner I (1978) Cytoplasmic filaments and gap junctions in epithelial cells and myofibroblasts during wound healing. J Cell Biol 76:561–568

14. Garner WL, Karmiol S, Rodriguez JL, Smith, DJ, Phan SH (1993) Phenotypic differences in cytokine responsiveness of hypertrophic scar versus normal dermal fibroblasts. J Invest Dermatol 101:875–879

15. Garner WL, Rittenberg T, Ehrlich HP, Karmiol S, Rodriguez JL, Smith DJ, Phan SH (1995) Hypertrophic scar fibroblasts accelerate collagen gel contraction. Wound Rep Regen 3:185–191

16. Garrel DR, Gaudreau P, Zhang L, Reeves I, Brazeau P (1991) Chronic administration of growth hormo-releasing factor increases wound strength and collagen maturation in granulation tissue. J Surg Res 51:297–302

17. Germain L, Jean A, Auger FA, Garrel DR (1994) Human wound healing fibroblasts have greater contractile properties than dermal fibroblasts. J Surg Res 57:268–273

18. Gillery P, Serpier H, Polette M, Bellon G, Clavel C, Wegroski Y, Birembaut P, Kalis B, Cariou R, Maquart F-X (1992) Gamma-interferon inhibits extracellular matrix synthesis and remodeling in collagen lattice cultures of normal and scleroderma skin fibroblasts. Eur J Cell Biol 57:2444–2253

19. Harrop AR, Gharary A, Scott PG, Forsyth N, Uji-Friedland A, Tredget EE (1995) Regulation of collagen synthesis and mRNA expression on normal and hypertrophic scar fibroblasts in vitro by interferon γ. J Surg Res 58:471–477

20. Krummel TM, Nelson J, Diegelmann R (1987) Fetal response to injury in the rabbit. J Pediatr Surg 33:601–644

21. Lin RY, Sullivan KM, Argenta PA, Lorenz HP, Adzick NS (1994) Scarless human fetal skin repair is intrinsic to the fetal fibroblast and occurs in the absence of an inflammatory response: in situ hybridization and immunochemical studies. Wound Rep Regen 2:297–305

22. Mast BA, Nelson JM, Krummel TM (1992) Tissue repair in the mammalian fetus. In: Cohen IK, Diegelmann RF, Lindblad WJ (eds) Wound healing: biochemical and clinical aspects. Saunders, Philadelphia, pp 326–343

23. Moulin V, Castilloux G, Jean A, Garrel DR, Auger FA, Germain L (1996) In vitro models to study wound healing fibroblasts. Burns 22:359–362

24. Moulin V, Auger FA, O'Connor-McCourt M, Germain L (1997) Fetal and postnatal differentially modulate human dermal fibroblast phenotypic and functional features in vitro. J Cell Physiol 171:1–10

25. Moulin V, Castilloux G, Auger FA, Garrel D, O'Connor-McCourt M, Germain L (1997) Modulated response to cytokines of human wound healing myofibroblasts compared to dermal fibroblasts Exp Cell Res 238:283–293

26. Nath RK, LaRegina M, Markham H, Ksander GA, Weeks PM (1994) The expression of TGF type beta in fetal and adult rabbit skin wounds. J Pediatr Surg 29:416–421

27. O'Connor-McCourt MD, Wakefield LM (1987) Latent transforming growth factor beta in serum: a specific complex with $\alpha$2-macroglobulin. J Biol Chem 262:14090–14099

28. Piscatelli SJ, Michaels BM, Gregory P, Jennings RW, Longaker MT, Harrison MR, Siebert JW (1994) Fetal fibroblast contraction of collagen matrices in vitro: the effects of EGF and TGF$\beta$. Ann Plast Surg 33:38–45

29. Reed MJ, Vernon RB, Abrass IB, Sage EH (1994) TGF$\beta$1 induces the expression of type 1 collagen and SPARC, and enhances contraction of collagen gels, by fibroblasts from young and aged donors. J Cell Physiol 158:169–179

30. Rompré P, Auger FA, Germain L, Bouvard V, Lopez Vallé CA, Thibault J, Le Duy A (1990) Influence of initial collagen and cellular concentrations on the final surface area of dermal and skin equivalents: a Box-Behnken analysis. In Vitro Cell Dev Biol 26:983–990

31. Ronnov-Jessen L, Petersen OW (1993) Induction of $\alpha$-smooth muscle actin by transforming growth factor $\beta$1 in quiescent human breast gland fibroblasts. Lab Invest 68:696–707

32. Rudolph R, Vande Berg J, Ehrlich PH (1992) Wound contraction and scar contracture. In: IK Cohen, RF Diegelmann, WJ Lindblad (eds) Wound healing: biochemical and clinical aspects 6. Saunders, Philadelphia, pp 96–114

33. Schürch W, Seemayer TA, Gabbiani G (1992) Myofibroblast. In: SS Sternberg (ed) Histology for pathologists 5. Raven, New York, pp 109–144

34. Shah M, Foreman D, Ferguson MWJ (1994) Neutralising antibody to TGF-$\beta$1,2 reduces cutaneous scarring in adult rodents. J Cell Sci 107:1137–1157

35. Tingström A, Heldin C-H, Rubin K (1992) Regulation of fibroblast-mediated collagen gel contraction by PDGF, IL1 and TGF$\beta$1. J Cell Sci 102:315–322

# The Myofibroblast in Neoplasia

W. Schürch

## 1 Discovery of the Myofibroblast

Since its discovery in granulation tissue of healing wounds, now over a quarter of a century ago [22], the myofibroblast has been described in: (1) normal tissue; (2) diverse responses to injury and repair phenomena; (3) quasi-neoplastic proliferative conditions; (4) the stromal response to certain forms of neoplasia; and (5) benign and malignant neoplasms (for review [49]). In practical terms, the surgical pathologist is a daily witness to this panoply of myofibroblastic proliferation. An appropriate evaluation of the myofibroblast with regard to neoplasia is impossible without identifying briefly where these cells occur, and without defining this unique cell.

## 2 Settings in which Myofibroblasts Occur

The first group of settings in which myofibroblasts occur relates to stromal cells with myoid features, present in many normal tissues. On the basis of putative ultrastructural and/or immunohistochemical evidence of smooth muscle differentiation, some of these stromal cells have been identified as myofibroblasts [14, 42]. Such stromal cells have been described in the intestinal mucosa, pulmonary alveolar septa, umbilical cord, lymph nodes, liver, spleen, bone marrow and glomerular mesangium, to cite principal locations.

The second group involves granulation tissue and diverse tissue responses, such as burn contractures, pulmonary sarcoidosis, interstitial lung fibrosis, localized and systemic scleroderma, atherosclerotic plaques, liver cirrhosis, sinus tracts and ischemic ulcer beds to cite but a few (for review [42, 48]).

The third group embodies the fibromatoses (superficial and deep musculoaponeurotic variants) and other soft tissue proliferations mimicking sarcomas, such as

Current Topics in Pathology, Volume 93
A. Desmoulière, B. Tuchweber (Eds.)
© Springer-Verlag Berlin Heidelberg 1999

nodular and proliferative fasciitis, proliferative myositis, cutaneous fibrous histiocytoma (dermatofibroma), elastofibroma and others, also defined as quasi-neoplastic proliferations [45].

The fourth group addresses the stromal response to neoplasia. Many invasive and
metastatic carcinomas, especially those characterized by hard consistency, retraction and fixation to adjacent tissues, elicit a desmoplastic stromal reaction that is
rich in myofibroblasts [47, 50]. Myofibroblasts have also been described in certain
sarcomas, where they generally constitute a small fraction of the cell population.
Myofibroblasts are regularly identified in sarcomas that are characterized by
stromal sclerosis [29]. Myofibroblasts are also consistently identified at the nodule-
stromal interphase in nodular sclerosing Hodgkin's disease [44].

Finally, the fifth group, deals with numerous benign and malignant neoplasms
of myofibroblasts – named myofibroblastomas and myofibrosarcomas, respectively – and with tumors of like substance, under an assortment of designations
(for review [49]).

## 3 Definition of the Myofibroblast

A precise definition of the myofibroblast is an issue of major importance for the daily practice of the surgical pathologist, since certain myofibroblastic soft-tissue proliferations might mimic sarcomas and vice versa. The myofibroblast is defin-
able essentially by ultrastructure as a highly differentiated cell with specialized
organelles, having features in common with smooth muscle cells and fibroblasts,
i.e., bundles of microfilaments with dense bodies running parallel to the long axis
through the cytoplasm (stress fibers), well-developed rough endoplasmic reticulum
and Golgi apparatus, notched nucleus, pinocytotic vesicles, partial investment by
external lamina (basal lamina), plasmalemmal attachment plaques, well-developed
fibronexuses (microtendons) and intercellular intermediate and gap junctions.
Myofibroblasts are generally also surrounded by relatively important amounts of
extracellular matrix. The three essential morphological elements which define
a myofibroblast are: stress fibers, i.e., bundles of actin micro(myo)filaments
with interspersed dense bodies running parallel to the long axis of the cell, usually
located beneath the cell membrane, well-developed cell-to-stroma attachment
sites (fibronexuses), and intercellular intermediate and gap junctions (Fig. 1 a–d).
The differences between smooth muscle cells and myofibroblasts may be subtle.
Smooth muscle cells generally lack typical isolated stress fibers since their cytoplasm is filled with bundles and aggregates of microfilaments and associated dense
bodies, but they are connected by intermediate and gap junctions and may also
develop attenuated fibronexuses [27]. The distinction between smooth muscle cells
is often made with difficulty. Nonetheless, the myofibroblast is defined by ultrastructure.

Myofibroblasts, smooth muscle cells and stromal cells with myoid features disclose heterogeneous cytoskeletal phenotypes with regard to intermediate filament,
actin isoform and smooth-muscle-myosin heavy-chain expression [48]. Thus, to
categorize a cell as a myofibroblast by immunohistochemical staining, pattern
alone is doubtful, given the cytoskeletal heterogeneity of such cells. Myofibro-

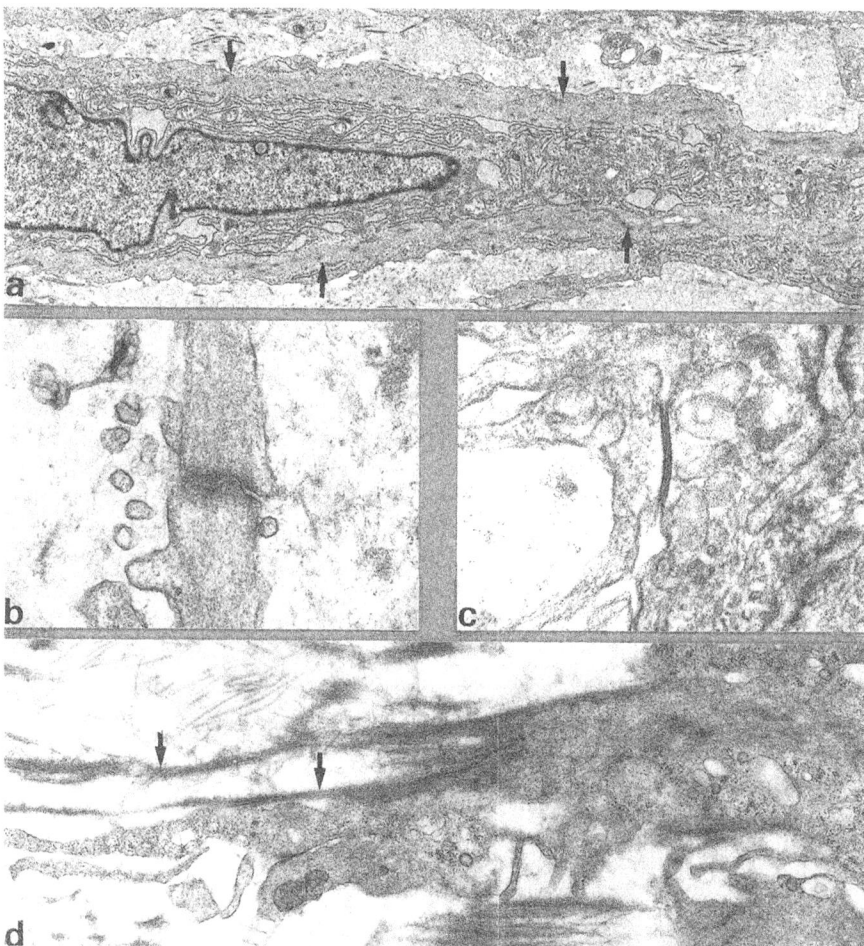

Fig. 1a–d. Ultrastructural characterization of the myofibroblast. a Typical myofibroblast from Dupuytren's disease with notched nucleus, well-developed rough endoplasmic reticulum and two stress fibers (*arrows*) running through the entire length of the subplasmalemmal cytoplasm. b Intermediate junction between two myofibroblasts from deep musculoaponeurotic fibromatosis. c Gap junction between two myofibroblasts from nodular fasciitis. d Well-developed fibronexus (cell-to-stroma attachment site) of myofibroblast from human granulation tissue. Uranyl acetate and lead citrate: a × 8000; b × 37,500; c × 90,000; d × 15,700

blastic phenotypes include: phenotype V, represented by cells expressing vimentin; phenotype VA, represented by cells positive for vimentin and $\alpha$-smooth muscle actin; phenotype VAD, represented by cells expressing vimentin, $\alpha$-smooth muscle actin and desmin; phenotype VD, represented by cells positive for vimentin and desmin; and phenotype VA(D)M, represented by cells reactive for vimentin, $\alpha$-smooth muscle actin and smooth-muscle-myosin heavy chains with and without desmin. Phenotypes V, VA, VAD, VD and VA(D)M also express cytoplasmic actin isoforms ($\beta$ and $\gamma$) [49].

Most vascular smooth muscle cells contain vimentin as there sole detectable intermediate filament, and a smaller proportion also express desmin [16, 23, 36, 40, 55]. In contrast, parenchymal smooth muscle cells of the respiratory, gastrointestinal and genitourinary tracts represent a homogeneous cell population in which desmin tends to be the exclusive intermediate filament [17, 31, 41]. With regard to muscle actin expression, vascular smooth muscle cells are characterized by a predominance of the $\alpha$-smooth muscle actin isoform. In contrast, parenchymal smooth muscle cells contain large amounts of the $\gamma$-smooth muscle actin isoform [48].

Stromal cells with myoid features occurring in normal tissues also disclose heterogeneous cytoskeletal phenotypes, the most frequent being VD and VA(D)M followed by VA and VAD phenotypes [11]. This cytoskeletal heterogeneity among these stromal cells could reflect different functional needs, since all of these stromal cells seem to participate in visceral contraction or extracellular matrix remodeling [39]. Another interpretation, recently advanced, proposes that most examples of spindle cells in normal tissues, cited in the literature as being myofibroblasts, might be closer to pericytes or smooth muscle cells [14], or simply represent stromal cells with myoid features of variable degree, according to a functional demand. In addition, stromal cells with myoid features do not exhibit the essential ultrastructural features of myofibroblasts. That said, myofibroblasts, as defined by the essential ultrastructural criteria indicated above, are not observed in normal tissue and, therefore, might not exist within the first group. There is, however, no doubt that myofibroblasts, as defined, are also observed in granulating healing wounds and in other tissue responses belonging to the second group.

## 4 Quasi-Neoplastic Proliferations

The superficial and deep musculoaponeurotic fibromatoses, nodular and proliferative fasciitis, proliferative myositis, cutaneous fibrous histiocytoma (dermatofibroma), elastofibroma, plasma cell granuloma of the lung, digital fibroma of infancy, and juvenile nasopharyngeal angiofibroma belong to the third group. In these conditions, the proliferating cells disclose heterogeneous cytoskeletal phenotypes which, in decreasing order, follow the VA, the VAD, the VD, and the VA(D)M types. All these conditions are replete with myofibroblasts, disclosing the typical and essential ultrastructural traits, including stress fibers, intercellular intermediate and gap junctions as well as fibronexuses [48]. Proper recognition of these quasi-neoplastic proliferations is of prime importance, since some may mimic sarcomas and vice versa.

## 5 Stromal Response to Neoplasia

Many invasive and metastatic carcinomas are characterized by wooden hard consistency, retraction and fixation to adjacent tissues. Typical examples are invasive breast carcinomas associated with skin dimpling and/or nipple retraction, annular stenosing colon carcinomas, gastric linitis plastica, the "frozen pelvis"

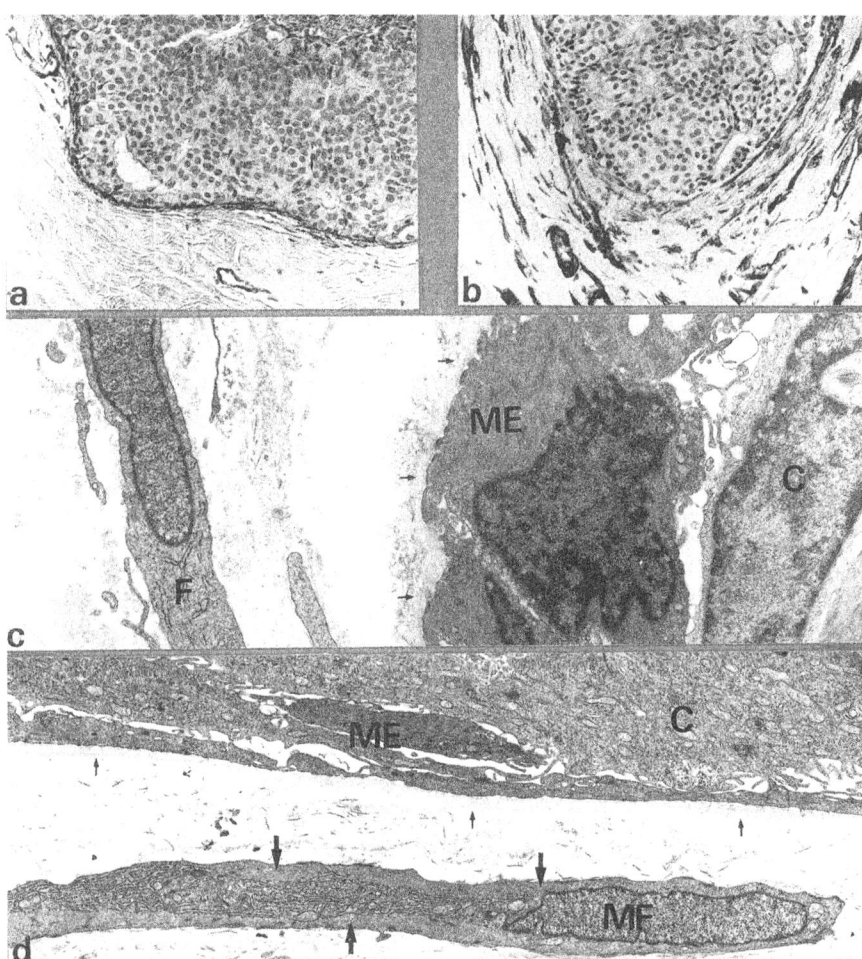

Fig. 2a–d. Ductal in-situ breast carcinoma. (same case). **a, b** Light-microscopic aspects of different areas from the same in-situ carcinoma, revealing continuous layer of α-smooth-muscle-actin-positive myoepithelial cells at the periphery of the carcinomatous duct without α-smooth-muscle-actin-positive stromal cells, except for vascular smooth muscle cells (**a**) and discontinuous myoepithelial cell layer as revealed by α-smooth-muscle-actin-reactive myo-epithelial cells, as well as numerous α-smooth muscle actin-positive stromal cells within periductal tissue (**b**). **c** Ultrastructural aspect of in situ ductal carcinoma with myopepithelial cells at the periphery of the duct (*ME*), filled with carcinoma cells (*C*), continuous basal lamina (*arrows*), and smooth contoured fibroblast (*F*) within periductal stroma. **d** Ductal in-situ carci-noma with continuous layer of myoepithelial cells (*ME*), filled with carcinoma cells (*C*) and developing myofibroblast (*MF*) with stress fibers in formation (*arrows*) in subplasmalemmal cytoplasm within periductal stroma. Avidin-biotin-complex-peroxidase staining for α-smooth muscle actin: **a** × 300; **b** × 300. Uranyl acetate and lead citrate: **c** × 10,0000; **d** × 8,250

accompanying advanced gynecological carcinomas, crateriform pleural retraction associated with pulmonary carcinomas, and metastatic carcinomas to lymph nodes that are fixed to surrounding tissues and overlaying skin. Myofibroblasts are absent or equivocally present in carcinomas lacking significant stromal desmoplasia, e. g., small cell undifferentiated carcinomas of the lung [48]. All these retraction phenomena have been attributed to the contractile forces generated by stromal myofibroblasts [46, 50, 54]. Well-developed myofibroblasts are only rarely observed within the stroma that, according to ultrastructure, is contiguous with in-situ breast carcinomas (Fig. 2a–d); this would suggest that invasion beyond the basal lamina is required to evoke a myofibroblastic stromal reaction. However, stromal cells expressing α-smooth muscle actin are observed around in situ ductal breast carcinomas (personal observation, Fig. 2b) and have been described in squamous intra-epithelial lesions of the uterine cervix, close to the basal lamina, in increasing numbers and intensity of staining – using immunohistochemical techniques – from low-grade to high-grade variants [9]. Thus, it is very likely that the initiation of the myofibroblastic stromal reaction around sites of high-grade dysplasia and in situ carcinomas might begin before stromal invasion is observed – quite likely mediated by cytokines [48, 49]. The epithelial stromal interactions in incipient carcinomas are complex and currently under investigation.

Myofibroblasts are not uniformly distributed within the stroma of invasive carcinomas. In breast carcinomas, for instance, they tend to be most numerous and best-developed within the young mesenchymal stroma, areas corresponding to early stromal invasion or, more consistently, within the peripheral invasive cellular front of such neoplasms (Fig. 3a, b). This too, denotes the reactive nature of this cell. The central sclerotic area of such carcinomas, in contrast, is devoid of myofibroblasts (Fig. 3c, d) or α-smooth-muscle-actin-positive cells [47], possibly a reflection of apoptosis. Three types of myofibroblastic stromal reaction have been described within infiltrating ductal breast carcinomas: (1) precocious, in which myofibroblasts precede the carcinoma cells by some distance into adjacent tissue; (2) synchronous, in which myofibroblasts appear spatially among carcinoma cells; and (3) late, in which myofibroblasts are identified central to the peripheral invasive cellular front [47]. The three types of myofibroblastic stromal reaction (precocious, synchronous and late) might coexist in the same breast carcinoma, with the synchronous usually being predominant [47].

When the collagenous matrix is analyzed, increased amounts of type-III collagen are present within the "young" mesenchyme, an area containing numerous myofibroblasts; in contrast, type-I collagen is most prominent within the central sclerotic zone of breast carcinomas [28], an area in which myofibroblasts are replaced by fibroblasts [47, 50].

Many pulmonary carcinomas, especially peripheral adenocarcinomas, are associated with some degree of scarring and are often associated with pleural retraction. If this process is pronounced, the term "scar carcinoma" is applied to these neoplasms. Earlier it was suggested that the presence of elastic fibers and anthracotic pigment in scars indicated that they had been present prior to the development of the neoplasm [7]. More recent literature suggests that scarring represents a desmoplastic stromal reaction in response to neoplastic invasion, rather than a preexisting condition. In favor of this latter interpretation is the presence of increased amounts of type-III collagen within pulmonary carcinomas [33], ana-

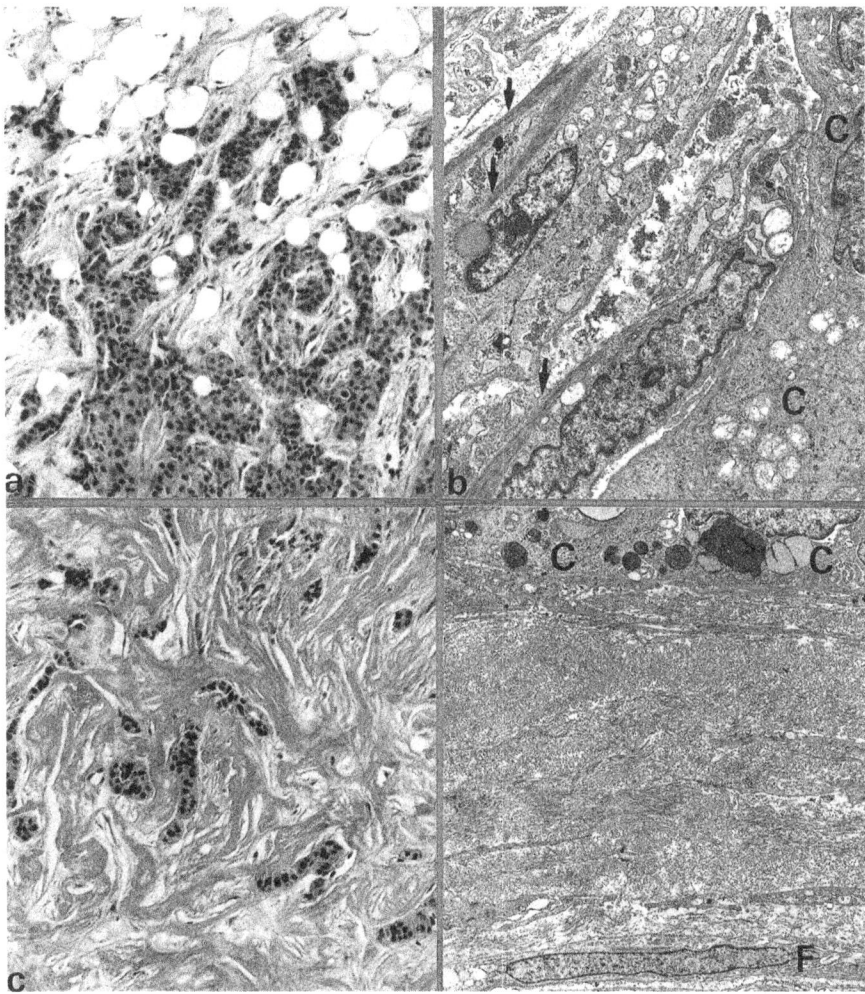

**Fig. 3a–d.** Invasive ductal breast carcinoma. **a** Light-microscopic aspect of peripheral invasive cellular front illustrating precocious stromal reaction, i.e., stromal cells which precede clusters of invasive carcinoma cells into adjacent fatty tissue. **b** Ultrastructural appearance of typical stromal myofibroblasts with stress fibers (*arrows*) adjacent to carcinoma cells (*C*). **c** Light-microscopic aspect of central sclerotic zone disclosing thick bands of collagen separating small clusters of carcinoma cells. **d** Ultrastructural appearance of central sclerotic zone with slender smooth-contoured fibroblast (*F*) and clusters of carcinoma cells (*C*) embedded in a densely collagenous matrix. Haematoxylin-Phloxine-Saffron: **a** × 300; **c** × 300. Uranyl acetate and lead citrate: **b** × 7500; **d** × 6600

logous to early invasive areas of ductal breast carcinomas [28]. In addition, ultra-structure demonstrates that the majority of stromal cells in "scar carcinomas" of the lung reveal typical features of myofibroblasts [3, 48], suggesting that scarring in pulmonary carcinomas represents a desmoplastic stromal reaction, analogous to many invasive and metastatic carcinomas elsewhere.

Cytoskeletal phenotypes with regard to expression of intermediate filaments, actin isoforms and smooth-muscle-myosin heavy chains reveal heterogeneity of stromal cells in invasive and metastatic carcinomas. Areas corresponding to early stromal invasion of ductal breast carcinomas contain myofibroblasts with a predominance of the VA type admixed with variable numbers of VAD, VA(D)M and V types [48], suggesting that certain stromal cells undergo definitive smooth-muscle metaplasia [VA(D)M cells]. Contrariwise, sclerotic areas of such carcinomas disclose numerous V cells with occasional VA cells. VA and VA(D)M cells are no longer observed, possibly as a result of apoptotic disappearance.

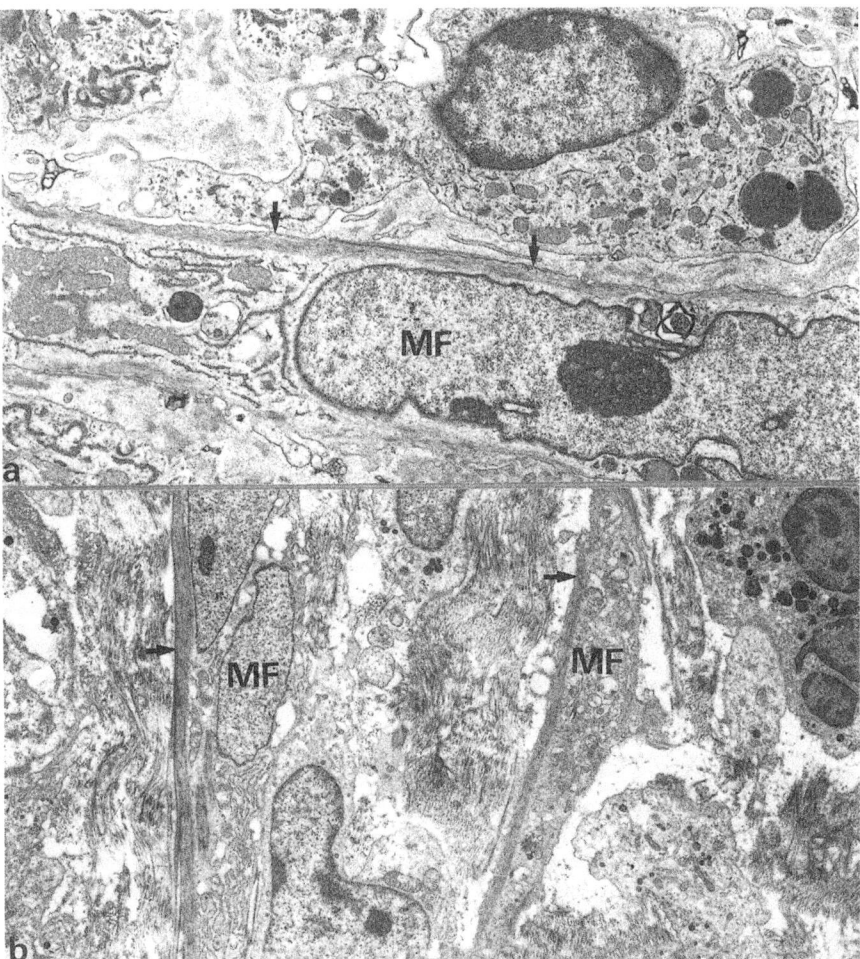

**Fig. 4a, b.** Malignant soft-tissue tumors with stromal myofibroblasts. **a** Typical myofibroblast (*MF*) with stress fiber (*arrows*) from malignant fibrous histiocytoma (storiform-pleomorphic variant). **b** Typical myofibroblasts (*MF*) with stress fibers (*arrows*) at nodule-stromal interphase from nodular sclerosing Hodgkin's disease. Uranyl acetate and lead citrate: **a** × 11,250; **b** × 11,250

With regard to malignant, non-epithelial neoplasms, myofibroblasts have been described in a limited number of sarcomas in which they generally constituted a small fraction of the cell population [20, 21, 29]. In the extensive and meticulous study of Lagacé et al. [29], they were identified in a large number of malignant fibrous histiocytomas (Fig. 4a) and well-differentiated sclerosing liposarcomas. Yet, in these sarcomas, the myofibroblasts never represented the dominant cellular element; in fact, they constituted a minor component and have been viewed as reactive elements, analogous to those observed in carcinomas with desmoplasia. No myofibroblasts were observed in an assortment of diverse sarcomas in which desmoplasia was absent [29]. In another study [44], myofibroblasts were consistently defined at the nodule–stromal interphase in nodular sclerosing Hodgkin's disease; this also was interpreted as another instance of myofibroblastic proliferation as a cellular stromal response to malignancy (Fig. 4b).

Originally, it was reasoned that the myofibroblastic stromal response in cancer represented a host response to the malignant neoplasm [45, 46], possibly to contain invasion. Recent work, however, suggests that in invasive carcinomas, stromal myofibroblasts secrete extracellular matrix-degrading enzymes, which would favor cancer invasion [2, 34]. In contrast, it was shown that lysyl oxidase, an enzyme responsible for extracellular matrix stabilization (cross-linking of collagen and elastin), was secreted by host cells (myofibroblasts and myoepithelial cells) around in situ breast carcinomas and in the precocious myofibroblastic stromal reaction of invasive ductal breast carcinomas [37]. Stromal reactions in carcinomas are not uniform. It is very likely that, even within the same neoplasm, mechanisms facilitating tumor invasion and others preventing or delaying invasion might operate.

# 6  Neoplasms of Myofibroblasts

Finally, several reports describe myofibroblastic neoplasms. Neoplastic transformation of the myofibroblasts – in the extreme – is possible [52], but certainly remains an uncommon event; the plethora of articles related to this matter (particularly in recent years) stems from the vague criteria employed to define this cell. The myofibroblast is a precisely defined cell at the ultrastructural level; its definition at the light microscopic and immunohistochemical levels is decisively less precise and, on occasion, imprecise. A significant number of reports describe myofibroblastic neoplasms; a few were considered as sarcomas [8, 10, 13, 14, 24, 52], and many more were described as benign myofibroblastomas or tumors of similar substance according to an assortment of designations [15, 19, 26, 30, 35, 38, 51, 53, 56, 57].

The benign myofibroblastic proliferations reported in the literature are generally well-circumscribed lesions, contrary to the poorly circumscribed and often infiltrating quality of reactive and quasineoplastic proliferative conditions, e.g., fibromatoses, nodular and proliferative fasciitis, proliferative myositis, and all lesions replete with typical myofibroblasts. Although thought to be composed of myofibroblasts, the majority of the benign myofibroblastomas was not examined by ultrastructure and, in the few cases for which this technique was performed, no typical myofibroblasts, as defined earlier, were found (Fig. 5a–c). For similar reasons, one might cast a jaundiced eye on the dominance of myofibroblasts in

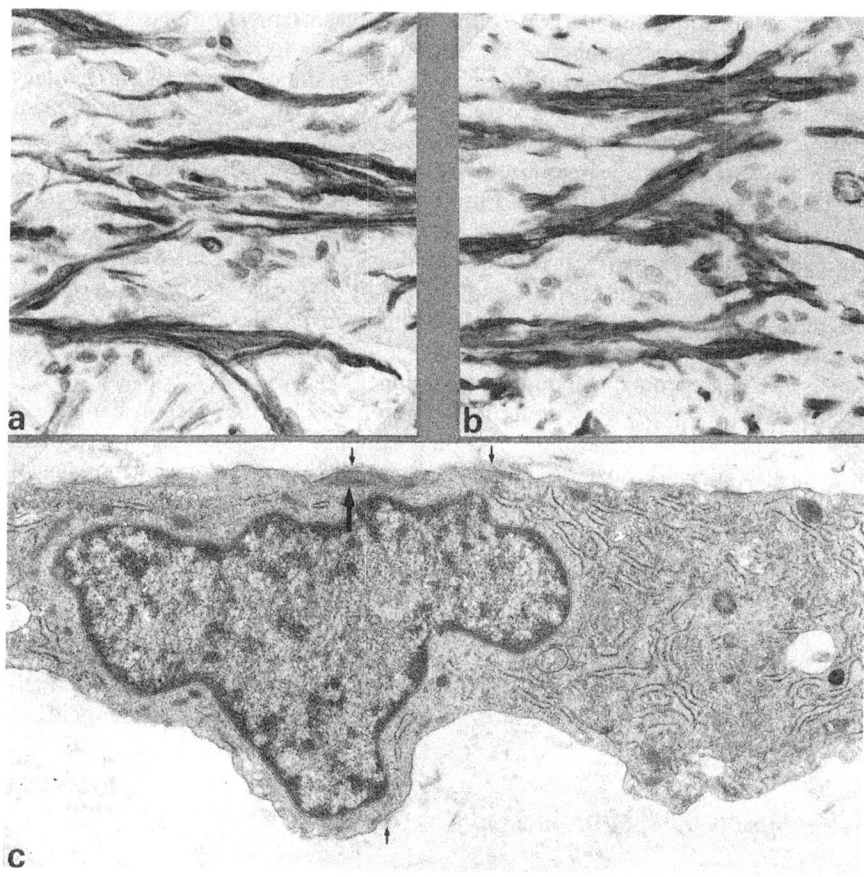

**Fig. 5 a–c.** So-called benign breast myofibroblastoma (courtesy of Dr. Louis R. Bégin, Montréal).
**a,b** Immunostaining of tumor cells for α-smooth muscle actin (**a**) and desmin (**b**). **c** Ultra-structural aspect of typical tumor cell disclosing fragments of external lamina (*small arrows*), pinocytotic vesicles, well-developed rough endoplasmic reticulum and subplasmalemmal short bundles of microfilaments with attenuated dense bodies (*large arrow*). Avidin-Biotin-Complex-Peroxidase reaction: **a** × 400; **b** × 400. Uranyl acetate and lead citrate: **c** × 18,900

mammary myofibroblastomas [53, 56], the palisaded myofibroblastomas and the intranodal hemorrhagic spindle-cell tumors with amianthoid fibers of lymph nodes [51, 57], soft-tissue myofibroblastomas [26], angiomyofibroblastomas of the vulva [15, 19, 35], angiomyofibroblastoma-like tumors of the male genital tract [30], meningeal myofibroblastomas [38], and pulmonary myofibroblastic tumors [1]. Immunohistochemically, the proliferating cells composing the so-called myo-fibroblastomas and all the related neoplasms disclose heterogeneous cytoskeletal phenotypes, e. g., positive reaction for muscle actin and absence of reactivity for desmin in the palisaded myofibroblastoma [57] and intranodal hemorrhagic spindle-cell tumors of lymph nodes [51], and staining for desmin associated with a negative reaction for muscle actins in angiomyofibroblastoma of the vulva [15]. The so-called myofibroblastomas and all other related neoplasms most likely represent myogenic stromal tumors (a designation proposed by Bégin [4]), possibly derived from myogenic stromal cells that have variable degrees of smooth muscle differentiation, rather than myofibroblastic neoplasms, because myofibroblasts, using strict ultrastructural criteria, were not observed.

Sarcomas composed entirely or partially of cells that disclose evidence of morphologic or immunohistochemical differentiation of myofibroblasts but lack the typical traits of myofibroblasts, as defined earlier, could well belong to the group of myogenic sarcomas [48]. It has to be remembered that many sarcomas, and also myogenic variants, may contain well-developed reactive stromal myofibroblasts [29, 48]. Occasionally, leiomyosarcomas may disclose rather well-developed fibronexuses and also well-developed rough endoplasmic reticulum, but they lack stress fibers (personal observation, 1997).

Accepting the concept that the myofibroblast is principally a reactive cell, the following has to be addressed: the literature cites cytogenetic and molecular genetic reports of clonality in desmoid tumors known to be composed, at least in part, of typical myofibroblasts [6, 32]. This presents a new twist to the tale, because it suggests that some myofibroblastic proliferations may be clonal, i. e., neoplastic. Yet, upon reflection, human atherosclerotic plaques also have been ascribed to monoclonal subintimal myocyte-like responses to injury [5, 25, 43]. This raises the issue of the significance of clonality, a matter well beyond this review.


# 7 Conclusion

Resting fibroblasts and, to a lesser extent, vascular smooth muscle cells, pericytes, and stromal cells with myoid features, are thought to be triggered by diverse cytokines to assume a myofibroblastic phenotype in granulation tissue, various reparative and reactive processes, quasineoplastic proliferations, and the stroma of certain neoplastic proliferations [48, 49]. In the granulating (healing) wound, genes that encode for apoptotic proteins are expressed to initiate myofibroblastic cell death when wound closure is accomplished. This would imply that the myofibroblast, at least in these settings, is a terminally differentiated cell with a finite lifespan. Commensurate with this, collagen synthesis shifts from type-III to type-I to provide necessary strength to the wound. Whether similar mechanisms are operative in the quasi-neoplastic proliferations or stroma of invasive carcinomas is not known. It is likely that scar formation (desmoplasia) in cancer results from myofibroblastic apoptosis and that keloids, hypertrophic scars and Dupuytren's type contractures result from imperfections of this normal apoptotic mechanism. This seems plausible because massive apoptosis has been reported as a putative mechanism of tumor regression in infantile myofibromatosis [18]. With regard to neoplasia, the proliferation of myofibroblasts initially was regarded to represent a host stromal response to invasive carcinomas characterized by desmoplasia [45, 46]. At the time, the myofibroblastic stromal reaction was regarded as beneficial to the host [45, 46]. Now some studies suggest that the myofibroblast in these conditions secretes extracellular matrix-degrading enzymes, thereby facilitating tumor invasion and progression [2, 34]. In contrast, extracellular matrix stabilization, as an enzymatic cellular host response preventing invasion, was also reported [37].

Carcinomas are not uniform with regard to stromal reactions. It is very likely that even within the same neoplasm, mechanisms facilitating tumor invasion and others preventing or delaying invasion might operate.

The issue of the myofibroblast as a neoplastic cell remains open. Lastly, some time ago [50], it was proposed that similarities might exist between the process of wound healing and the stromal response to neoplastic invasion. This assumption may also be extended to quasi-neoplastic proliferative conditions, e.g., Dupuytren's disease and related proliferative conditions. During normal wound-healing and within nodules of Dupuytren's disease and possibly in other quasi-neoplastic proliferations, the myo-fibroblastic/fibroblastic reaction appears to be centripetal, whereas with neoplastic invasion, this reaction is centrifugal [48], indicating that cancers are wounds which heal partially or, more often, wounds which do not heal [12]. The underlying cellular/molecular mechanisms explaining these fundamental differences, including the presence, delay or absence of apoptosis, remain to be explored.

# References

1. Alobeid B, Beneck D, Sreekantaiah C, Abbi RK, Slim MS (1997) Congenital pulmonary myo-fibroblastic tumor: a case report with cytogenetic analysis and review of the literature. Am J Surg Pathol 21:610–614
2. Basset P, Bellocq JP, Wolf C, Stoll I, Hutin P, Limacher JM, Podhajcer OL, Chenard MP, Rio MC, Chambon P (1990) A novel metalloproteinase gene specifically expressed in stromal cells of breast carcinomas. Nature 348:699–704
3. Barsky SH, Huang SJ, Bhuta S (1986) The extracellular matrix of pulmonary scar carcinomas is suggestive of a desmoplastic origin. Am J Pathol 124:412–419
4. Bégin LR (1991) Myogenic stromal tumor of the male breast (so-called myofibroblastoma). Ultrastruct Pathol 15:613–622
5. Benditt EP (1988) Origins of human atherosclerotic plaques. The role of altered gene expression. Arch Pathol Lab Med 112:997–1001
6. Bridge JA, Sreekantaiah C, Mouron B, Neff JR Sandberg AA, Wolman SR (1992) Clonal chromosomal abnormalities in desmoid tumors: implications for histopathogenesis. Cancer 69:430–436
7. Carrol R (1962) Influence of lung scars on primary lung cancer. J Pathol Bacteriol 83: 293–297
8. Churg AM, Kahn LB (1977) Myofibroblasts and related cells in malignant fibrous and fibro-histiocytic tumors. Hum Pathol 8:205–218
9. Cintorino M, Bellizzi de Marco E, Leoncini P, Tripodi SA, Xu LJ, Sappino AP, Schmitt-Gräff A, Gabbiani G (1991) Expression of α-smooth muscle actin in stromal cell of the uterine cervix during epithelial neoplastic changes. Int J Cancer 47:843–846
10. D'Andrian G, Gabbiani G (1980) A metastasizing sarcoma of the pleura composed of myo-fibroblasts. In: Fenoglio CM, Wolf M (eds) Progress in surgical pathology. Masson Publishing, New York, pp 31–40
11. Desmoulière A, Gabbiani G (1994) Modulation of fibroblastic cytoskeletal features during pathological situations: the role of extracellular matrix and cytokines. Cell Motil Cytoskeleton 29:195–203
12. Dvorak HF (1986) Tumors: wounds that do not heal. Similarities between tumor stroma generation and wound healing. New Engl J Med 315:1650–1659
13. Eyden BP, Christensen L, Tagore V, Harris M (1992) Myofibrosarcoma of subcutaneous soft tissue of the cheek. J Submicrosc Cytol Pathol 24:307–313
14. Eyden BP, Ponting J, Davies H, Bartley C, Torgersen E (1994) Defining the myofibroblast: normal tissues, with special reference to the stroma cells of the Warton's jelly in human umbilical cord. J Submicrosc Cytol Pathol 26:347–355

15. Fletcher CDM, Tsang WYW, Fisher C, Lee KC Chan JKC (1992) Angiomyofibroblastoma of the vulva. A benign neoplasm distinct from aggressive angiomyxoma. Am J Surg Pathol 16:373–382
16. Frank ED, Warren L (1981) Aortic smooth muscle cells contain vimentin instead of desmin. Proc Natl Acad Sci U S A 78:3020–3024
17. Franke WW, Schmid E, Freudenstein C, Appelhans B, Osborn M Weber K, Keenan TW (1980) Intermediate-sized filaments of the prekeratin type in myoepithelial cells. J Cell Biol 84:633–654
18. Fukasawa Y, Ishikura H, Takada A, Yokoyama S, Imamura M, Yoshiki T, Sato H (1994) Massive apoptosis in infantile myofibromatosis. A putative mechanism of tumor regression. Am J Pathol 144:480–485
19. Fukunaga M, Nomura K, Matsumoto K, Doi K, Endo Y, Ushigome S (1997) Vulval angiomyofibroblastoma. clinicopathologic analysis of six cases. Am J Clin Pathol 107:45–51
20. Gabbiani G, Fu YS, Kaye GI, Lattes R, Majno G (1972) Epithelioid sarcoma. A light and electron microscopic study suggesting a synovial origin. Cancer 30:486–499
21. Gabbiani G, Kaye GI Lattes R, Majno G (1971) Synovial sarcoma. Electron microscopic study of a typical case. Cancer 28:1031–1039
22. Gabbiani G, Ryan GB, Majno G (1971) Presence of modified fibroblasts in granulation tissue and their possible role in wound contraction. Experientia 27:549–550
23. Gabbiani G, Schmid E, Winter S, Chaponnier C, de Chastonay C, Vanderkerckhove J, Weber K, Franke WW (1981) Vascular smooth muscle cells differ from other smooth muscle cells: predominance of vimentin filaments and a specific $\alpha$-type actin. Proc Natl Acad Sci U S A 78:298–302
24. Ghadially FN, McNaughton JD, Lalonde JM (1983) Myofibroblastoma: a tumor of myofibroblasts. J Submicrosc Cytol 15:1055–1063
25. Gordon D, Reidy MA, Benditt EP, Schwartz SM (1990) Cell proliferation in human coronary arteries. Proc Natl Acad Sci U S A 87:4600–4604
26. Herrera GA, Johnson WW, Lockard VG, Walker BL (1991) Soft tissue myofibroblastomas. Mod Pathol 4:571–577
27. Hüttner I, Kocher O, Gabbiani G (1989) Endothelial and smooth muscle cells. In: Camilleri JP, Berry CL, Fiessinger JL, Bariéty J (eds) Disease of the arterial wall. Springer Verlag, Berlin Heidelberg New York, pp 3–41
28. Lagacé R, Grimaud JA, Schürch W, Seemayer TA (1985) Myofibroblastic stromal reaction of the breast and variations of collageneous matrix and structural glycoproteins. Virchows Arch A 408:49–59
29. Lagacé R, Schürch W, Seemayer TA (1980) Myofibroblasts in soft tissue sarcomas. Virchows Arch 389:1–11
30. Laskin WB, Fetsch JF, Mostofi FK. Angiomyofibroblastoma-like tumor of the male genital tract: analysis of 11 cases with comparison to the female angiomyofibroblastoma and spindle cell lipoma. Am Surg Pathol 22:6–16
31. Lazarides E (1980) Intermediate filaments as mechanical integrators of cellular space. Nature 293:249–256
32. Lucas DR, Shroyer KR, McCarthy PJ Markham NE, Fujita M, Enomoto TE (1997) Desmoid tumor is a clonal cellular proliferation: PCR amplification of HUMARA for analysis of patterns of X-chromosome inactivation. Am J Surg Pathol 21:306–311
33. Madri JA, Carter D (1984) Scar cancers of the lung: origin and significance. Hum Pathol 15:625–631
34. Nielsen BS, Sehested M, Timshel S, Pyke C, Dano K (1996) Messenger RNA for urokinase plasminogen activator is expressed in myofibroblasts adjacent to cancer cells in human breast cancer. Lab Invest 74:168–177
35. Ockner DM, Sayadi H, Swanson PE, Ritter JH, Wick MR (1997) Genital angimyofibroblastoma. Comparison with aggressive angiomyxoma and other myxoid neoplasms of skin and soft tissue. J Clin Pathol 107:36–44
36. Osborn M, Caselitz J, Weber K (1981) Heterogeneity of intermediate filament expression in vascular smooth muscle: a gradient in desmin positive cells from the rat aortic arch to the level of the arteria iliaca communis. Differentiation 20:196–202

37. Peyrol S Raccurt M, Gerard F, Gleyzal C, Grimaud JA, Sommer P (1997) Lysyl oxidase gene expression in the stromal reaction to the in situ and invasive breast cacinoma. Am J Pathol 150:497–507
38. Prayson RA, Estes ML, McMahon JT, Kalfas I, Sebek BA (1993) Meningeal myofibroblastoma. Am J Surg Pathol 19:931–936
39. Sappino AP, Schürch W, Gabbiani G (1990) Differentiation repertoire of fibroblastic cells: expression of cytoskeletal proteins as markers of phenotypic modulations. Lab Invest 63:144–161
40. Schmid E, Osborn M, Rungger-Brändle E, Gabbiani G, Weber K, Franke WW (1982) Distribution of vimentin and desmin filaments in smooth muscle tissue of mammalian and avian aorta. Exp Cell Res 137:329–334
41. Schmid E, Tapscott S, Bennett GS, Croop J, Fellini SA, Holtzer H, Franke WW (1979) Differential location of different types of intermediate-sized filaments in various tissues of the chicken embryo. Differentiation 15:27–40
42. Schmitt-Gräff A, Desmoulière A, Gabbiani G (1994) Heterogeneity of myofibroblast phenotypic features: an example of fibroblastic cell plasticity. Virchows Arch 425:3–24
43. Schwartz SM, Majeski MW, Murry CE (1995) The intima development and monoclonal responses to injury. Atherosclerosis 118:S125–140
44. Seemayer TA, Lagacé R, Schürch W (1980) On the pathogenesis of sclerosis and nodularity in nodular sclerosing Hodgkin's disase. Virchows Arch A 385:283–291
45. Seemayer TA, Lagacé R, Schürch W, Thelmo WL (1980) The myofibroblast: biologic, pathologic and theoretical considerations. Pathol Annu 15:443–470
46. Seemayer TA, Schürch W, Lagacé R, Tremblay G (1979) Myofibroblasts in the stroma of invasive and metastatic cacinoma: a possible host response to neoplasia. Am J Surg Pathol 3:525–533
47. Schürch W, Lagacé R, Seemayer TA (1982) Myofibroblastic stromal reaction in retracted scirrhous carcinoma of the breast. Surg Gynecol Obstet 154:351–358
48. Schürch W, Seemayer TA, Gabbiani G (1997) Myofibroblast. In: Sternberg SS (ed) Histology for pathologists. Lippincott-Raven, Philadelphia, pp 129–165
49. Schürch W, Seemayer TA, Gabbiani G (1998) The myofibroblast. A quarter century after its discovery (editorial). Am J Surg Pathol 22:141–147
50. Schürch W, Seemayer TA, Lagacé R (1981) Stromal myofibroblasts in primary invasive and metastatic carcinoma. A combined immunological, light and electron microscopic study. Virchows Arch A 391:125–139
51. Suster S, Rosai J (1989) Intranodal hemorrhagic spindle-cell tumor with "amianthoid" fibers. Report of six cases with a distinctive mesenchymal neoplasm of the inguinal region that simulates Kaposi's sarcoma. Am J Surg Pathol 13:347–357
52. Taccagni G, Rovere G Masullo M, Christensen L, Eyden B (1997) Myofibrosarcoma of the breast. Review of the literature on myofibroblastic tumors and criteria for defining myofibroblastic differentiation. Am J Surg Pathol 21:489–496
53. Thomas TMM, Myint A, Mak CKL, Chan JKC (1997) Mammary myofibroblastoma with leimyomatous differentiation. Am J Clin Pathol 107:52–55
54. Tremblay G (1979) Stromal aspects of breast carcinoma. Exp Mol Pathol 31:52–55
55. Travo P, Weber K, Osborn M (1982) Co-existence of vimentin and desmin type intermediate filaments in a subpopulation of adult rat vascular smooth muscle cells growing in primary culture. Exp Cell Res 139:87–94
56. Wargotz ES, Weiss SW, Norris HJ (1987) Myofibroblastoma of the breast. Sixteen cases of a distinct benign mesenchymal tumor. Am J Surg Pathol 11:493–502
57. Weiss SW, Gnepp DR, Bratthauer GL (1989) Palisaded myofibroblastoma. A benign mesenchymal tumor of lymph node. Am J Surg Pathol 13:341–346

# The Concept of Organizing Pneumonia*

J.-F. CORDIER

## 1 Unresolved Pneumococcal Pneumonia

At the beginning of the 19th century, LAENNEC described the sequential gross pathological stages of acute lobar pneumonia, which was later related to pneumococcal infection [27]. The first stage is congestion, in which the involved lobe is heavy and congested. During the next stage, called red hepatization, the lobe becomes red and dense, much like the liver. After a stage of gray and airless lung (grey hepatization), resolution of pneumonia usually occurs with eventual complete healing.

Histologically, congestion in pneumococcal pneumonia is characterized by the presence of edema containing many pneumococci, red cells and neutrophils. During red hepatization, the most conspicuous finding is the filling of alveoli by fibrin exudates. Next, the resolution of pneumonia corresponds to liquefaction of the fibrinous deposits, which are further removed by both expectoration and the action of macrophages. Resolution of pneumonia is usually complete with no sequelae.

However, before the era of antibiotics, some patients with pneumococcal pneumonia had an unfavorable course characterized by unresolved pneumonia, which often resulted in death. The concept of organizing pneumonia progressively emerged when pathologists, at the beginning of the century, described the failure of resolution of pneumococcal pneumonia in detail with progressive organization of the inflammatory exudates in the alveoli and resulting fibrosis [18, 30]. FLOYD [18] observed that "cells with elongated nuclei, exhibiting all transitions to fibroblasts, appear within the substance of the fibrin plugs and on their surface", and that fibrin was progressively replaced by connective tissue. Organizing pneumonia was thereafter long considered merely a consequence of unresolved infectious pneumonia before it was recently reconsidered as a more general type of pulmonary inflammation.

* Supported by grant HCL-PHRC 93-97.005.

Current Topics in Pathology, Volume 93
A. Desmoulière, B. Tuchweber (Eds.)
© Springer-Verlag Berlin Heidelberg 1999

## 2 Organization of Diffuse Alveolar Damage

The diffuse alveolar damage underlying adult respiratory-distress syndrome (ARDS) comprises an early acute exudative stage, with the formation of intra-alveolar hyaline membranes along the alveolar walls, followed by a chronic organizing stage. Since intraalveolar organization takes place in the process of fibrogenesis of ARDS, studies on the acute exudative stage are instructive for understanding the initial mechanisms preceding the organization of alveolar exudates.

The first step of alveolar damage is the injury to both the capillary endothelial cells and alveolar epithelial cells, resulting in high-permeability edema with leakage into alveoli of plasma fluid and especially coagulation proteins. Normally, there is a balance between procoagulant activity (mainly factor VII and tissue factor) and fibrinolytic activity (plasminogen activator) in the alveolar lumen and on alveolar surfaces. However, in ARDS, both increased procoagulant activity and decreased fibrinolytic activity [6, 20, 40] result in intraalveolar coagulation of exudated coagulation proteins, leading to widespread fibrin deposits in alveoli. Experimental studies have established the role of local abnormalities of coagulation and fibrinolytic pathways in animal models of acute lung injury [21, 22, 37]. Hyperoxia-induced lung disease in mice results in prominent intraalveolar fibrin deposition, with overproduction of plasminogen-activator inhibitor-1 (PAI-1), which impairs fibrinolytic activity in the alveolar compartment [3]. During bleomycin-induced lung injury in the mouse, whole-lung PAI-1 is dramatically induced, and in situ hybridization shows that PAI-1 messenger ribonucleic acid (mRNA) is induced within the fibrin-rich fibroproliferative lesions, primarily in fibroblast-like and macrophage-like cells [33]. Mice genetically deficient in PAI-1 fail to develop intra-alveolar deposits of fibrin in response to hyperoxia [3], and transgenic mice over-expressing PAI-1 experience greater bleomycin-induced pulmonary fibrosis than mice that are homozygous deficient for PAI-1 [15]. Clearly, enhanced intraalveolar coagulation and impaired intraalveolar fibrinolysis favor the development of intraalveolar fibrosis by providing and maintaining a fibrin matrix, which may be further invaded by fibroblasts. In addition to being part of the coagulation cascade, coagulation factors may also act as an interface between coagulation and inflammation, as demonstrated for factor Xa, which may promote recruitment of mast cells and rapid release of vasoactive mediators through effector-cell protease receptor-1 [8].

Fibrin degradation products are potent chemotactic factors for pre-stimulated neutrophils. However, peptides digested from fibrin by human neutrophil elastase are more potent than digestion products by plasmin, thus suggesting an auto-amplification of neutrophilic inflammation [28]. The migration and invasion of fibrin by fibroblasts involves the cell-surface matrix receptor CD44 [38] that has possible complex biological activities [1]. Patients dying from acute alveolar fibrosis after lung injury have CD44-expressing mesenchymal cells throughout newly formed fibrotic tissue [38]. The 85-kDa CD44 is expressed by lung-injury fibroblasts, and anti-CD44 antibodies block the invasion of a fibrin matrix by the fibroblasts [38].

At the beginning of the chronic organization stage, hyaline membranes and fibrin deposits are progressively replaced by intraalveolar fibrosis with several possible lesions: individualized intraalveolar buds in the lumen of airspaces, diffuse intraalveolar fibrosis and fibrotic masses apposed to the alveolar walls [19]. Myofibroblasts involved in these processes are found in the interstitium and some alveolar spaces [19]. Intraalveolar fibrosis may be further incorporated in the alveolar wall, resulting in extensive and severe pulmonary fibrosis. The outcome of ARDS is either death ensuing from irreversible extensive fibrosis, or complete recovery with no or minimal sequelae. It is quite uncommon that patients surviving ARDS have significant residual fibrosis. Corticosteroids may have a beneficial role in some patients with ARDS at the chronic stage [29]. However, the factors influencing the evolution toward lethal fibrosis or complete healing are presently unknown.

## 3 Cryptogenic Organizing Pneumonia

Organizing pneumonia may result from several determined causes, such as drug-induced lung disease [9]. Cryptogenic organizing pneumonia (COP), also called idiopathic bronchiolitis obliterans organizing pneumonia (BOOP), is a recently described clinicopathological disorder, distinct from the other idiopathic fibrosing interstitial pneumonias [10, 12, 17]. It is characterized by a subacute onset of symptoms with fever, cough and moderate dyspnea. The most typical imaging pattern consists of several areas of patchy alveolar opacities with a peripheral distribution. Bronchoalveolar lavage shows a mixed pattern with increased lymphocytes, neutrophils and eosinophils. The pathological hallmark of COP is the presence of organizing pneumonia at lung biopsy, with or without accompanying bronchiolitis obliterans of the proliferative type. Although COP may occasionally heal spontaneously, most patients require corticosteroid treatment, which produces a dramatic effect within a few days with complete clinical and imaging recovery. However, relapses are extremely frequent while reducing or after stopping corticosteroids, thus suggesting an active and sustained inflammatory process only transiently interrupted by treatment. Corticosteroids may be necessary for more than 1 year to obtain the final resolution of the inflammatory process.

Although intraalveolar fibrosis is, in no way, specific for this condition, in COP the intraluminal buds are the most conspicuous and represent the major pathological finding; in other disorders, they are generally only accessory findings of little clinical interest. By definition, the cause of COP is unknown, but whatever the cause, the pathological lesions of COP are not blurred by associated factors such as infection or ventilation of patients with high concentrations of oxygen, as occurs in pneumococcal pneumonia and ARDS, respectively. The study of COP is, therefore, really a unique model of inflammatory-lung disease with organizing pneumonia [11].

The sequence of changes leading to the typical intraalveolar fibrosis of COP has been established and demonstrates a crucial role for myofibroblasts in this inflammatory and fibrosing process [4, 24, 26, 31, 34].

Alveolar epithelial injury is the first event, with necrosis and detachment of pneumocytes I and II, resulting in the denudation of epithelial basal laminae. Damage to the endothelial cells may also be present, but it is usually mild. The epithelial basal laminae are not destroyed, but they are locally ruptured with the formation of gaps. No hyaline membranes are present, in contrast with the lesions of diffuse alveolar damage. At this stage, inflammatory cells (lymphocytes, and neutrophil and eosinophil polymorphonuclears) are present within the alveolar interstitium. The fibroblasts in the interstitium show morphological signs of activation, with an electron-dense cytoplasm and conspicuous rough endoplasmic reticulum and Golgi apparatus. Nevertheless, there is no increase in the number of interstitial fibroblasts and no interstitial collagen deposition.

Three distinct sequential intraalveolar cell-matrix patterns characterize the intraalveolar fibrogenesis, starting with alveolar epithelial injury.

Fibrinoid inflammatory cell clusters within the lumen of alveoli consist of large bundles of fibrin associated with inflammatory cells (mainly lymphocytes and plasma cells, and occasionally mast cells and polymorphonuclears). Conspicuous macrophages are seen engulfing and degrading fibrin bundles. Coagulation factors VII and X and fibrinogen are associated with the fibrin deposits. Immunoglobulins and fibronectin are also present. These proteins are likely exudated from plasma for their major part. There is almost no intraluminal reticulin framework at this stage.

Fibroinflammatory buds represent the next stage, with the progressive disappearance of fibrin deposits that become fragmented. Inflammatory cells are less numerous. Type-II pneumocytes proliferate and cover areas of the epithelial basal laminae. However, the most important finding, at this stage, is the intraalveolar migration of fibroblasts from the interstitium through the gaps of the epithelial basal laminae. Fibroblasts colonize and circumscribe the fibrinoid inflammatory cell clusters, and further proliferate, as shown by occasional mitotic figures. The presence of intracytoplasmic filaments is conspicuous beneath their cytoplasmic membrane, and immunostaining demonstrates the presence of desmin and smooth-muscle actin. At this stage, a reticulin intraalveolar framework may be identified.

Mature fibrotic buds progressively replace the fibroinflammatory buds. The intraalveolar buds are composed of a fibrotic matrix, consisting of a sequential deposition of fibronectin, procollagen III, collagen III, collagen I and other matricial proteins. Concentric cellular rings of fibroblasts are separated by the loose polymorphic matrix deposits, thus forming the typical mature intraalveolar buds characteristic of COP. The fibroblasts, especially at the periphery of the bud (where they are spindle shaped), are typical myofibroblasts with bundles of cytoplasmic filaments oriented along the axis of the cells, with dense condensations similar to those of smooth-muscle cells. The rough endoplasmic reticulum is abundant. The study of the anti-adhesive glycoproteins has demonstrated that tenascin is present through the entire extracellular matrix of the buds, SPARC (also called osteonectin) is present intracellularly in the fibroblasts, and thrombospondin is localized in the extracellular matrix immediately beneath reparative epithelium [25].

An animal model of respiratory reovirus 1/L induction of intraluminal fibrosis in CBA/J mice has been recently developed, which closely resembles the temporal sequence of human BOOP [5]. It suggests that both genetic factors and the degree of severity of the initial injury are determinants in the progression toward intraluminal fibrosis.

Thus, meticulous and comprehensive morphological analysis identifies several biopathological processes in COP, mainly consisting of epithelial injury, intraalveolar coagulation, intraalveolar migration of fibroblasts with further proliferation and phenotypic modulation into myofibroblasts, and intraalveolar fibrogenesis. It may seem clear that many proteins (as fibronectin and coagulation-cascade components) involved in these processes may be exudated from plasma as a consequence of the permeability edema induced by the epithelial injury. However, several studies in experimental models of fibrosis have demonstrated the intraalveolar production of proteins, especially cytokines which play a role on chemotaxis, activation and replication of the fibroblasts, and the further organization and control of pulmonary fibrosis. For example, transfer of the granulocyte–macrophage colony stimulating factor gene to rat lung both induces transforming growth factor beta (TGF-$\beta$1) and myofibroblast accumulation in the rat [41]. The role of the myofibroblast in several types of pulmonary and extrapulmonary fibrosis has been emphasized in several studies [13, 23, 32, 36, 42–44].

In COP, the expression of interleukin 8 and fibronectin genes is increased in alveolar macrophages [7]. Platelet-derived growth factor (PDGF) antibody immunostaining shows that tissue monocytes or macrophages positive for PDGF are scattered in the buds, as well as within the alveolar interstitium [2].

## 4 Organizing Pneumonia as a Model of Reversible Fibrosis

Whereas usual interstitial pneumonia inexorably progresses to widespread pulmonary fibrosis and subsequent death despite therapeutic attempts, the usual complete resolution of intraalveolar fibrosis in COP treated by corticosteroids (and less consistently in ARDS or acute interstitial pneumonia) suggests that a complete degradation of the collagen and associated matricial components occurs.

This degradation requires the action of specific enzymes and especially the matrix metalloproteinases (MMP), the gelatinases and the stromelysins. Other proteinases, such as elastase and plasmin, also participate in the degradation of the fibrotic matrices. Many cells in the pulmonary distal airspaces are capable of producing these enzymes, including polymorphonuclears, monocyte macrophages and the fibroblasts themselves. Cytokines may modulate the production of collagenase by fibroblasts [14, 35], and the composition of the fibrotic matrix itself may modulate the production of proteases [16]. Relaxin, a cytokine/growth factor, in addition to inhibiting the TGF-$\beta$-mediated overexpression of collagens I and III by human-lung fibroblasts, stimulates the expression of MMP-1 in a biphasic, dose-dependent manner [39]. The induction of a matrix-degradative phenotype in human-lung fibroblasts may, thus, play a role in the reversibility of pulmonary fibrosis. Although the possible mechanisms of reversibility of intraalveolar fibrosis are many, their respective role in organizing pneumonia is unknown.

## 5 Conclusion

Organizing pneumonia is a fascinating model of pulmonary fibrosing inflammation, entirely reversible with corticosteroids in its archetype of COP. Since the alveolar lumen is devoid of fibroblasts and connective matrix in the normal lung, it allows the study of pathohistophysiological events, leading to the organization of buds of granulation tissue and fibrosis where the myofibroblasts play a crucial role. Understanding the biopathology of organizing pneumonia may provide useful information for a better approach and treatment of the many fibrosing pulmonary disorders.

## References

1. Aruffo A (1996) CD44: one ligand, two functions. J Clin Invest 98:2191–2192
2. Aubert JD, Pare PD, Hogg JC, Hayashi S (1997) Platelet-derived growth factor in bronchiolitis obliterans-organizing pneumonia. Am J Respir Crit Care Med 155:676–681
3. Barazzone C, Belin D, Piguet PF, Vassalli JD, Sappino AP (1996) Plasminogen activator inhibitor-1 in acute hyperoxic mouse lung injury. J Clin Invest 98:2666–2673
4. Basset F, Ferrans VJ, Soler P, Takemura T, Fukuda Y, Crystal RG (1986) Intraluminal fibrosis in interstitial lung disorders. Am J Pathol 122:443–461
5. Bellum SC, Dove D, Harley RA, Greene WB, Judson MA, London L, London SD (1997) Respiratory reovirus 1/L induction of intraluminal fibrosis. A model for the study of bronchiolitis obliterans organizing pneumonia. Am J Pathol 150:2243–2254
6. Bertozzi P, Astedt B, Zenzius L, Lynch K, Lemaire F, Zapol W, Chapman HAJ (1990) Depressed bronchoalveolar urokinase activity in patients with adult respiratory distress syndrome. N Engl J Med 322:890–897
7. Carre PC, King TE Jr., Mortensesen R, Riches DWH (1994) Cryptogenic organizing pneumonia: increased expression of interleukin-8 and fibronectin genes by alveolar macrophages. Am J Respir Cell Mol Biol 10:100–105
8. Cirino G, Cicala C, Bucci M, Sorrentino L, Ambrosini G, DeDominicis G, Altieri DC (1997) Factor Xa as an interface between coagulation and inflammation. Molecular mimicry of factor Xa association with effector cell protease receptor-1 induces acute inflammation in vivo. J Clin Invest 99:2446–2451
9. Cordier JF (1993) Cryptogenic organizing pneumonitis. Bronchiolitis obliterans organizing pneumonia. Clin Chest Med 14:677–692
10. Cordier JF, Loire R, Brune J (1989) Idiopathic bronchiolitis obliterans organizing pneumonia. Definition of characteristic clinical profiles in a series of 16 patients. Chest 96: 999–1004
11. Cordier JF, Peyrol S, Loire R (1994) Bronchiolitis obliterans organizing pneumonia as a model of inflammatory lung disease. In: Epler GR (ed) Diseases of the bronchioles. Raven Press, New York, pp 313–345
12. Davison AG, Heard BE, McAllister WAC, Turner-Warwick ME (1983) Cryptogenic organizing pneumonitis, Q J Med 52:382–394
13. Desmouliere A, Gabbiani G (1994) Modulation of fibroblastic cytoskeletal features during pathological situations: the role of extracellular matrix and cytokines. Cell Motil Cytoskeleton 29:195–203
14. Edwards DRG, Murphy G, Reynolds JJ, Whitham SE, Docherty AJP, Angel P, Heath JK (1987) Transforming growth factor beta modulates the expression of collagenase and metalloproteinase inhibitor. Embo J 6:1899–1904
15. Eitzman DT, McCoy RD, Zheng X, Fay WP, Shen T, Ginsburg D, Simon RH (1996) Bleomycin-induced pulmonary fibrosis in trangenic mice that either lack or overexpress the murine plasminogen activator inhibitor-1 gene. J Clin Invest 97:232–237
16. Emonard H, Takiya C, Dreze S, Cordier JF, Grimaud JA (1989) Interstitial collagenase (MMP-1), gelatinase (MMP-2) and stromelysin (MMP-3) released by human fibroblasts cultured on acellular sarcoid granulomas (sarcoid matrix complex, SMC). Matrix 9:382–388
17. Epler GR, Colby TV, McLoud TC, Carrington CB, Gaensler EA (1985) Bronchiolitis obliterans organizing pneumonia. N Engl J Med 312:152–158
18. Floyd R (1922) Organization of pneumonic exudates. Am J Med Sci 163:527–548

19. Fukuda Y, Ishizaki M, Masuda Y, Kimura G, Kawanami O, Masugi Y (1987) The role of intra-alveolar fibrosis in the process of pulmonary structural remodeling in patients with diffuse alveolar damage. Am J Pathol 126:171-182
20. Idell S, Gonzalez K, Bradford H, MacArthur CK, Fein AM, Maunder RJ, Garcia JG, Griffith DE, Weiland J, Martin TR (1987) Procoagulant activity in bronchoalveolar lavage in the adult respiratory distress syndrome: contribution of tissue factor associated with factor VII. Am Rev Respir Dis 136:1466-1474
21. Idell S, Peters J, James KJ, Fair DS, Coalson JJ (1989) Local abnormalities of coagulation and fibrinolytic pathways that promote alveolar fibrin deposition in the lungs of baboons with diffuse alveolar damage. J Clin Invest 84:181-193
22. Idell S, Peterson BT, Gonzalez KK, Gray LD, Bach R, McLarty J, Fair DS (1988) Local abnormalities of coagulation and fibrinolysis and alveolar fibrin deposition in sheep with oleic acid-induced lung injury. Am Rev Respir Dis 138:1282-1284
23. Kapanci Y, Desmouliere A, Pache JC, Redard M, Gabbiani G (1994) Cytoskeletal protein modulation in pulmonary alveolar myofibroblasts during idiopathic pulmonary fibrosis. Possible role of transforming growth factor beta and tumor necrosis factor alpha. Am J Respir Crit Care Med 152:2163-2169
24. Katzenstein AL, Myers JL, Prophet WD, Corley LS III, Shin MS (1986) Bronchiolitis obliterans and usual interstitial pneumonia. A comparative clinicopathologic study. Am J Surg Pathol 10:373-381
25. Kuhn C, Mason RJ (1995) Immunolocalization of SPARC, tenascin, and thrombospondin in pulmonary fibrosis. Am J Pathol 147:1759-1769
26. Kuhn C, McDonald JA (1991) The roles of the myofibroblast in idiopathic pulmonary fibrosis. Ultrastructural and immunohistochemical features of sites of active extracellular matrix synthesis. Am J Pathol 138:1257-1265
27. Laennec RTH (1826) Traité de l'Auscultation Médiate et des Maladies des Poumons et du Coeur. Chaudet 2nd edn, Paris
28. Leavell KJ, Peterson MW, Gross TJ (1996) The role of fibrin degradation products in neutro-phil recruitment to the lung. Am J Respir Cell Mol Biol 14:53-60
29. Meduri GU, Belenchia JM, Estes RJ, Wunderink RG, El Torky M, Leeper KVJ (1991) Fibro-proliferative phase of ARDS. Clinical findings and effects of corticosteroids, Chest 100:943-952
30. Milne LS (1911) Chronic pneumonia (including a discussion of two cases of syphilis of the lung). Am J Med Sci 142:408-438
31. Myers JL, Katzenstein AL (1988) Ultrastructural evidence of alveolar epithelial injury in idiopathic bronchiolitis obliterans organizing pneumonia. Am J Pathol 132:102-109
32. Ohta K, Mortenson RL, Clark RAF, Hirose N, King TE, Jr (1995) Immunohistochemical identification and characterization of smooth muscle-like cells in idiopathic pulmonary fibrosis. Am J Respir Crit Care Med 152:1659-1665
33. Olman MA, Mackman N, Gladson CL, Moser KM, Loskutoff DJ (1995) Changes in pro-coagulant and fibrinolytic gene expression during bleomycin-induced lung injury in the mouse. J Clin Invest 96:1621-1630
34. Peyrol S, Cordier JF, Grimaud JA (1990) Intra-alveolar fibrosis of idiopathic bronchiolitis obliterans-organizing pneumonia. Cell-matrix patterns. Am J Pathol 137:155-170
35. Postlethwaite AE, Lachman LB, Mainardi CL, Kang AH (1983) Interleukin 1 stimulation of collagenase production by cultured fibroblasts. J Exp Med 157:801-806
36. Schmitt-Graff A, Desmouliere A, Gabbiani G (1994) Heterogeneity of myofibroblast pheno-typic features: an example of fibroblastic cell plasticity. Virchows Arch 425:3-24
37. Sitrin RG, Brubaker PG, Fantone JC (1987) Tissue fibrin deposition during acute lung injury in rabbits and its relationship to local expression of procoagulant and fibrinolytic activi-ties. Am Rev Respir Dis 135:930-936
38. Svee K, White J, Vaillant P, Jessurun J, Roongta U, Krumwiede M, Johnson D, Henke C (1996) Acute lung injury fibroblast migration and invasion of a fibrin matrix is mediated by CD44. J Clin Invest 98:1713-1727
39. Unemori EN, Pickford LB, Salles AL, Piercy CE, Grove BH, Erikson ME, Amento EP (1996) Relaxin induces an extracellular matrix-degrading phenotype in human lung fibroblasts in vitro and inhibits lung fibrosis in a murine model in vivo. J Clin Invest 98:2739-2745

40. Vassali JD, Sappino AP, Belin D (1991) The plasminogen activator/plasmin system. J Clin Invest 1067–1072

41. Xing Z, Tremblay GM, Sime PJ, Gauldie J (1997) Overexpression of granulocyte-macrophage colony-stimulating factor induces pulmonary granulation tissue formation and fibrosis by induction of transforming growth factor-$\beta$1 and myofibroblast accumulation. Am J Pathol 150:59–66

42. Zhang H-Y, Gharaee-Kermani M, Zhang K, Karmiol S, Phan SH (1996) Lung fibroblast $\alpha$-smooth muscle actin expression and contractile phenotype in bleomycin-induced pulmonary fibrosis. Am J Pathol 148:527–537

43. Zhang K, Flanders KC, Phan SH (1995) Cellular localization of transforming growth factor-$\beta$ expression in bleomycin-induced pulmonary fibrosis. Am J Pathol 147:352–361

44. Zhang K, Rekhter MD, Gordon D, Phan SH (1994) Myofibroblasts and their role in lung collagen gene expression during pulmonary fibrosis. A combined immunohistochemical and in situ hybridization study. Am J Pathol 145:114–125

# Endothelial Repair in Atherogenesis

A. I. Gotlieb, T.-Y. Joseph Lee

## 1 Introduction

The pathogenesis of an atherosclerotic plaque is a complex and chronic process that is closely associated with the structure and function of endothelial cells [12, 13, 21]. Although the sequence of events that lead to the initiation and progression of fibrofatty atherosclerotic plaques is not fully understood, there is much support for the theory that disruption of both structural and functional endothelial integrity plays an important role in atherogenesis; both in the initiation of the lesion and the growth of the plaque as it causes lumenal stenosis (Table 1). Once viewed as simply a passive barrier between blood and the vessel wall, the endothelium is now recognized: (1) as playing a dynamic biological role in the regulation of normal vascular function, (2) in the regulation of coagulation and fibrinolysis, (3) in platelet and leukocyte activation, (4) in the repair of the arterial wall following injury, and (5) in the pathogenesis of vascular diseases. In addition to acting as a thromboresistant surface and macromolecular barrier [7], endothelial cells are very active metabolically. Endothelial cells also act as signal transducers for the cells within the wall, thus regulating smooth muscle cell function via paracrine processes, including vasomotion, cell proliferation, and matrix secretion. Many endothelial functions are inducible, and important interactions that regulate endo-thelial activity occur at the vessel wall–blood interface and at the endothelial- sub-

Table 1. Disruption of endothelial barrier integrity

Disruption leads to an imbalance of factors resulting in vascular disease:
  Dysfunction of endothelial cell–cell interaction
  Dysfunction of endothelial cell-substratum interaction
  Dysfunctional endothelial repair

Current Topics in Pathology, Volume 93
A. Desmoulière, B. Tuchweber (Eds.)
© Springer-Verlag Berlin Heidelberg 1999

endothelial matrix interface. Thus, modulation of endothelial phenotype may lead to endothelial dysfunction and promote vascular disease.

## 2 Endothelial Cells and Structural Integrity

The walls of large- and medium-sized arteries consist of three layers; the intima, media and the adventitia. With respect to the pathogenesis of atherosclerosis, intimal integrity is most important. The intima is bounded on its inner surface by the endothelium and its outer surface by the internal elastic lamina [36]. This part of the intima, just beneath the endothelium, is often referred to as the subendo-thelium. In addition to endothelial cells, the intima contains some smooth muscle cells and the occasional macrophage. These smooth muscle cells may proliferate over time to produce mild eccentric or diffuse intimal thickening, especially at branch points. The endothelial cells of normal arteries form a continuous single layer of flattened cells, orientated with the long axis in the direction of blood flow. In areas of turbulent flow or altered shear, the cells are altered in shape [23, 27]. In high shear they are elongated. In low shear they are cobblestone in shape. The shape of the cells is maintained by the endothelial-cell cytoskeleton consisting of microfilaments and microtubules. Cell–cell interactions are the function of tight junctions and adhesion junctions which regulate permeability [19, 20, 32, 37]. Cell–cell contact between endothelial cells is maintained via unique calcium-dependent adhesion molecules of the cadherin family in adherens junctions [18]. Neural (N) and vascular endothelial (VE) cadherin are found in endothelial cells; the latter is specific to endothelium. VE cadherin forms complexes with catenins, some of which link the catenin/cadherin complex to actin microfilaments [22]. A change in calcium levels can affect both the shape and the degree of contact between the cells. Vinculin is co-localized with peripheral F-actin microfilament bundles at sites of cell–cell contact. In addition, adhesion plaques containing vinculin are important sites for the anchoring of endothelial cells to the subendo-thelium at focal adhesion sites [1]. Disruption of these junctions and/or adhesion plaques results in an immediate loss of endothelial integrity due to subtle changes in intercellular adhesion, actual retraction of adjacent cells leaving small gaps in the endothelium or frank loss of endothelial cells. There is normally very little turnover of endothelial cells in the aorta, except at a few specific sites that are predisposed to atherosclerotic plaques [3, 30], thus suggesting that endothelial integrity is strictly maintained in the normal resting state by quiescent endo-thelial cells.

## 3 Cytoskeletal Fiber Systems and In Vitro Repair

Dynamic cytoskeletal fiber systems are important in regulating endothelial repair [42, 44] once endothelial integrity is disrupted. Microfilaments appear to play a role in the force generation needed for migration [25] and in cell–substratum adhesion and cell–cell adhesion [35, 40], while the centrosomes and its associated microtubules play an important role in directional cell migration [14, 16, 26, 42]. We have previously shown that endothelial cells in normal confluent monolayers are characterized by a dense peripheral band (DPB) of actin microfilament bundles and few central microfilament bundles [45]. The centrosomes are normally found randomly distributed around the nucleus with no specific orientation [14, 16].

Using large- and small-wound in vitro models [6, 13, 15, 16, 42, 44], we have described the sequence of cellular events that occur at the initiation of repair. Adjacent endothelial cells attempt to repair a denuded area by rapidly extruding lamellipodia into this area. This extrusion of lamellipodia depends on the presence of intact actin microfilaments. In small wounds, repair occurs rapidly by lamellipodia extrusion by the cells surrounding the denuded area [41]. If repair is incomplete, such as in larger wounds, then a second set of events occurs that leads to cell migration and eventual proliferation. This is characterized by the redistribution of the centrosome toward the front of the cell and elongation of the endothelial cell in preparation for translocation of the cell. DPB breakdown ensues, which also results in decreased cell–cell adhesion, and directed migration follows to continue the process of re-endothelialization [46]. In large wounds, repair by cell proliferation is required and proliferation itself is dependent on cell migration [6].

## 4 Three Stages of Early In Vitro Repair

The endothelial cell is unique because it must undergo a transition from a resting cell with a cytoskeleton organized for barrier function, to one that promotes cell translocation following denuding endothelial injury. Since we had shown that actin microfilaments are critical for both maintaining the integrity of the resting monolayer and for optimum re-endothelialization, we carried out a detailed study of the organization of microfilaments as the cell undergoes the transition from a resting to a translocating cell. We used an in vitro model, in which a linear wound was made with a spatula in a confluent monolayer of porcine aortic endothelial cells. The complex reorganization of actin microfilament bundles following injury and their relationship to microtubules and vinculin was studied in cells at the wound edge using immunofluorescent scanning laser confocal microscopy and time-lapse videomicroscopy. As noted above, in the resting confluent monolayer microfilaments were present as a DPB located toward the upper part of the cell and as central microfilament bundles at the substratum.

Three distinct stages of microfilament reorganization occurred sequentially during early repair. Stage I followed wounding and involved the reduction of the DPB of microfilaments and associated peripheral cell–cell vinculin plaques. This was associated with rapid forward actin-based lamellipodia extrusions and cell elongation. Low-dose cytochalasin, which did not disrupt the morphology of microfilament bundles, reduced elongation. Stage II, occurring within 2 h after wounding, was characterized by central microfilaments behind the lamellipodia distributed parallel to the wound edge with vinculin plaques at their tips (Fig. 1). This was associated with prominent spreading at the front of the cell, which enhanced the extent of coverage of the denuded wound area. Stage III, occurring between 6 h and 8 h, was characterized by the orientation of central microfilaments

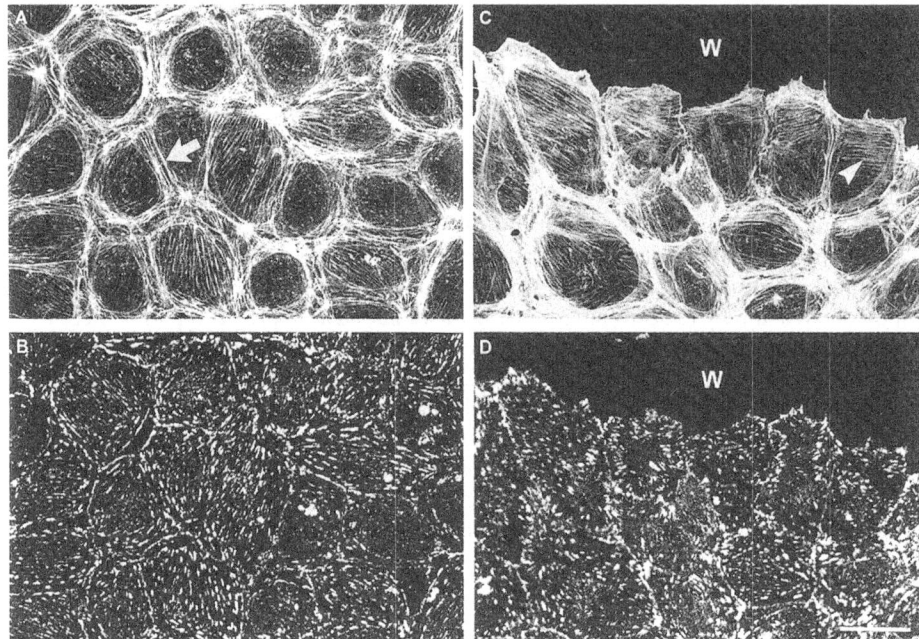

**Fig. 1 A–D.** Photomicrograph of endothelial cells double stained at confluency (**A, B**) and 2 h following wounding (**C, D**) for F-actin with rhodamine-phalloidin (**A, C**) and vinculin with an anti-vinculin antibody (**B, D**). The wound at 2 h is at the top (*W*). Note the dense peripheral band (*DPB*) of actin microfilaments at confluency (*arrow*) and the presence of central microfilaments parallel to the wound edge (*arrowhead*) in cells along the wound at 2 h following injury. Bar = 25 μm

perpendicular to the wound edge with vinculin plaques at their tips, and was associated with the initiation of cell translocation. There was no specific structural association between central microfilaments and microtubules, as the former were located toward the substratum, while the latter were located toward the center and upper part of the cell. Thus, the sequential appearance of the three patterns of microfilament distribution define the cytoskeletal events that regulate the reestablishment of endothelial integrity following denuding endothelial injury [28]. The molecular mechanisms that regulate these cytoskeletal changes are not yet understood.

## 5 Actin Microfilament Organization in Endothelial Cells In Vivo in Health and Atherosclerosis

Using double-labeling fluorescence-microscopy techniques to localize both F-actin and cell nuclei in situ [23], we showed that endothelial actin microfilaments are organized into central and peripheral bundles as seen in vitro [4, 15]. The distribution of microfilaments is important since central microfilaments, also referred to as stress fibers, and peripheral microfilaments are considered to be essential in cell-substratum adhesion [13]) and cell–cell adhesion [34, 42, 43], respectively. We have shown previously that the distribution and organization of endothelial microfilaments in the rabbit aorta are functions of the location of cells [24] and the hemodynamic stress exerted on them [23]. Profound variations in the extent of peripheral actin at the cell boundaries and the amount, length and thickness of central microfilaments were seen. Current evidence indicates that an elongated cell shape and prominent central microfilament bundles are indications that the cells were exposed to elevated hemodynamic shear stress, while a cobblestone morphology and prominent peripheral actin bundles are characteristic of cells exposed to static-flow conditions or low shear stress.

Since actin microfilaments are essential in the maintenance of endothelial integrity and in the repair of injured endothelium, we have carried out a detailed study of the distribution of microfilaments in the immediate vicinity of aortic branches. Branches are of major interest because there is a predilection for atherosclerotic lesions near branch ostia. We made an extensive, systemic examination of branches of the aorta and iliac arteries using in situ staining of perfusion-fixed arteries. Microfilaments were localized using rhodamine phalloidin. Three patterns of staining were observed. Some endothelial cells showed prominent central stress fibers. Others had few central stress fibers, but prominent peripheral fibers. Still others showed an intermediate pattern with some central and some peripheral fibers present. At small-branch sites, the lip of the divider was more blunt, and there were more cells with peripheral actin. At large branches, cells with peripheral actin were confined mainly to the lip, while there were many more cells with prominent central fibers. We also found that major differences can occur over very small distances, therefore, adjacent cells may show strikingly different patterns of microfilament distribution. These patterns appear to reflect the geometry of the flow divider and local variations in hemodynamic shear stress. The differences in microfilament distribution may reflect differences in endothelial functions, which are essential in maintaining endothelial integrity.

We carried out studies to test whether hypercholesterolemia influences the distribution of endothelial-cell microfilaments during the initiation and growth of fatty streak-type lesions [5]. We classified the lesions occurring over a 20-week period into four types, based on the location and extent of macrophage infiltration observed microscopically. The earliest lesion was characterized by macrophages adherent to the endothelial surface. Minimal lesions were characterized by a few cells in the subendothelium. Intermediate lesions consisted of numerous subendothelial macrophages in a minimally raised lesion. Advanced fatty streak lesions were elevated with several layers of macrophages. The organization of peripheral junctional actin (the DPB) and of central endothelial-cell actin-microfilament bundles was studied in each of these lesions using fluorescent microscopy. We found that in the aorta away from branch sites and in areas away from lesions the central microfilament distribution was unaffected by hypercholesterolemia. The macrophages entered the wall without any identifiable reorganization in the microfilaments. During the accumulation of subendothelial macrophages in minimal and intermediate lesions stress fibers were initially increased in comparison with lesion-free areas. In raised advanced lesions, however, the central microfilaments became thinner and disappeared. However, at flow dividers, where central stress fibers are normally prominent, endothelial cells on the surface of inter-mediate lesions showed a reduction in central fibers, and peripheral bands became prominent. This was associated with changes in cell shape from elongated to cobblestone cells. Thus, actin microfilament bundles in endothelial cells underwent substantial changes in distribution during the accumulation of subendothelial macrophages, forming hypercholesterolemia-induced fatty streak-type lesions. These changes may influence repair after injury and promote atherogenesis.

## 6 Hemodynamic Effects on Endothelial Wound Repair

We decreased blood flow rates and shear stresses in common carotid arteries of rabbits by ligating the ipsilateral external carotid artery [39]. After 24 h of decreas-ed flow, endothelial cells were less elongated, contained fewer central microfila-ment bundles and showed less polarity of the centrosome toward the heart when compared with endothelial cells in carotid arteries with normal flow. To examine endothelial wound repair, we made narrow longitudinal intimal wounds at the time of flow reduction using a nylon monofilament device. In arteries with normal blood flow, endothelial cells at the edge of the wound initially spread and elongat-ed in the direction of the wound. The DPB of actin was attenuated and central microfilaments became more prominent. Endothelial cells remained in close contact with their neighbors in the monolayer. The centrosome of cells adjacent to the wound was redistributed toward the wound side of the nucleus at 6 h and 12 h. Complete closure occurred by 24 h, at which time the elongated endothelial cells covering the wound were organized in a herringbone pattern with their down-stream ends at the center of the wound. With decreased flow and shear stress, the cells at the wound edge spread less than those in normal vessels at 12 h after wounding and were randomly oriented and polygonal in shape. Also, re-endo-thelialization proceeded more slowly and there was a marked reduction of central microfilaments in cells at the wound edge. At 24 h, the wounds were still open, the endothelial cells covering the central portion of the wound did not maintain inti-mate contact with their neighbors, and orientation of the centrosome toward the wound was reduced. We hypothesize that loss of cell–cell contact during repair at low flow rates and low shear stress disrupts intercellular communication and results in disruption of cytoskeletal reorganization during repair, thereby, slowing the repair process [38].

## 7 Regulation of Endothelial Wound Repair

It is likely that there are numerous soluble factors that regulate repair in addition to the hemodynamic shear stress we described above. In the face of small denuding injuries, the large-vessel endothelium undergoes a process of rapid repair involv-ing actin microfilaments, microtubules, and centrosomes, to re-establish an intact monolayer. It was hypothesized that increased susceptibility to atherosclerosis in diabetes mellitus may be due, in part, to delayed re-endothelialization following endothelial injury. To test this, the effects of high insulin concentrations on the re-endothelialization of small wounds was examined using an in vitro porcine aortic endothelial-cell wound model. Elevated concentrations of insulin did not disrupt the confluent endothelial monolayer or alter endothelial cell shape. Insulin also did not induce detectable alterations in the distribution of microtubules and microfilaments in the confluent monolayer. High insulin did not reduce the extent of re-endothelialization of a linear wound made in the confluent monolayer. Centrosomal reorientation was similar to that of control wounded cultures, as was the reorganization of the microfilaments and microtubules. The data suggest that the atherogenic effects of hyperinsulinemia may not be due to disruption of endothelial repair.

Matrix composition is also an important regulator of large-vessel endothelial migration. Fibronectin reduces the rate of wound repair, while collagen I and III promote it [31].

Fibroblast growth factor (FGF-2) has been shown to be an endogenous regulator, but not the only regulator of endothelial migration in repairing wounds [2]. Exogenous FGF-2 has been shown to embrace migration and repair as well [33]. It has been shown that endothelial cell movement stimulated by FGF-2 is mediated by a pertussis toxin-sensitive pathway regulating phospholipase $A_2$ activity.

Rapid, efficient repair of the endothelium following focal endothelial wounding and denudation is regulated by a complex series of cellular processes. Directed cell migration, an early essential event in repair, is thought to be initiated by centrosome redistribution towards the front of the cell prior to the onset of migration. Therefore, centrosomal polarity may be an important regulatory event in directed endothelial cell migration. We have shown that transient inhibition of translation and transcription at the time of wounding disrupts rapid repair by interfering with centrosome redistribution to the front of the cell [9]. One of the signals that promotes transcription is the release of FGF-2 from the cells at the time of wounding [10].

To study this, in vitro wounds were created down the middle of confluent porcine aortic endothelial monolayers by mechanical denudation. Conditioned media collected at 1 h, but not at 24 h, after wounding contained FGF-2 (bFGF). Antibodies directed against FGF-2, added to the cultures at the time of wounding, significantly inhibited cell migration and transiently inhibited centrosome redistribution. When transcription was transiently inhibited with actinomycin D, present at 1 h before and for 1 h after wounding, the cells moved more slowly taking five times longer for the wound to close. Throughout this period, centrosomes did not reorient to the front of the cells. When either recombinant FGF-2 or conditioned media collected from control cultures at 1 h after wounding was added at 23 h after actinomycin D was washed out (at which time RNA synthesis returned to control levels), the centrosomes redistributed to the front of the cells and cells migrated at a rapid rate similar to control. However, the recombinant FGF-2 or conditioned media had no effect when added immediately after actinomycin D was removed, when RNA synthesis was still inhibited. Thus, FGF-2 initiates centrosome redistribution by stimulating processes that lead to the transcription of an as yet unknown essential gene(s) that is induced immediately following wounding. This appears to be at least one mechanism by which FGF-2 enhances aortic endothelial migration and repair at the site of an endothelial wound.

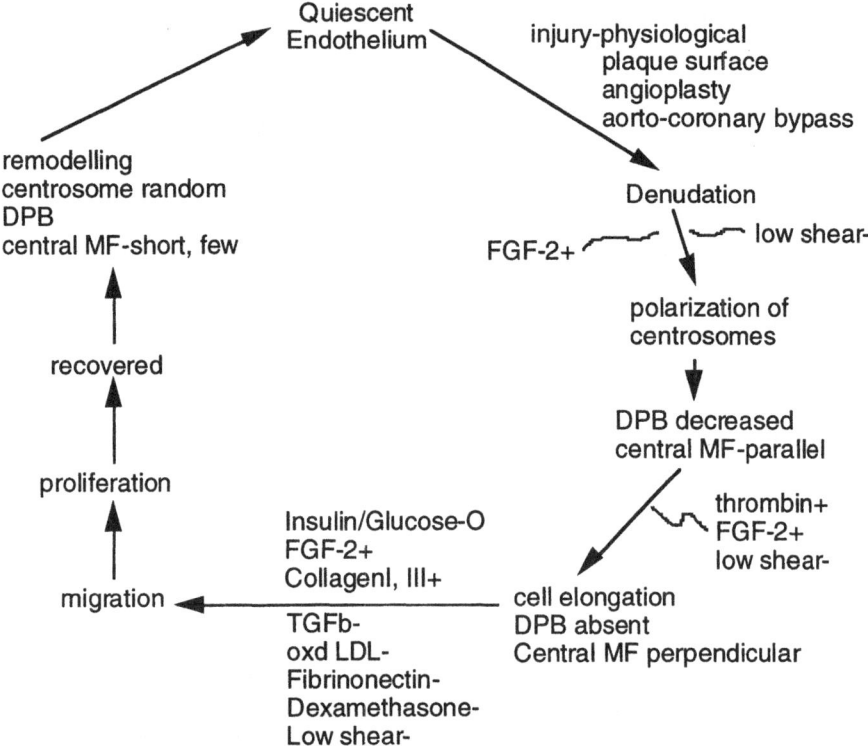

**Fig. 2.** Series of steps characterizing the repair of the vascular endothelium and the restoration of the confluent monolayer and endothelial integrity

Thrombin [8], prednisolone [11], transforming growth factor-$\beta$ (TGF$\beta$) and low-density lipoprotein (LDL) have been reported to delay in vitro endothelial repair [17]. Thrombin inhibited human iliac artery endothelial-cell monolayer repair and proliferation after in vitro denuding mechanical injury [8].

We have also found that genistein, a tyrosine kinase inhibitor, and sodium orthovandate, a tyrosine phosphatase inhibitor, inhibited both cell elongation and progression of endothelial cells through the three early stages of endothelial repair described above. Genistein did not have an effect on endothelial cell progression through stage I or II, but had dramatic inhibitory effects on the formation of central microfilaments perpendicular to the wound edge during stage III [29]. Sodium orthovanadate resulted in inhibiting early endothelial repair by disrupting proper actin central-microfilament formation in each of the early stages (unpublished data). Thus, tyrosine kinase and phosphatase activity may be critical in the regulation and progression of early endothelial wound repair.

Our studies have shown that endothelial repair (Fig. 2) is a complex dynamic process, which is closely associated with the cytoskeleton and is regulated by several soluble extracellular factors, as well as the matrix on which the cells reside.

# References

1. Albelda SM, Buck CA (1990) Integrins and other cell adhesion molecules. FASEB J 4: 2868–2880
2. Biro S, Yu Z-X, Fu Y-M, Smale G, Sasse J, Sanchez J, Ferrans VJ, Casscells W (1994) Expression of subcellular distribution of basic fibroblast growth factor are regulated during migration of endothelial cells. Circ Res 74:485–494
3. Caplan BA, Schwartz CJ (1973) Increase endothelial turnover in areas of in vivo Evans blue uptake in the pig aorta. Atherosclerosis 17:401–417
4. Colangelo S, Langille BL, Gotlieb AI (1994) Endothelial microfilament distribution in the immediate vicinity of arterial branch sites. Cell Tissue Res 278:235–242
5. Colangelo S, Langille BL, Steiner G, Gotlieb AI (1998) Alterations in endothelial F-actin microfilaments in rabbit aorta in hypercholesterolemia. Arterioscler Thromb Vasc Biol 18:52–56
6. Coomber BL, Gotlieb AI (1990) In vitro endothelial wound repair: interaction of cell migration and proliferation. Arteriosclerosis 10:215–222
7. Dejana E, Corada M, Lampugnani MG (1995) Endothelial cell-to-cell junctions. FASEB J 9:910–918
8. DiMuzio PJ, Pratt KJ, Park PK, Carabasi RA (1994) Role of thrombin in endothelial cell monolayer repair in vitro. J Vasc Surg 20:621–628
9. Ettenson D, Gotlieb AI (1993) In vitro large-wound re-endothelialization. Arterioscler Thromb 13:1270–1281
10. Ettenson D, Gotlieb AI (1995) Basic fibroblast growth factor is a signal for the initiation of centrosome redistribution to the front of migrating endothelial cells at the edge of an in vitro wound. Arterioscler Thromb Vasc Biol 15:515–521
11. Fyfe AI, Rosenthal A, Gotlieb AI (1995) Immunosuppresive agents and endothelial repair: prednisolone delays migration and cytoskeletal rearrangement in wounded porcine aortic monolayers. Arterioscler Thromb Vasc Biol 15:1166–1171
12. Garlanda C, Deja E (1997) Heterogeneity of endothelial cells. Arterioscler Thromb Vasc Biol 17:1193–1202
13. Gotlieb AI, Langille BL, Wong MKK, Kim DW (1991) Structure and function of the endothelial cytoskeleton. Lab Invest 65:123–127
14. Gotlieb AI, McBurnie-May LM, Subrahmanyan L, Kalnins VI (1981) Distribution of microtubule organizing centers in migrating sheets of endothelial cells. J Cell Biol 91:589–594
15. Gotlieb AI, Spector W, Wong MKK, Lacey C (1984) In vitro reendothelialization: microfilament bundle redistribution in a migrating sheet of porcine endothelial cells. Arteriosclerosis 4:91–96
16. Gotlieb AI, Subrahmanyan L, Kalnins VI (1983) Microtubule organizing centers and cell migration: effects of inhibition of migration and microtubule disruption in endothelial cells. J Cell Biol 96:1266–1272
17. Heimark RL, Twardzki DR, Schwartz S (1986) Inhibition of endothelial regeneration by type-beta transforming growth factor from platelet. Science 233:1078–1080
18. Heimark RL, Degner M, Schwartz SM (1990) Identification of a Ca$^{2+}$-dependent cell-cell adhesion molecule in endothelial cells. J Cell Biol 110:1745–1756
19. Hinsbergh VWM (1997) Endothelial permeability for macromolecules. Arterioscler Thromb Vasc Biol 17:1018–1023
20. Hüttner I, Boutet M, More RH (1973) Studies on protein passage through arterial endothelium: II. regional differences in permeability to fine structural protein tracers in arterial endothelium of normotensive rat. Lab Invest 28:678–685
21. Introna M, Mantovani A (1997) Early activation signals in endothelial cells; stimulation by cytokines. Arterioscler Thromb Vasc Biol 17:423–428
22. Kemler R (1993) From cadherins to catenins: cytoplasmic protein interactions and regulation of cell adhesion. Trends Genet 9:317–321
23. Kim DW, Gotlieb AI, Langille BL (1989a) In vivo modulation of endothelial F-actin microfilaments by experimental alterations in shear stress. Arteriosclerosis 9:439–445

24. Kim DW, Langille BL, Wong MKK, Gotlieb AI (1989b) Patterns of endothelial microfilament distribution in the rabbit aorta in situ. Circ Res 64:21–31
25. Kreis TE, Birchmeier W (1980) Stress fibre sarcomeres of fibroblasts are contractile. Cell 22:555–561
26. Kupfer A, Louvard D, Singer SJ (1982) Polarization of the Golgi apparatus and the micro-tubule-organizing center in cultured fibroblasts at the edge of an experimental wound. Proc Natl Acad Sci U S A 79:2603–2607
27. Langille BL, Adamson SL (1981) Relationship between blood flow direction and endothelial cell orientation at arterial branch sites in rabbits and mice. Circ Res 48:481–488
28. Lee TYJ, Rosenthal A, Gotlieb AI (1996) The transition of aortic endothelial cells from resting to migrating cells is associated with three sequential patterns of microfilament organization. J Vasc Res 33:13–24
29. Lee T-Y J, Gotlieb AI (1996) Genistein inhibits cell elongation during the initiation of endo-thelial wound repair (abstract). FASEB J 10:A1001
30. Lin S-J, Jan K-M, Weinbaum S, Chien S (1989) Transendothelial transport of low density lipoprotein in association with cell mitosis in rat aorta. Arteriosclerosis 9:230–236
31. Madri JA, Bell L, Marx M, Mervin JR, Basson C, Prinz C (1991) Effects of soluble factors and extracellular matrix components on vascular cell behavior in vitro and in vivo: models of de-endothelialization and repair. J Cell Biochem 45:123–130
32. Rojanasakul Y, Robinson JR (1991) The cytoskeleton of the cornea and its role in tight junc-tion permeability. Int J Pharm 68:135–149
33. Sato Y, Rafkin DB (1988) Autocrine activities of basic fibroblast growth factor: regulation of endothelial cell movement, plasminogen, activator synthesis, and DNA synthesis. J Cell Biol 107:1199–1205
34. Shasby DM, Shasby SS, Sullivan JM, Peach MJ (1982) Role of endothelial cell cytoskeleton in control of endothelial permeability. Circ Res 51:657–661
35. Singer I (1982) Association of fibronectin and vinculin with focal contacts and stress fibers in vascular endothelial cells in vivo. J Cell Biol 92:398–408
36. Stary HC, Blankenhorn D, Chandler AB, Glagov S, Insull W Jr, Richardson M, Rosenfeld ME, Schaffer SA, Schwartz CJ, Wagner WD, Wissler RW (1992) A definition of the intima of human arteries and its atherosclerotic-prone regions. Circulation 85:391–405
37. Volk T, Geiger B (1984) A 135-kd membrane protein of intercellular adherens junctions. EMBO J 3:2249–2260
38. Vyalov S, Langille BL, and Gotlieb AI (1996) Low shear stress disrupts repair processes and slows in vivo reendothelialization: effects of shear stress. Am J Pathol 149:2107–2118
39. Walpola PL, Gotlieb AI, Langille BL (1993) Monocyte adhesion and changes in endothelial cell number, morphology and F-actin distribution elicited by low shear stress in vivo. Am J Pathol 142:1392–1400
40. Wong AJ, Pollard TD, Herman IM (1983) Actin filament stress fibers in vascular endothelial cells in vivo. Science 219:867–869
41. Wong MKK, Gotlieb AI (1984) In vitro reendothelialization of single cell wound: role of microfilament bundles in rapid lamellipodia- mediated wound closure. Lab Invest 51:75–81
42. Wong MKK, Gotlieb AI (1988) The reorganization of microfilaments, centrosomes, and microtubules during in vitro small wound reendothelialization. J Cell Biol 107:1777–1783
43. Wong MKK, Gotlieb AI (1990) Endothelial monolayer integrity: perturbation of F-actin filaments and the DPB vinculin network. Arteriosclerosis 10:76–84
44. Wong MKK, Gotlieb AI (1984) In vitro reendothelialization of a single cell wound: Role of microfilament bundles in rapid lamellipodia mediated wound closure. Lab Invest 51:75–81
45. Wong MKK, Gotlieb AI (1986) Endothelial cell monolayer integrity I. Characterization of dense peripheral band of microfilaments. Arteriosclerosis 6:212–219
46. Wong MKK, Gotlieb AI (1988) The reorganization of microfilaments, centrosomes, and microtubules during in vitro small wound reendothelialization. J Cell Biol 107:1777–1783

# Glomerulosclerosis: The Role of Interstitial Myofibroblasts in its Progression

M. El Nahas, E. C. Muchaneta-Kubara, N. Tamimi, D. Goumenos

## 1 Introduction

The progression of chronic renal failure (CRF) and the associated renal scarring often lead inexorably to end-stage renal insufficiency with patients requiring dialysis replacement therapy. Considerable research has focused over the last quarter century on the study and understanding of the mechanisms of renal scarring, in particular glomerulosclerosis. Less research and emphasis have been put on the study and the relevance of tubulointerstitial scarring leading to the progression of CRF, not to mention vascular sclerosis, which has received scanty attention.

In this review, I would like to explore the possibility that glomerulosclerosis evolves through and under the influence of renal interstitial and vascular factors. In particular, I will put forward a hypothesis linking the progression of glomerulosclerosis to the proliferation of interstitial myofibroblasts, including those derived from the perivascular adventitia, thus linking vascular sclerosis, interstitial fibrosis and glomerulosclerosis.

## 2 Glomerulosclerosis: The Intrinsic Pathway

Glomerulosclerosis takes place following a wide range of glomerular injuries; immune and non-immune mediated. Glomerulosclerosis is likely to be initiated by damage to the glomerular endothelial lining [20]. Endothelial injury would lead to phenotypic and functional changes of endothelial cells, leading to the attraction of platelets and leukocytes into the glomerular capillaries, their activation, adhesion and infiltration of glomerular tufts [20]. Interactions would then be initiated between infiltrating cells and resident ones through the paracrine and juxtacrine release of cytokines, chemokines and growth factors [20]. This may contribute to the proliferation of mesangial cells and the expansion of the mesangial extracellular matrix (ECM) leading to mesangiosclerosis [13]. It is also likely that

Current Topics in Pathology, Volume 93
A. Desmoulière, B. Tuchweber (Eds.)
© Springer-Verlag Berlin Heidelberg 1999

glomerulosclerosis is precipitated by damage to the glomerular epithelial cells with their distortion, stretching and the denudation of the underlying basement membrane favouring excessive trafficking of macromolecules [18].

The progression of glomerulosclerosis and the associated damage to its cell lines (endothelial, mesangial and epithelial) is associated with the neo-expression or upregulation of a range of cytoskeletal proteins including $\alpha$-smooth muscle actin ($\alpha$-SMA) [9]. We and others have observed that experimental diabetic nephropathy is associated with the neo-expression of vimentin within glomerular endothelial cells [19]. Some have suggested that vimentin plays an important role in the regulation of the glomerular response to injury [24]. Vimentin-null mice seem to be incapable of glomerular vasodilatation in response to renal ablation, suggesting a heightened vasoconstrictive response to endothelin [24]. We also noted the neo-expression of $\alpha$-SMA by mesangial cells in the course of experimental and clinical nephropathies [9]. Such expression is associated with progressive glomerulosclerosis in an experimental model of accelerated glomerulonephritis [30]. Similarly, epithelial cells appear to express cytoskeletal proteins, such as vimentin and desmin, in response to injury [9]. The expression of these cytoskeletal proteins and filaments by glomerular cells is likely to reflect phenotypic changes [9]. The full implication of these changes and their contribution to the progression of glomerulosclerosis remain to be elucidated.

Glomerulosclerosis is not invariably progressive though, as there are examples to suggest that it can be reversible. This is certainly the case in the anti-thy 1.1 model of experimental glomerulonephritis, in which the accumulation of mesangial matrix is reversible, probably under the influence of glomerular collagenases (matrix metalloproteinases; MMPs) [17]. It is only when repeated injections of the anti-mesangial (thy 1.1) antibody are given, that progressive glomerulosclerosis takes place in association with tubulointerstitial changes [29]. This is consistent with other observations in experimental models of renal diseases, where the progression of CRF only takes place when there is associated tubulointerstitial changes, including inflammation and fibrosis [8]. This suggests that glomerulosclerosis in the absence of tubulointerstitial fibrosis may be self-limited and even irreversible. This raises the question as to how is the progression of glomerulosclerosis influenced by tubulointerstitial fibrosis.

## 3 Glomerulosclerosis: The Extrinsic Pathway

The extrinsic pathway of glomerulosclerosis stipulates an invasion of scarred glomeruli by interstitial myofibroblasts. This would give a primary role for interstitial fibrosis in the pathogenesis of glomerulosclerosis. This is consistent with the relevance of tubulointerstitial changes to the progression of CRF; it is well known that parameters of tubulointerstitial changes, such as tubular atrophy, interstitial inflammation and fibrosis, are all strong predictors of renal function and its decline [1]. Progressive renal failure is associated with severe tubular atrophy. Such tubular changes are characterised by necrosis and apoptosis of tubular cells [21]. Ultimately, these cells slough off into the tubular lumen. We and others have noted that tubular injury, atrophy and regeneration are associated with the dedifferentiation of tubular cells with the associated expression of vimentin [16]. However, the relevance of vimentin to these changes has been questioned through the observations that vimentin-null mice have a normal tubular regeneration in response to injury [25]. A major role for tubular cells in the initiation and progression of tubulointerstitial fibrosis may be mediated by the capacity of these cells to act as antigen-presenting cells. Furthermore, they are capable of releasing chemokines, cytokines and growth factors, as well as activating adjacent interstitial fibroblasts [15]. Tubular cells also have the capacity to respond to autacoids, such as angiotensin II [28], and growth factors, such as platelet-derived growth factor (PDGF) and transforming growth factor-$\beta$ (TGF-$\beta$) [28], by increasing their synthesis and release of collagen. They have also been shown to respond to exposure to serum proteins, as in proteinuric states, by enhanced synthesis of growth factors and ECM components [3].

Tubular cells are also capable of modulating the behaviour of adjacent quiescent interstitial fibroblasts. They have been shown in co-culture conditions to stimulate [14] and inhibit [11] the proliferation of interstitial renal fibroblasts. The activation of quiescent renal fibroblasts stimulates their acquisition of myofibroblastic characteristics, including the expression of $\alpha$-SMA and that of cytoskeletal proteins [9, 10].

Vascular adventitia may be another source of activated interstitial fibroblasts. In experimental models of interstitial renal fibrosis, it has been demonstrated that these cells produce interstitial collagen and seem to diffuse out of renal vessels into the interstitium [27]. A link between renal interstitial fibrosis and vascular injury and sclerosis is tempting as hypertensive and ischemic renal injury are both associated with interstitial renal fibrosis. Damage to vascular endothelial cells, in the presence of optimal growth factors in the adventitia, leads to the expansion and proliferation of vascular pericytes [7]. These may, in turn, contribute to renal interstitial fibrosis and ultimately to glomerulosclerosis, as they seem to diffuse into the interstitium and, subsequently, to accumulate around renal tubules and glomeruli [9, 10]. These cells are also capable of the synthesis of fibrogenic growth factors, collagens and their regulating enzymes [23]. Interstitial fibrosis would lead to the strangulation of renal arterioles, causing further ischemia and renal fibrosis [2].

But how would interstitial myofibroblasts cause glomerulosclerosis? This is done through direct and indirect pathways; directly, by invading the Bowman's space through breaks in Bowman's capsule [26]. This was described many years ago in a variety of chronic glomerular diseases in humans, where breaks in Bowman's capsule and adhesions allowed the infiltration of the glomerular tuft by interstitial fibroblasts and the deposition of interstitial collagen type III within scarred glomeruli [26]. These observations have since been confirmed in experimental and clinical nephropathies [9, 26]. Fibroblasts may be attracted into Bowman's space by chemotactic growth factors or even chemotactic components of the ECM such as fibronectin. Indirectly, interstitial myofibroblasts could accelerate glomerulosclerosis through the narrowing of renal arterioles, including those feeding the glomeruli contributing to their ischemia and sclerosis.

It is, therefore, important to appreciate that glomerulosclerosis is unlikely to evolve in isolation. More plausible is the possibility that glomerulosclerosis is the end product of complex interactions between the glomeruli, renal tubules, interstitium and vessels. Such a concept may open the way to novel therapeutic approaches based on the manipulation of interstitial myofibroblasts and aimed at the prevention of renal scarring and glomerulosclerosis.

## 4 Therapeutic Implications

Interventions aimed directly or indirectly at myofibroblast activation and proliferation are worthy of investigation. Indirectly, the inhibition of autacoids (angiotensin II) [12] and growth factors (PDGF [22] and TGF-$\beta$1 [5]) known to activate myofibroblasts have been proved protective in experimental models. Similarly, heparin administration has been proved to be protective in experimental renal disease, an effect possibly mediated by the inhibitory action of this proteoglycan on myofibroblasts [4]. Gamma-interferon is also a potent inhibitor of myofibroblasts' activation [4]. Preliminary data from our research laboratory suggest a protective effect during the course of experimental renal scarring through a reduction in the number of activated myofibroblasts [31]. Finally, a better understanding of the control of myofibroblasts' proliferation, survival and death [6] may open the way to therapies based on the manipulation of apoptosis.

## References

1. Bohle A, Strutz F, Muller GA (1994) On the pathogenesis of chronic renal failure in primary glomerulopathies: a view from the interstitium. Exp Nephrol 2:205–210
2. Bohle A, von Gise H, Mackensen-Haen S, Stark-Kakob B (1981) The obliteration of postglomerular capillaries and its influence upon the function of both glomeruli and tubules. Klinische Wochenschrift 59:1043–1051
3. Burton C, Walls J (1994) Proximal tubular cells, proteinuria and tubulointerstitial scarring. Nephron 68:287–293
4. Desmouliere A, Gabbiani G (1994) Modulation of fibroblastic cytoskeletal features during pathological situations: the role of extracellular matrix and cytokines. Cell Motil Cytoskeleton 29:195–203
5. Desmouliere A, Geinoz A, Gabbiani F, Gabbiani G (1993) Transforming growth factor-$\beta$1 induces a-smooth muscle actin expression in granulation tissue myofibroblasts and in quiescent and growing fibroblasts. J Cell Biol 112:1103–1111
6. Desmouliere A, Redard M, Darby I, Gabbiani G (1995) Apoptosis mediates the decrease in cellularity during the transition between granulation tissue and scar. Am J Pathol 146:56–66
7. Edelman ER, Nugent MA, Smith LT, Karnovsky MJ (1992) Basic fibroblast growth factor enhances the coupling of intimal hyperplasia and proliferation of vasa vasorum in injured rat arteries. J Clin Invest 89:465–473
8. El Nahas AM (1997) Mechanisms of experimental and clinical renal scarring. In: Oxford Textbook of Clinical Nephrology, Oxford University Press, pp 1749–1788
9. El Nahas AM, Muchaneta-Kubara EC, Zhang G-Z, Adam A, Goumenos D (1996) Phenotypic modulation of renal cells during experimental and clinical renal scarring. Kidney Int 49[suppl 54]:S23–S27
10. Goumenos D, Brown CB, Shortland J, El Nahas AM (1994) Myofibroblasts and the progression of IgA nephropathy. Nephrol Dial Transpl 9:1418–1425
11. Grupp C, Lottermoser J, Cohen DI, Begher M, Franz H-E, Muller GA (1997) Transformation of rat inner medullary fibroblasts to myofibroblasts in vitro. Kidney Int 52:1279–1290

12. Johnson RJ, Alpers CE, Yoshimura A, Lombardi D, Pritzl P, Floege J, Schwartz SM (1992) Renal injury from angiotensin II-mediated hypertension. Hypertension 19:464–474
13. Kashgarian M, Sterzel RB (1992) The pathobiology of the mesangium. Kidney Int 41: 524–529
14. Knecht A, Fine LG, Kleinman KS (1991) Fibroblasts of rabbit kidney in culture.II. Paracrine stimulation of papillary fibroblasts by PDGF. Am J Physiol 261:F292–F299
15. Kuncio GS, Neilson EG, Haverty T (1991) Mechanisms of tubulointerstitial fibrosis. Kidney Int 39:550–556
16. Muchaneta-Kubara EC, El Nahas AM (1997) Myofibroblast phenotypes expression in experimental renal scarring. Nephrol Dial Transpl 12:904–915
17. Okuda S, Languino LR, Ruoslahti E, Border WA (1990) Elevated expression of transforming growth factor-$\beta$ and proteoglycan production in experimental glomerulonephritis. J Clin Invest 86:453–462
18. Rennke HG (1993) How does glomerular epithelial cell injury contributes to progressive glomerular damage? Kidney Int 45[suppl 45]:S58–S63
19. Sanai T, Muchaneta-Kubara EC, Oldroyd S, Thomas G, Sobka T, El Nahas AM (1998) Expression of intermediate filament proteins during the course of experimental diabetic nephropathy. Nephrol Dial Transpl (in press)
20. Savage COS (1994) The biology of the glomerulus: endothelial cells. Kidney Int 45:314–319
21. Sugiyama H, Kashihara N, Makino H, Yamazaki Y, Ota Z (1996) Apoptosis in glomerular sclerosis. Kidney Int 49:103–111
22. Tang WW, Hill DC, Tarpley JE, Van GY, Qi M (1995) PDGF-B is associated with myofibroblast formation in a-GBM Ab tubulointerstitial nephritis (TIN) (abstract). J Am Soc Nephrol 6:913
23. Tang WW, Van GY, Qi M (1997) Myofibroblasts and $\alpha$1 (III) collagen expression in experimental tubulointerstitial nephritis. Kidney Int 51:926–931
24. Terzi F, Henrion E, Colucci-Guyon E, Babinet C, Briand P, Levy B, Friedlander G (1996) Subotal nephrectomy (Nx) is lethal in vimentin-null mice: role of endothelin. J Am Soc Nephrol 7:1574
25. Terzi F, Maunoury R, Colucci-Guyon E, Friedlander G (1997) Normal tubular and differentiation of the post-ischemic kidney in mice lacking vimentin. Am J Pathol 150:1361–1371
26. Striker L M-M, Killen PD, Chi E, Striker GE (1984) The composition of glomerulosclerosis: 1. studies in focal sclerosis, crescentic glomerulonephritis and membranoproliferative glomerulonephritis. Lab Invest 51:181–192
27. Wiggins RC, Goyal M, Merritt SE, Killen PD (1993) Vascular adventitial expression of collagen I messenger ribonucleic acid in anti-glomerular basement membrane antibody-induced nephritis in the rabbit. A cellular source for interstitial collagen synthesis in inflammatory renal disease. Lab Invest 68:557–565
28. Wolf G, Zahner G, Schroeder R, Stahl RAK (1996) Transforming growth factor-$\beta$ mediated angiotensin II-induced stimulation of collagen type IV synthesis in cultured murine proximal tubular cells. Nephrol Dial Transpl 11:263–269
29. Yamamoto T, Noble NA, Miller DE, Border WA (1994) Sustained expression of TGF-$\beta$1 underlies development of progressive kidney fibrosis. Kidney Int 45:916–927
30. Zhang G, Moorhead PJ, El Nahas AM (1995) Myofibroblasts and the progression of experimental glomerulonephritis. Exp Nephrol 3:308–318
31. Oldroyd S, Thomas G, El Nahas M (1998) Manipulation of experimental renal fibrosis by intra-renal administration of interferon-$\gamma$. J Am Soc Nephrol 9:618(a)

# The Myofibroblast as an Inflammatory Cell in Pulmonary Fibrosis

S. H. Phan, K. Zhang, H. Y. Zhang, M. Gharaee-Kermani

## 1 Introduction

Pulmonary fibrosis is commonly characterized by some degree of inflammation and abnormal tissue repair, resulting in the replacement of normal functional tissue with scar or connective tissue. Current understanding of the pathogenesis of pulmonary fibrosis revolves around the complex interaction of inflammatory and lung structural cells, as mediated by their products, including cytokines, as well as by intimate cell-to-cell interactions that, in turn, are mediated by adhesion molecules and other receptors. As originally envisioned, the inflammatory and, in certain cases, the immune cells are thought to be the source of mediators that are targeted at structural cells (which respond by proliferating and producing extracellular matrix). Progress during the past decade, however, has made untenable this view that structural cells are passive targets. There is now mounting evidence of a more active role for these cells, including that of regulating the inflammatory and immune responses themselves. This paper will review and discuss some of this evidence, in the context of the role of the myofibroblast in pulmonary fibrosis.

## 2 The Myofibroblast in Pulmonary Fibrosis

The appearance de novo of an activated fibroblast phenotype during pulmonary fibrosis is not dissimilar to that at other sites of tissue repair and fibrosis. Thus, lung tissue from patients with pulmonary fibrosis is characterized by the presence of myofibroblast cells that actively synthesize extracellular matrix and cytokines with inflammatory, as well as fibrogenic, activities, such as transforming growth factor beta (TGF$\beta$) [22, 26, 27]. Immunohistochemical evidence suggests an association between the presence of $\alpha$-smooth muscle actin-positive cells within the

Current Topics in Pathology, Volume 93
A. Desmoulière, B. Tuchweber (Eds.)
© Springer-Verlag Berlin Heidelberg 1999

fibrotic foci, and increased cellular collagen expression in these lesions [1, 20, 32]. The circumstantial evidence is strengthened by the demonstration of a correlation between peak collagen gene expression and peak $\alpha$-smooth muscle actin expression in these cells [24, 32, 39]. Furthermore, fibroblasts from fibrotic lesions are known to have greater collagen synthetic capacity than those from control, non-fibrotic, sites [4, 19, 23, 25, 40, 49], although their actin phenotype is unclear. Studies of granulation-tissue myofibroblasts show these cells to express vimentin and $\alpha$-smooth muscle actin, while at the same time exhibiting elevated collagen synthetic capacity [37]. The first direct in vivo evidence that the lung myofibroblast is the primary source of increased procollagen-I gene expression during pulmonary fibrosis comes from studies using combined in situ hybridization to detect collagen and cytokine expression, and immunohistochemistry to detect $\alpha$-smooth muscle actin expression in the same tissue section. These studies unequivocally identify the myofibroblast as the predominant, if not the sole, cellular source of these proteins at distinct stages during the evolution of the response to bleomycin-induced lung injury [53–55, 57]. The pathogenetic significance of the myofibroblast is further supported by the presence of these cells in lung fibrotic lesions induced by the transfection of certain cytokines into rodent lungs [39, 50, 53–55, 57].

In successful tissue repair after injury, subsidence of the synthetic/proliferative phase is accompanied by the gradual disappearance of the myofibroblast. This is also seen in a model of lung injury with self-limiting pulmonary fibrosis. In this rodent model of bleomycin-induced pulmonary fibrosis, the active fibrosis phase lasts for approximately 3 weeks after induction of lung injury, after which it subsides, sparing enough residual unaffected lung tissue for the animal to survive [39, 50, 53–55, 57]. As the fibrosis subsides, the myofibroblasts, and cytokine and collagen expression subside [55, 57], thus providing further association between myofibroblasts and active fibrosis.

The myofibroblast has also been identified as the cell responsible for wound contraction. Increased contractility or decreased lung compliance is another known feature of fibrotic lung tissue, whose development also correlates with the emergence of myofibroblasts [1, 32]. This property can be manifested in vitro by the enhanced ability of myofibroblasts to contract collagen gels when compared with cells expressing lower levels of $\alpha$-smooth muscle actin [52].

Taken together, these findings strongly implicate the myofibroblast as a key cell in the pathogenesis of pulmonary fibrosis; it appears de novo at fibrotic sites, and has the capacity to regulate, directly and indirectly, many of the hallmarks of this process, including inflammation, elevated cytokine expression, excessive extracellular matrix deposition and increased contractility. In addition to elaboration of cytokines and other inflammatory/immune mediators, the myofibroblast also responds to many of these same mediators. Its demise is associated with resolution of the active fibrosis phase. Many of these properties resemble those attributed to cells of the inflammatory system; hence, a comparative analysis of these properties in myofibroblasts and inflammatory cells may be instructive in further delineating the in vivo role of the myofibroblast in pulmonary fibrosis. The following discussion will examine each of these aspects to highlight the similarities.

## 3 The Emergence of the Myofibroblast

Considering the potential importance of the myofibroblast in pulmonary fibrosis, understanding the mechanism for its emergence should provide some insight into the initiation and propagation of the fibrotic process. The presence of the myofibroblast has already been shown to signify likely progression to renal failure in membranous nephropathy [42]. The de novo emergence of this cell is, in some ways, similar to the recruitment of inflammatory cells to sites of tissue injury, in the sense that they are not normally present at such tissue sites. Furthermore, the recruited inflammatory cells undergo certain phenotypic alterations when recruited to such sites, in a manner that resembles the differentiation of fibroblasts to myofibroblasts – namely, the induction of cytokine/chemokine expression. Presumably, this activation or differentiation event is under the influence of the cytokines that these cells are, themselves, capable of producing. However, there are certain features of the myofibroblast phenotype that are helpful in understanding the genesis of this cell.

This discussion hinges on the frequent observation that fibroblasts are heterogeneous with respect to a number of parameters [41]. Of relevance to this discussion is the existence of a type of fibroblast, referred to as a myofibroblast on the basis of its ultrastructural features, that contains elements found in both smooth muscle cells and fibroblasts [14, 15, 30]. Ultrastructurally, these cells exhibit dense aggregates of microfilaments and specialized contacts with adjacent myofibroblasts and the extracellular matrix [15]. Cells with similar characteristics have been identified in other fibrotic conditions, including pulmonary fibrosis [1, 20, 32, 45]. These cells emerge with a distinct time course that correlates with the proliferative phase and contraction of the wound, after which they gradually disappear [6, 45]. The cytoskeletal phenotype described in fibrotic lungs is reported to be positive for $\alpha$-smooth muscle actin and vimentin, but negative for desmin, i. e., they possess the VA phenotype. This is in contrast to the lung smooth muscle cells, which also express desmin [27, 46].

In normal rat lungs, the smooth muscle cells surrounding blood vessels and airways represent the major cell type positive for the $\alpha$-smooth muscle actin isotype, with some staining also seen in septal tip cells and pericytes [27, 32]. In both animal models and human patients, pulmonary fibrosis is associated with the appearance of a new population of $\alpha$-smooth muscle actin positive cells (VA phenotype), in the interstitium and in the intra-alveolar foci of fibrosis [1, 13, 32]. These myofibroblasts have been isolated from the bronchoalveolar lavage fluid of patients with scleroderma, but not from fluid from healthy control subjects [29]. In bleomycin-induced pulmonary fibrosis, significant numbers of these cells become prominent toward the end of the first week, when increased collagen gene expression has also been noted [1, 32].

Despite these suggestive observations, the genesis of the myofibroblast in fibrotic tissues remains an unresolved issue. The possible cells of origin include the fibroblast, the smooth muscle cells of adjacent blood vessels or airways, and the pericyte [28, 45]. More definitive in vitro studies favor the fibroblast as the likely originating cell for the myofibroblast, on the basis of biochemical and morphological evidence [8, 9, 38]. The lack of desmin staining in myofibroblasts of fibrotic lungs argues against the smooth muscle cell as the cell of origin, and favors the fibroblast – and perhaps the pericyte – as the cell of origin [28].

Other studies indicate that myofibroblast cells likely emerge from fibroblasts in the adventitial areas surrounding the small airways and adjacent blood vessels [55, 57]. This conclusion is based on the lack of $\alpha$-smooth muscle actin expression in these cells prior to day 3 after induction of pulmonary fibrosis by endotracheal bleomycin injection, which argues against the pericyte as the cell of origin. This is supported by a recent study of hyperoxic pulmonary hypertension, in which the contractile cells appearing in the walls of lung microvessels appear to be derived from interstitial fibroblasts that migrate from adjacent adventitia [21]. These cells subsequently acquire contractile properties consistent with myofibroblasts. The time course of appearance of these cells and their clear distinction from pre-existing pericytes and smooth muscle cells in the vessel wall support the conclusion that myofibroblasts emerge from pre-existing adventitial fibroblasts [55, 57].

More convincing evidence comes from in vitro studies. Fibroblasts, including cell lines, in tissue culture are heterogeneous with respect to $\alpha$-smooth muscle actin staining, with a range of 0–50% of cells being positive in recent studies [8, 52]. This heterogeneity is initially interpreted as being due to contamination by smooth muscle cells. However, when these cells are cloned, the cloned subpopulations still maintain this heterogeneity with respect to expression of the actin isotype [8]. This is consistent with the suggestion that environmental factors associated with the cell culture conditions may be important for expression of $\alpha$-smooth muscle actin [34] and, hence, for the emergence of the myofibroblast phenotype. It also indicates that these actin-positive cells do not result from contamination by smooth muscle cells during the isolation procedures. Taken together, the evidence thus suggests that activation of the fibroblasts by certain regulatory factors can induce their differentiation to myofibroblasts. In the next section, the role of cytokines are considered in this differentiation event.

## 4 Cytokines as Regulators of Myofibroblasts

Inflammatory cells are activated by cytokines and, in the context of highlighting the similarity between myofibroblasts and inflammatory cells, the question that needs to be addressed is whether and how the myofibroblast responds to cytokines. As discussed in the preceding sections, myofibroblasts appear to have several distinct properties that are important in the pathogenesis of pulmonary fibrosis. First, with respect to the differentiation event itself, in vitro studies have shown environmental factors to be important in the emergence of the myofibroblast. Among these factors are cytokines, such as TGF$\beta$ and granulocyte-macrophage colony-stimulating factor (GM-CSF), which are known to upregulate $\alpha$-smooth muscle actin expression, and interferon gamma (IFN$\gamma$) and interleukin (IL)-1$\beta$, which downregulate such expression [7, 8, 33, 34, 43, 51, 52]. Extracellular matrix components, in conjunction with tumor necrosis factor alpha (TNF$\alpha$) treatment, can also affect actin expression [9]. When examined in vivo, neutralization of TNF$\alpha$ inhibits lung TGF$\beta$1 expression, bleomycin-induced pulmonary fibrosis, and the emergence of myofibroblasts [56], thus confirming the importance of TGF$\beta$1 in the genesis of the myofibroblast. Another study found that, despite its ability to stimulate the appearance of myofibroblasts in vivo, GM-CSF is ineffective in vitro for promoting the differentiation of fibroblasts to myofibroblasts [43], suggesting that other factors are involved in the GM-CSF effect on fibroblast actin expression. The available evidence is thus relatively convincing in terms of implicating a role for certain cytokines in the genesis of the myofibroblast.

The presence of myofibroblasts is associated with increased contractility of affected lung tissue, thus implicating these cells in causation of this physiologic alteration [1, 11]. This altered functional property in myofibroblasts is due to elevated endogenous TGFβ1 expression [52], and is consistent with the ability of TGFβ1 to upregulate expression of α-smooth muscle actin [7, 52]. Thus, responsiveness to cytokines can be manifested in enhanced contractility of the fibrotic lung tissue. Other well-characterized responses of fibroblasts to cytokines, which are of special relevance to the pathogenesis of pulmonary fibrosis, include the following. First, there are proliferative effects of many of these cytokines, some of which are known growth factors. Second, there are stimulatory effects on extracellular matrix production. Both of these are key features of the active fibrotic lesion and, with regard to the increased matrix production, in vivo data have already identified the myofibroblast as the predominant cell responsible for collagen gene expression in bleomycin-induced pulmonary fibrosis [55, 57]. A third effect is the chemotactic recruitment of fibroblasts by cytokines such as TGFβ and platelet-derived growth factor (PDGF). Thus, the myofibroblast/fibroblast responds to cytokines in a fashion that is, in many ways, comparable with that of inflammatory cells. Furthermore, these responses are of direct relevance to fibrosis.

## 5  The Myofibroblast as a Source of Cytokines

What is the significance of cytokine production in terms of the similarities between myofibroblasts and inflammatory cells? Inflammatory cells are recruited to sites of tissue injury where, upon activation, they are known to secrete cytokines and other mediators that can enhance the inflammation, tissue injury and recruit other cells. Myofibroblasts are, in a manner of speaking, also recruited to similar sites after the acute inflammatory response. The role of the myofibroblast in elaboration of cytokines is well documented [53, 54] and, as mentioned previously, some of these cytokines appear to be involved in regulating the emergence of the myofibroblast phenotype itself [52]. However, localization of myofibroblasts with respect to fibroblasts is not clear from such studies, since the isolated fibroblasts are likely to be heterogeneous [23, 34, 41, 46]. Nevertheless, in vivo data have shown that cytokine expression is primarily a property of the myofibroblast [53, 54], suggesting that the situation may be comparable in vitro.

Expression of chemotactic cytokines or chemokines, such as monocyte chemo-attractant protein-1 (MCP-1), by isolated fibroblasts can be induced by treatment with inflammatory cytokines such as TNFα [48]. Secretion of such chemokines in vivo would contribute toward the recruitment of leukocytes, such as monocytes and other mononuclear cells, and thus promote inflammation with consequent enhancement of fibrogenic cytokine and growth factor production by the recruited cells. This, in turn, may promote the emergence of additional myofibroblasts, resulting in a positive feedback loop, which would amplify and prolong the fibrosis. Autocrine and paracrine effects of the myofibroblast-derived fibrogenic cytokines, e. g., TGF$\beta$ would, themselves, be expected to play similar amplifying roles as well. These cellular interactions via such complex cytokine networking may be the basis for the progressive disease, resulting in end-stage lung and a fatal outcome. Hence, this property of cytokine expression, which is shared by both inflammatory cells and myofibroblasts, is an important component of the fibrotic process.

## 6 Disappearance of the Myofibroblast

Successful wound repair and self-limited pulmonary fibrosis are characterized by the disappearance of myofibroblasts as the inflammatory and proliferative/synthetic phases subside. In this sense, the myofibroblast also resembles the inflammatory cell, in that the resolution of inflammation is characterized by the disappearance of the inflammatory cells. The mechanism for this disappearance is now known to be due to apoptosis of the inflammatory cells (which are terminally differentiated), although the process can be retarded by the presence of certain cytokines that promote their survival. Does this apply to the mechanism of myofibroblast disappearance? The answer to this question is addressed by recent studies of the role of apoptosis in the disappearance of myofibroblasts [51, 56]. Resolving fibrotic lesions are accompanied by the gradual disappearance of the myofibroblast, presumably by apoptosis [56]. Treatment of fibroblasts with antibodies to the adhesion receptor CD44 induces apoptosis [18]. Even more convincing is the demonstration that the myofibroblast is selectively (with respect to the fibroblast) susceptible to apoptosis when treated with IL-1$\beta$ under serum-free conditions [51]. The same study also suggests that IL-1$\beta$-induced downregulation of $\alpha$-smooth muscle actin expression in isolated lung fibroblasts is due to selective depletion of actin-expressing cells by apoptosis [51]. Such a possibility has parallels in the disappearance of inflammatory cells from resolving sites of inflammation. For example, eosinophils at inflammatory sites undergo apoptosis, which can be prevented by providing a source of certain cytokines, e. g., IL-5 [47].

The apoptotic process is incompletely understood, but is thought to occur via distinct pathways that culminate in a cascade of proteases and in the activation of nucleases that cause DNA degradation [36, 44]. Especially well understood are the mechanisms initiated by binding of Fas ligand (FasL) to its receptor, Fas – a member of the TNF$\alpha$ receptor family – which triggers activation of IL-1$\beta$-converting-enzyme-like (ICE-like) proteases, including cysteine protease P-32 (CPP-32) [36, 44]. Bleomycin-induced apoptosis in hepG2 cells is mediated via this Fas/FasL-initiated pathway [35]. This is consistent with a recent study showing elevated Fas and FasL expression in the lungs of animals with bleomycin-induced pulmonary fibrosis, which was associated with the detection of large numbers of apoptotic nuclei [17].

Of special significance to this discussion is evidence that actin and other cytoskeletal proteins may serve as substrates for apoptotic pathway-associated proteases [5, 16, 31]; this may provide an explanation for the increased susceptibility of actin-expressing cells to apoptosis [51]. The role of inducible NO synthetase (iNOS) in apoptosis has been documented in fibroblasts and in other cells [2, 3, 12, 51], but where it stands relative to these other proteins is unclear. Recent studies also show a yin-yang-type regulation of apoptosis by the Bcl-2 family of proteins with anti-apoptotic activity, and Bax with apoptotic-promoting properties. They appear to be acting upstream of the activation of the apoptotic protease cascade [36, 44]. The significance of this Bcl-2 versus Bax balance in vivo is illustrated by the fact that a balance in favor of Bcl-2 predominance leads to hypertensive vascular wall thickening, presumably by inhibiting apoptosis in the cells comprising this wall [10]. This brief overview clearly indicates that more work needs to be done in this area to fully delineate the apoptotic pathway involved in myofibroblast apoptosis.

## 7 Conclusion

The emergence of myofibroblasts in pulmonary fibrosis accompanies or follows the onset of inflammation, and the subsidence of active fibrosis is associated with the disappearance of these cells. The thesis of this paper is that this behavior and other characteristics of the myofibroblast are reminiscent of cells in the inflammatory system. The recruitment of leukocytes to the site of tissue injury by chemokines and other chemoattractants, their activation/differentiation by these factors as manifested by changes in morphological appearance and production of cytokines, and their disappearance by apoptotic mechanisms, are defining properties of the inflammatory cell. Fibroblasts can clearly be recruited by chemotactic mechanisms in response to certain factors, including cytokines, although their numbers can also increase by cellular proliferation. Their activation or differentiation to myofibroblasts is promoted by cytokines, and results in morphological changes and upregulation with respect to cytokine expression. With regard to their disappearance, there is now mounting evidence for apoptosis as a mechanism for myofibroblast disappearance. Given these similarities, the myofibroblast may therefore be considered an inflammatory cell, based on its ability to elaborate and respond to inflammatory cytokines, the suggestion of terminal differentiation and disappearance via apoptosis. Such a concept may be useful in guiding future studies of the role of the myofibroblast in pulmonary fibrosis.

## References

1. Adler KB, Low RB, Leslie KO, Mitchell J, Evans JN (1989) Biology of disease. Contractile cells in normal and fibrotic lung. Lab Invest 60:473–485
2. Ankarcrona M, Dypbukt J, Brune MB, Nicotera P (1994) Interleukin-1β-induced nitric oxide production activates apoptosis in pancreatic RINm5F cells. Exp Cell Res 213:172–181
3. Blanco FJ, Ochs RL, Schwarz H, Lotz M (1995) Chondrocyte apoptosis induced by nitric oxide. Am J Pathol 146:75–82
4. Breen E, Falco V, Absher M, Cutroneo KR (1990) Subpopulations of rat lung fibroblasts with different amounts of type I and type III collagen mRNAs. J Biol Chem 265:6286–6290

5. Cryns VL, Bergeron L, Zhu H, Li H, Yuan J (1996) Specific cleavage of α-fodrin during Fas- and tumor necrosis factor-induced apoptosis is mediated by an interleukin-1β-converting enzyme/Ced-3 protease distinct from the poly(ADP-ribose) polymerase protease. J Biol Chem 271:31277–31282

6. Darby I, Skalli O, Gabbiani G (1990) α-smooth muscle actin is transiently expressed by myofibroblasts during experimental wound healing. Lab Invest 63:21–29

7. Desmoulière A, Geinoz A, Gabbiani F, Gabbiani G (1993) Transforming growth factor-β1 induces α-smooth muscle actin expression in granulation tissue myofibroblasts and in quiescent and growing cultured fibroblasts. J Cell Biol 122:103–111

8. Desmoulière A, Rubbia-Brandt L, Abdiu A, Walz T, Maciera-Coelho A, Gabbiani G (1992) α-Smooth muscle actin is expressed in a subpopulation of cultured and cloned fibroblasts and is modulated by γ-interferon. Exp Cell Res 201:64–73

9. Desmoulière A, Rubbia-Brandt L, Grau G, Gabbiani G (1992) Heparin induces α-smooth muscle actin expression in cultured fibroblasts and in granulation tissue myofibroblasts. Lab Invest 67:716–725

10. Diez J, Panizo A, Hernandez M, Pardo J (1997) Is the regulation of apoptosis altered in smooth muscle cells of adult spontaneously hypertensive rats? Hypertension 29:776–780

11. Evans JN, Kelly J, Low RB, Adler KB (1982) Increased contractility of isolated lung parenchyma in an animal model of pulmonary fibrosis induced by bleomycin. Am Rev Respir Dis 125:89–94

12. Fehsel K, Kroncke K, Meyer KL, Huber H, Wahn V, Kolb-Bachofen V (1995) Nitric oxide induces apoptosis in mouse thymocytes. J Immunol 155:2858–2866

13. Fukuda Y, Ishizaki M, Masuda Y, Kimura G, Kawanami O, Masugi Y (1987) The role of intraalveolar fibrosis in the process of pulmonary structural remodeling in patients with diffuse alveolar damage. Am J Pathol 126:171–182

14. Gabbiani G, Hirschel BJ, Ryan GB, Statkow PR, Majno G (1972) Granulation tissue as a contractile organ. A study of structure and function. J Exp Med 135:719–734

15. Gabbiani G, Ryan GB, Majno G (1971) Presence of modified fibroblasts in granulation tissue and their possible role in wound contraction. Experientia 27:549–550

16. Guenal I, Risler Y, Mignotte B (1997) Down-regulation of actin genes precedes microfilament network disruption and actin cleavage during p53-mediated apoptosis. J Cell Sci 110:489–495

17. Hagimoto N, Kuwano K, Nomoto Y, Kunitake R, Hara N (1997) Apoptosis and expression of Fas/Fas ligand mRNA in bleomycin-induced pulmonary fibrosis in mice. Am J Respir Cell Mol Biol 16:91–101

18. Henke C, Bitterman PB, Roongta U, Ingbar D, Polunovsky V (1996) Induction of fibroblast apoptosis by anti-CD44 antibody. Implications for the treatment of fibroproliferative lung disease. Am J Pathol 149:1639–1650

19. Ikeda H, Wu GY, Wu CH (1993) Lipocytes from fibrotic rat liver have an impaired feedback response to procollagen propeptides. Am J Physiol 264:G157–G162

20. Johnson RJ, Iida H, Alpers CE, Majesky MW, Schwartz SM (1991) Expression of smooth muscle cell phenotype by rat mesangial cells in immune complex nephritis. α-Smooth muscle actin is a marker of mesangial cell proliferation. J Clin Invest 87:847–858

21. Jones R (1992) Ultrastructural analysis of contractile cell development in lung microvessels in hyperoxic pulmonary hypertension. Fibroblasts and intermediate cells selectively reorganize nonmuscular segments. Am J Pathol 141:1491–1505

22. Kapanci Y, Desmoulière A, Pache JC, Redard M, Gabbiani G (1995) Cytoskeletal protein modulation in pulmonary alveolar myofibroblasts during idiopathic pulmonary fibrosis. Possible role of transforming growth factor beta and tumor necrosis factor alpha. Am J Respir Crit Care Med 152:2163–2169

23. Karmiol S, Phan SH (1992) Phenotypic changes in lung fibroblast populations in pulmonary fibrosis. In: Phipps RP (ed) Pulmonary fibroblast heterogeneity. CRC Press, Boca Raton, pp 1–26

24. Kelley J, Chrin L, Shull S, Rowe DW, Cutroneo KR (1985) Bleomycin selectively elevates mRNA levels for procollagen and fibronectin following acute lung injury. Biochem Biophys Res Commun 131:836–843

25. Kikuchi K, Hartl CW, Smith EA, LeRoy EC, Trojanowska M (1992) Direct demonstration of transcriptional activation of collgen gene expression in systemic sclerosis fibroblasts: Insensitivity to TGF$\beta_1$ stimulation. Biochem Biophys Res Commun 187:45–50

26. Kuhn C, McDonald JA (1991) The roles of the myofibroblast in idiopathic pulmonary fibrosis. Ultrastructural and immunohistochemical features of sites of active extracellular matrix synthesis. Am J Pathol 138:1257–1265

27. Leslie KO, Mitchell J, Low R (1992) Lung myofibroblasts. Cell Motil Cytoskeleton 22:92–98

28. Leslie KO, Mitchell J, Low R (1992) Lung myofibroblasts. Cell Motil Cytoskel 22:92–98

29. Ludwicka A, Trojanowska M, Smith EA, Baumann M, Strange C, Korn JH, Smith T, Leroy EC, Silver RM (1992) Growth and characterization of fibroblasts obtained from broncho-alveolar lavage of patients with scleroderma. J Rheumatol 19:1716–1723

30. Majno G, Gabbiani G, Hirschel BJ, Ryan GB, Statkov PR (1971) Contraction of granulation tissue in vitro: similarity to smooth muscle. Science 173:548–550

31. Mashima T, Naito M, Noguchi K, Miller DK, Nicholson DW, Tsuruo T (1997) Actin cleavage by CPP-32/apopain during the development of apoptosis. Oncogene 14:1007–1012

32. Mitchell J, Woodcock-Mitchell J, Reynolds S, Low R, Leslie KO, Adler K, Gabbiani G, Omar S (1989) $\alpha$-Smooth muscle actin in parenchymal cells of bleomycin-injured rat lung. Lab Invest 60:643–650

33. Mitchell JJ, Woodcock-Mitchell J, Low RB, Absher M (1991) Modulation of $\alpha$ smooth muscle actin by growth state and TGF$\beta$ in lung myofibroblasts. J Cell Biol 15:161a

34. Mitchell JJ, Woodcock-Mitchell JL, Perry L, Zhao J, Low RB, Baldor L, Absher PM (1993) In vitro expression of the alpha-smooth muscle actin isoform by rat lung mesenchymal cells: regulation by culture condition and transforming growth factor-beta. Am J Respir Cell Mol Biol 9:10–18

35. Muller M, Strand S, Hug H, Heinemann EM, Walczak H, Hofmann WJ, Stremmel W, Krammer PH, Galle PR (1997) Drug-induced apoptosis in hepatoma cells is mediated by the CD95 (APO-1/Fas) receptor/ligand system and involves activation of wild-type p53. J Clin Invest 99:403–413

36. Nagata S (1997) Apoptosis by death factor. Cell 88:355–365

37. Oda D, Gown AM, Berg JSV, Stern R (1990) Instability of the myofibroblast phenotype in culture. Exp Mol Pathol 52:221–224

38. Oda D, Gown AM, Berg JSV, Stern R (1988) The fibroblast-like nature of myofibroblasts. Exp Mol Pathol 49:316–329

39. Phan SH, Kunkel SL (1992) Lung cytokine production in bleomycin-induced pulmonary fibrosis. Exp Lung Res 18:29–43

40. Phan SH, Varani J, Smith D (1985) Rat lung fibroblast collagen metabolism in bleomycin-induced pulmonary fibrosis. J Clin Invest 76:241–247

41. Phipps RP (ed) (1992) Pulmonary fibroblast heterogeneity. CRC Press, Boca Raton

42. Roberts ISD, Burrows C, Shanks JH, Venning M, McWilliam LJ (1997) Interstitial myofibro-blasts: predictors of progression in membranous nephropathy. J Clin Pathol 50:123–127

43. Rubbia-Brandt L, Sappino A, Gabbiani G (1991) Locally applied GM-CSF induces the accu-mulation of $\alpha$-smooth muscle actin containing myofibroblasts. Virchows Arch B Cell Pathol 60:73–82

44. Rudin CM, Thompson CB (1997) Apoptosis and disease: regulation and clinical relevance of programmed cell death. Annu Rev Med 48:267–281

45. Skalli O, Gabbiani G (1988) The biology of the myofibroblast. Relationship to wound con-traction and fibrocontractive diseases. In: Clark RAF, Henson PM (eds) The molecular and cellular biology of wound repair. Plenum, New York, pp 373–402

46. Skalli O, Schürch W, Seemayer T, Lagacé R, Montandon D, Pittet B, Gabbiani G (1989) Myofibroblasts from diverse pathologic settings are heterogeneous in their content of actin isoforms and intermediate filament proteins. Lab Invest 60:275–285

47. Stern M, Meagher L, Savill J, Haslett C (1992) Apoptosis in human eosinophils. Programmed cell death in the eosinophil leads to phagocytosis by macrophages and is modulated by IL-5. J Immunol 148:3543–3549

48. Strieter RM, Wiggins R, Phan SH, Wharram BL, Showell HJ, Remick DG, Chensue SW, Kunkel SL (1989) Monocyte chemotactic protein gene expression by cytokine-treated human fibroblasts and endothelial cells. Biochem Biophys Res Commun 162:694–700

49. Uitto J, Perejda AJ, Abergel RP, Chu M-L, Ramirez F (1985) Altered steady state ratio of type I/III procollagen mRNAs correlates with selectively increased type I procollagen biosynthesis in cultured keloid fibroblasts. Proc Natl Acad Sci U S A 82:5935–5939
50. Xing Z, Tremblay GM, Sime PJ, Gauldie J (1997) Overexpression of granulocyte-macrophage colony-stimulating factor induces pulmonary granulation tissue formation and fibrosis by induction of transforming growth factor-beta 1 and myofibroblast accumulation. Am J Pathol 150:59–66
51. Zhang H, Gharaee-Kermani M, Phan SH (1997) Regulation of lung fibroblast α-smooth muscle actin expression, contractile phenotype and apoptosis by IL-1β. J Immunol 158:1392–1399
52. Zhang H, Gharaee-Kermani M, Zhang K, Phan SH (1996) Lung fibroblast contractile and α-smooth muscle actin phenotypic alterations in bleomycin-induced pulmonary fibrosis. Am J Pathol 148:527–537
53. Zhang K, Flanders KC, Phan SH (1995) Cellular localization of transforming growth factor β expression in bleomycin-induced pulmonary fibrosis. Am J Pathol 147:352–361
54. Zhang K, Gharaee-Kermani M, Jones ML, Warren JS, Phan SH (1994) Monocyte chemoattractant protein-1 gene expression in bleomycin-induced pulmonary fibrosis. J Immunol 153:4733–4741
55. Zhang K, Gharaee-Kermani M, McGarry B, Phan SH (1994) In situ hybridization analysis of lung α1 (I) and α2 (I) collagen gene expression in bleomycin-induced pulmonary fibrosis in the rat. Lab Invest 70:192–202
56. Zhang K, Gharaee-Kermani M, McGarry B, Remick D, Phan SH (1997) TNFα mediated lung cytokine networking and eosinophil recruitment in pulmonary fibrosis. J Immunol 158:954–959
57. Zhang K, Rekhter MD, Gordon D, Phan SH (1994) Co-expression of α-smooth muscle actin and type I collagen in fibroblast-like cells of rat lungs with bleomycin-induced pulmonary fibrosis: a combined immuno-histochemical and in situ hybridization study. Am J Pathol 145:114–125

# Cell–Cell and Cell–Matrix Interactions During Breast Cancer Progression

A. Noel, F. Kebers, E. Maquoi, J. M. Foidart

## 1 Introduction

Cancer cells are not simply isolated islands of cells residing in a specific organ; they are surrounded by a modified extracellular matrix and by stromal cells of the host tissue, both of which influence tumor progression. The stroma peritumoral is different from the normal breast stroma and is critically involved in malignant growth.

The extracellular matrix is a complex meshwork of collagens, fibrillar glycoproteins and proteoglycans that determines tissue architecture and conditions many biological activities. Components of the extracellular matrix provide a large variety of specific signals that directly influence cell proliferation, migration, morphology, differentiation, and biosynthetic activities [22]. In addition, the extracellular matrix plays essential roles in cell survival, since loss of adhesive contact results in a form of apoptosis termed anoikis [14].

It has become clear that the extracellular matrix proteins are made up of structural modules that encode information that is interpreted by cells through interactions with plasma-membrane receptors, mostly of the integrin family [22]. Although the precise transduction of matrix signaling remains to be elucidated, there is considerable evidence that the extracellular matrix influences cell properties and behavior by modification of cytoskeletal organization and activation of second-messenger and protein-kinase pathways [22]. In addition, the extracellular matrix is a site of sequestration of various factors that are likely to affect cell activity, such as growth factors, mobility factors, natural proteases and their inhibitors. Finally, proteolytic fragments of the extracellular matrix, termed matrikines, may constitute new signals for connective tissue cells. Cryptic regulatory sequences of amino acids in extracellular matrix macromolecules may become accessible after partial proteolytic cleavage and convey new information to neighboring cells. These matrikines are thus able to regulate connective-tissue cell activities and represent a regulatory loop for fibroblasts or endothelial cells.

Current Topics in Pathology, Volume 93
A. Desmoulière, B. Tuchweber (Eds.)
© Springer-Verlag Berlin Heidelberg 1999

The extracellular matrix is involved in both normal and pathological processes. Recent studies have revealed the importance of the basement membrane for the morphogenesis and differentiation of mammary epithelial cells [22, 44, 53]. For example, laminin-1, one of the major components of basement membranes, acts synergistically with lactogenic hormones to activate transcription of a tissue-specific gene $\beta$-casein in normal mammary cells [24]. These experiments demonstrate the important role of the microenvironment in the control and maintenance of breast-specific function [53].

In tumors, alterations of the extracellular matrix might therefore lead to abnormal host and cancer cell functions and even to cancer progression. Perturbations in the production, deposition and degradation of matrix components have been observed in mammary carcinomas [24]. For example, transgenic mice overexpressing stromelysin-1, an extracellular-matrix-degrading enzyme, were shown to undergo premature involution of the mammary gland in pregnancy and, later, to develop mammary tumors [2]. These observations suggest that perturbation of the tissue microenvironment by proteases may be sufficient to induce tumor formation.

Breast carcinomas are often characterized by a stromal reaction that consists of modifications in the composition of both the cellular elements (myofibroblastic, endothelial, and inflammatory cells) and of the extracellular matrix. This reactive stroma (often termed desmoplastic reaction) actually constitutes a major part of the neoplasm [54].

For a long time, only the neoplastic cells were the focus of interest in cancer research and the stroma was considered a reactive component without major biological and clinical significance. However, it has become clear that the stromal cells and their products (matrix components, growth factors, proteases) condition the phenotype of cancer cells. Thus, tumors represent a complex ecosystem in which interactions between multiple host cells and the extracellular matrix, between tumor cells and the extracellular matrix, and between tumor cells and host cells lead to reciprocal influences resulting in tumor promotion, invasion and metastasis [9, 27, 32, 54].

In this study, we focus on the importance of the peritumoral microenvironment, particularly the fibroblasts and their proteases on tumor growth in vivo.

## 2 Stromal Reaction in Breast Carcinoma

Invasive or infiltrating ductal carcinomas, which represent the most common type of breast cancer, are characterized by pronounced desmoplasia and are often referred to as "scirrhous carcinomas". Desmoplasia is a common host response to epithelial tumor and is classically described as fibroblast proliferation in conjunction with extracellular-matrix remodeling. This reactive stroma exhibits many of the changes observed during wound healing, albeit in an uncontrolled fashion [9]. Stroma generation is essential to the growth of solid tumors, most obviously because of the stroma's supply of blood vessels, which are required for tumor progression [10, 16]. Therefore, the stroma is not a passive barrier to be penetrated by invasive tumors, but is an active player in cancer progression.

## 2.1 Extracellular Matrix Remodeling

Interstitial connective tissue is composed of interstitial collagens (mainly collagen types I and III), fibronectin and various proteoglycans. The "desmoplastic reaction" is characterized by both quantitative and qualitative modifications in the composition of the connective tissue matrix [21, 32, 34]. An excessive accumulation of extracellular matrix components, including different types of collagen (type I, III, V), fibronectin, elastin and proteoglycans, is often observed. In addition, non-basement-membrane type-IV collagen was shown to be present in elastotic fibers of breast tumor tissues [51]. Interestingly, trimer of $\alpha 1$ type-I collagen chain (I-trimer) and ED-B+ fibronectin resulting from alternative splicing of pre-mRNA (otherwise only found in embryonic tissues) were re-expressed in infiltrating ductal carcinomas [21]. Furthermore, breast tumor cells and stromal cells have been shown to re-express the laminin $\beta 2$ chain, which is widely distributed in embryonic basement membrane, but missing from mature tissue [21]. Bone sialoprotein (BSP), a bone-matrix protein involved in hydroxyapatite crystal formation, is ectopically expressed in human breast cancer and results in the formation of microcalcification which can be detected in early lesions [2].

Lysyl oxidase is involved in collagen and elastin crosslinking. While it is undetectable in normal breast, its expression was observed in newly formed stroma of benign lesions and in situ ductal breast carcinoma. It has been postulated to be part of an early host defense mechanism. In contrast, lysyl oxidase was not found in the stroma of invasive tumors [37]. This low level of lysyl oxidase crosslinking may be responsible for a loss of matrix organization and a higher sensitivity to metalloproteases, both of which could favor tumor invasion. Altogether, these observations underline both quantitative and qualitative modifications of the tumor stroma.

Quantitative changes in matrix components may be related to an imbalance between their synthesis and degradation. Tumor cells may directly alter the adjacent matrix by producing excessive matrix proteins or proteolytic enzymes. Alternatively, the desmoplastic response may depend on specific interactions between tumor cells and host fibroblastic cells. For example, breast adenocarcinoma cells in culture were shown to produce diffusible factors that were able to specifically stimulate the synthesis of proteoglycans, different types of collagen and fibronectin by human fibroblasts [28, 32, 34]. Indeed, while human breast tumoral MCF7 cells were unable to synthesize collagen in culture, they induced a three- to fourfold enhancement of collagen production by human fibroblasts [34]. Similarly, Nabeshima et al. isolated a tumor-cell-surface-associated protein that stimulates the production of interstitial collagenase by neighboring fibroblasts [29].

## 2.2 Modification of Cellular Composition

Breast neoplastic stroma contains a heterogeneous cell population composed of fibroblasts, myofibroblasts, endothelial cells and inflammatory cells. Those cells produce a variety of cytokines, growth factors, and proteases which may influence neoplastic cell properties.

The appearance of myofibroblasts expressing $\alpha$-smooth muscle actin is a prominent feature of the stromal reaction observed in wound healing and carcinomas. In ductal mammary carcinomas, for example, they constitute more than 70% of stromal cells. Ronnov-Jessen et al. [42] suggested that the myofibroblasts in breast carcinoma are formed primarily by differentiation from fibroblasts, but they may also be derived from vascular smooth muscle cells, and occasionally from pericytes. Cytokines such as transforming growth factor beta (TGF$\beta$), produced by cancer cells or released from the extracellular matrix, are likely to be involved in these differentiation processes [42]. In breast cancer, the myofibroblasts have been shown to produce enzymes involved in proteolysis of matrix components, such as urokinase plasminogen activator and stromelysin-3 [49].

## 3  Role of Basement Membrane in Tumorigenicity In Vivo

Much of our understanding of the role of the extracellular matrix in tumor growth has come through the use of Matrigel. Matrigel is a solubilized basement-membrane matrix extracted from the Engelbreth Holm Swarm tumor. Its major components are laminin-1, type-IV collagen ($\alpha 1$ and $\alpha 2$ chains), heparan sulfate proteoglycans, and entactin. It polymerizes at 37 °C to produce a reconstituted, biologically active matrix that aids adhesion and differentiation of cells [47]. Various growth factors also accumulate in Matrigel, including at least epidermal growth factor (EGF), insulin-like growth factor (IGF-1), platelet-derived growth factor (PDGF), TGF$\beta$ and basic fibroblast growth factor (bFGF) [47].

When various human cancer cells (lung, prostatic, mammary, colonic carcinomas and melanoma cells) are mixed with Matrigel and transplanted subcutaneously into nude mice, tumors develop rapidly [12, 13, 25, 31, 32, 34, 48]. In the absence of Matrigel, human breast adenocarcinoma MCF7 cells and MCF7/6 cells failed to produce tumor (Table 1). These findings indicate that interactions with basement-membrane components are required for breast tumor formation. For some other mammary cell lines tested (Table 1), Matrigel reduced the latency of tumor appearance. In addition, it increased or maintained the percentage of tumor-bearing animals at 100%.

It is difficult to determine whether tumor growth is induced by matrix molecules themselves or by other components present in Matrigel [4]. Indeed, the numerous active growth factors present in Matrigel may influence tumor cell properties [47]. However, Matrigel devoid of growth factors ("depleted" Matrigel) is as efficient as complete Matrigel in stimulating MCF7 cell growth (unpublished data) and B16.F10 melanoma growth in vivo [13].

Laminin-1 is the major glycoprotein of Matrigel. Its co-injection with submandibular carcinoma cells can reproduce the effect of Matrigel [15]. This may not be true for all tumor cell types, given that Fridman et al. [12] showed that the growth of human cell lung carcinoma cells was not stimulated by laminin. Thus, the tumor-promoting effect of laminin appeared to be dependent on the cell types tested. Nevertheless, different laminin-derived peptides have been shown to influence tumor cell growth. For example, the YIGSR site promoted cell adhesion and migration by binding to a 32/67-kDa laminin-binding protein (on the cell

**Table 1.** Effect of matrigel on the in vivo tumorigenicity of human breast adenocarcinoma cells

| Cells | Treatment[a] | Incidence | Latency period[b] (days) |
|---|---|---|---|
| MCF7 | None | 0/20 | – |
| | Matrigel | 20/20 | 16 |
| | "Depleted Matrigel" | 5/5 | 18 |
| MCF7/6 | None | 0/10 | – |
| | Matrigel | 5/5 | 39 |
| MCF7 gpt | None | 10/10 | 31 |
| | Matrigel | 10/10 | 8 |
| MCF7 ras | None | 9/10 | 27 |
| | Matrigel | 10/10 | 10 |
| MCF7 (AZ) | None | 10/10 | 54 |
| | Matrigel | 10/10 | 10 |
| MCF7 (AZ) TD5 | None | 10/10 | 54 |
| | Matrigel | 10/10 | 10 |
| MDA-MB231 | None | 5/10 | 46 |
| | Matrigel | 5/5 | 32 |

[a] $10^6$ Cells were injected in nude mice in the absence (none) or in the presence of matrigel.
[b] The latency period was estimated as the number of days needed to obtain tumors of 200 mm$^3$.

surface) that functions as one putative receptor [15]. The YIGSR peptide inhibits angiogenesis and the tumor-promoting effect of Matrigel on prostatic carcinoma cells [36]. When co-injected with melanoma cells, or fibrosarcoma HT1080 cells, the YIGSR peptide prevented tumor metastasis and growth in the presence of Matrigel [5, 19]. The RGD site is expected to be biologically active since it is part of the cell adhesion site to fibronectin, vitronectin and other proteins. Although its precise role in laminin has not been elucidated, it appears to promote adhesion of endothelial cell to Matrigel [1].

More numerous studies have focused on the SIKVAV peptide present at the end of the long arm just above the large globule on the $\alpha$1 chain. Peptides containing this sequence are angiogenic in several in vitro models [15]. In vivo, it increases the number of metastatic lesions by melanoma cells and colon cancer cells to the lung [5, 20]. This peptide also enhances plasminogen activation and gelatinase A activity [20, 43]. It is worth noting that the SIKVAV site is present at a region where the three chains form a coiled-coil structure and where laminin is known to bind to other extracellular matrix components, such as heparin and type-IV collagen. For this reason, it has been suggested that the SIKVAV site is cryptic under some conditions. If this is the case, laminin could possess alternative properties. It is likely that some laminin domains are neither active nor available at all times. In authentic tumors, this peptide could be released by proteolysis of subepithelial basement membrane by serine proteases or matrix metalloproteinases.

Altogether, these observations indicate that in the Matrigel tumor-promoting model, many factors can act in a cooperative way to facilitate tumor growth.

## 4 Role of Stromal Cells in In Vivo Tumorigenesis

The ability of tumor cells to grow and metastasize is affected by the presence of adjacent host cells, particularly fibroblasts or myofibroblasts [16]. Co-injection of fibroblasts and parental MCF7 cells in the presence of Matrigel increased tumor growth (Fig. 1) and shortened the latency period (14 days versus 26 days) (Table 2). In these conditions, the tumor incidence always reached 100% and the tumor volume was increased (Table 2 and Fig. 1). Such tumor-promoting effects of fibroblasts are also observed with breast cancer MDA-MB231 cells [31]. The co-inoculation of fibroblasts with tumoral cells is as efficient in ectopic sites (subcutaneous injection) as in orthotopic sites (in fat pad) [39].

Fibroblasts can affect mammary cells by secreting several classes of compound, including: (1) matrix proteins, (2) soluble chemokines, cytokines and growth factors, and (3) proteases. Together with growth factors, such matrix proteins could promote the proliferation of endothelial cells, tumor cells or both [31, 50]. In this regard, the co-injection of lethally irradiated fibroblasts with human cancer cells enhances their tumorigenic potential, supporting a role for the matrix itself [6]. In addition, fibroblast-conditioned medium injected weekly at the site of inoculation of MCF7 cells and Matrigel reproduced, partially, the effect of fibroblasts on tumor growth by affecting the rate of tumor growth, but not the latency period (Fig. 1). The failure of the conditioned medium to shorten the latency period may be

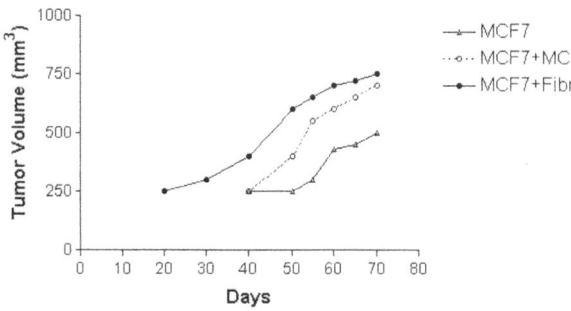

**Fig. 1.** Effect of fibroblasts on MCF7 cells' tumor growth. MCF7 cells ($2.5 \times 10^5$) were injected subcutaneously without fibroblasts (Δ), with fibroblasts (●, *continuous line*), or with medium conditioned with fibroblasts (○, *dashed line*)

**Table 2.** Effect of tissue inhibitor 2 of matrix metalloproteinases (TIMP2) on the tumor-promoting effect of fibroblasts on MCF7 cells in in vivo tumorigenicity

|  | Latency period (days)[a] | | Tumor volume at the end of the assay ($mm^3$)[b] | |
|---|---|---|---|---|
|  | Without fibroblasts | With fibroblasts | Without fibroblasts | With fibroblasts |
| Control MCF7 cells | 25 | 13 | 114 ± 10 | 208 ± 15 |
| MCF7 TIMP2 cells | 28 | 28 | 110 ± 10 | 101 ± 15 |

[a] Latency period, the number of days between injection and development of tumor larger than 80 $mm^3$ in 100% of injection sites.
[b] Mean volume of tumors at the end of the assay.

related to subcutaneous dilution of soluble factors before tumor take. This result suggests the involvement of soluble factors secreted by fibroblasts. Among the soluble factors, stromal matrix metalloproteinases (MMPs) represent putative contributors of the stromal involvement in tumor progression.

## 5 Role of Stromal Matrix Metalloproteinases

The MMPs are a family of zinc-dependent endopeptidases with a broad spectrum of proteolytic activities towards extracellular matrix components [3]. The collagenases (interstitial collagenase, neutrophil collagenase, collagenase-3) are characterized by their ability to cleave fibrillar interstitial collagens. The gelatinases A and B are particularly potent against denatured collagens and type-IV collagen of basement membranes. Stromelysins 1 and 2, as well as matrilysin have a broad substrate specificity and degrade proteoglycans and glycoproteins (laminin and fibronectins). In contrast, stromelysin-3 appears to have more restricted substrate specificity. The newly described membrane type (MT)-MMPs are able to activate progelatinase A by proteolytic cleavage of its pro-domain [40]. The proteolytic activity of MMPs is controlled by physiological inhibitors, the tissue inhibitors of matrix metalloproteinases (TIMP) [8].

An important aspect which was controversial for a long time, is to determine where MMPs are expressed in tumors. Results shedding light on this are the observations that stromelysin-3 mRNA and protein expression is localized specifically to the stroma of breast cancers, but not in tumor cells themselves [41]. Similarly, gelatinase A mRNAs are localized by in situ hybridization on tumor cells. The protein is however immunolocalized to the surface of breast tumor cells themselves [38], suggesting a binding at tumor cell surface of gelatinase A produced by fibroblasts. Together with the findings that interstitial collagenase and MT1-MMP mRNA are associated with the stroma, all these data demonstrate that stromal cell production of MMPs represents a major contribution to overall tumor metalloproteinase activity [17, 41].

The role of stromal proteases in cancer progression is supported by the fact that stromelysin-3 can promote the tumor formation of MCF7 cells transfected with cDNAs encoding either human or murine stromelysin-3 [33]. In addition, high ST3 expression levels are predictive of a poor clinical outcome in breast cancer [7].

Studies with natural MMP inhibitors, the TIMPs, and synthetic MMP inhibitors have demonstrated that MMP activity is required for tumor progression and metastasis in several model systems [8, 46]. In this context, reduction of tumor growth and local invasion is observed when TIMP2 was overexpressed in tumor cells, using either by transfection of TIMP2 cDNA [8] or retroviral-mediated gene transfer [18]. Batimastat, an inhibitor of MMPs, inhibited for example human breast cancer growth and metastasis in nude-mice models [26, 46]. The overexpression of TIMP-4 in human MDA-MB 435 breast carcinoma cells reduced in vivo tumor growth and angiogenesis [52].

We have infected MCF7 cells with a retroviral vector containing TIMP-2. No differences in tumor incidence or latency period were observed when MCF7 cells were transfected with vector alone (MCF7 *puro*) or TIMP2 producing MCF7 cells were injected with Matrigel (Table 2). This result is consistent with the lack of MMP production by MCF7 cells. However, the co-injection of these TIMP2-producing MCF7 cells with fibroblasts and Matrigel abolished the tumor-promoting effect of fibroblasts (Table 2). The main effect was to enhance the latency period, suggesting that stromal MMPs mainly affect early events of tumor progression.

One contribution of stromal proteases could be the release of biologically active factors from the extracellular matrix. Indeed, as mentioned above, various growth factors (IGFs, FGFs and TGF$\beta$s) are associated with matrix proteins or with heparan sulfate groups on proteoglycan [45]. Their release by MMPs from matrix and/or activation of their latent forms may result in their binding to and stimulation of tumor cells. MMPs are indeed able to cleave growth factor-controlling molecules, such as insulin-like growth factor-binding protein 3 (IGFBP-3) or the ecto domain of the fibroblast growth factor receptor 1 (FGFR1) [11, 23]. These activated growth factors could act indirectly on cancer cells by promoting migration of stromal cells, proliferation, and biosynthetic activities. Alternatively, some of these factors have angiogenic activities and contribute to the angiogenic effect of Matrigel. Together these data emphasize the importance of stromal cells and their products, such as proteases, during cancer progression.

# 6 Perspectives

Targeting stromal cells for therapeutic purpose rather than cancer cells themselves could be important since, if preventing the functions of the stroma can be abrogated, tumors should be deprived of important and essential support needed for angiogenesis, growth and metastasis. In this context, stromal MMPs are attractive targets since by their mode of action, the toxicity profile of MMP inhibitors, would differ markedly from cytotoxic drugs. Several synthetic MMP inhibitors have demonstrated anti-tumor activity in various experimental models developed in nude mice [46]. Phase-III clinical trials have been already initiated. The next step will be to identify more specific and/or more potent inhibitors for each MMPs expressed in human breast carcinomas.

**Acknowledgements.** We gratefully acknowledge Mrs. H. Brisy for her skillful secretarial assistance. This work was supported by grants from the Communauté Française de Belgique (Actions de Recherches Concertées 93/98–171 and 95/00–191); the Commission of European Communities (Biotech No. CT960464); the Fonds de la Recherche Scientifique Médicale (No. 3.4573.95); the Fonds National de la Recherche Scientifique (FNRS; Lotto 9.4561.94, 9.4556.95); the Association Sportive Contre le Cancer; the Centre Anticancéreux près l'Université de Liège; the CGER – Assurances 1996/1999; the Fondation Léon Frédéricq, University of Liège; the Fonds d'Investissements de Recherche Scientifique, CHU, Liège, Belgium; General RE-Luxembourg; and from industry – Boehringer Mannheim, Penzberg, Germany. A.N. is a permanent research fellow of the National Fund for Scientific Research (FNRS; Brussels, Belgium).

# References

1. Baatout S (1997) Endothelial differentiation using Matrigel (review). Anticancer Res 17: 451–456
2. Bellahcène A, Menard S, Bufalino R, Moreau L, Castronovo V (1996) Expression of bone sialoprotein in primary human breast cancer is associated with poor survival. Int J Cancer 69:350–353
3. Birkedal-Hansen H (1995) Proteolytic remodeling of extracellular matrix. Cur Opin Cell Biol 7:728–735
4. Bonfil RD, Vinyals A, Bustuoabad OD, Llorens A, Banavides FJ, Gonzales-Garrigues M, Fabra A (1994) Stimulation of angiogenesis as an explanation of Matrigel-enhanced tumorigenicity. Int J Cancer 58:233–239
5. Bresalier RS, Schwartz B, Kim YS, Duh QY, Kleinman HK, Sullam PM (1995) The laminin a1 chain Ile-Lys-Val-Ala-Val (IKVAV)-containing peptide promotes liver colonization by human colon cancer cells. Cancer Res 55:2476–2480
6. Camps JL, Chang SM, Hsu TC, Freeman MR, Hong SJ, Zhau HE, von Eschenbach AC, Chung LWK (1990) Fibroblast-mediated acceleration of human epithelial tumor growth in vivo. Proc Natl Acad Sci U S A 87:75–79
7. Chenard MP, O'Siorain L, Shering S, Rouyer N, Lutz Y, Wolf C, Basset P, Bellocq JP, Duffy MJ (1996) High levels of stromelysin-3 correlate with poor prognosis in patients with breast carcinoma. Int J Cancer 69:448–451
8. DeClerck YA, Perez N, Shimada H, Boone TC, Langley KE, Taylor SM (1992) Inhibition of invasion and metastasis in cells transfected with an inhibitor of metalloproteinases. Cancer Res 52:701–708
9. Dvorak HF (1986) Tumors: wounds that do not heal. Similarities between tumor stroma generation and wound healing. N Engl J Med 315:1650–1659
10. Folkman J (1995) Angiogenesis in cancer, vascular, rheumatoid, and other disease. Nat Med 1:27–31
11. Fowlkes JL, Enghild JJ, Suzuki K, Nagase H (1994) Matrix metalloproteinases degrade insulin-like growth factor-binding protein-3 in dermal fibroblast cultures. J Biol Chem 269:25742–25746
12. Fridman R, Giaccone G, Kanemoto T, Martin GR, Gazdar AF, Mulshine JL (1990) Reconstituted basement membrane (Matrigel) and laminin can enhance the tumorigenicity and the drug resistance of small cell lung cancer cell lines. Proc Natl Acad Sci U S A 87:6698–6702
13. Fridman R, Kibbey MC, Royce LS, Zain M, Sweeney TM, Jicha DL, Yannelli JR, Martin GR, Kleinman HK (1991) Enhanced tumor growth of both primary and established human and murine tumor cells in athymic mice after coinjection with Matrigel. J Natl Cancer Inst 83:769–775
14. Frisch SM, Ruoslahti E (1997) Integrin and anoikis. Curr Opin Cell Biol 9:701–706
15. Grant DS, Kibbey MC, Kinsella JL, Cid MC, Kleinman HK (1994) The role of basement membrane in angiogenesis and tumor growth. Pathol Res Pract 190:854–863
16. Grégoire M, Lieubeau B (1995) The role of fibroblasts in tumor behavior. Cancer Metastasis Rev 14:339–350
17. Heppner KJ, Matrisian LM, Jensen RA, Rodgers WH (1996) Expression of most matrix metalloproteinase family members in breast cancer represents a tumor-induced host response. Am J Pathol 149:273–282
18. Imren S, Kohn DB, Shimada H, Blavier L, DeClerck YA (1996) Overexpression of tissue inhibitor of metalloproteinases-2 by retroviral-mediated gene transfer in vivo inhibits tumor growth and invasion. Cancer Res 56:2891–2895
19. Iwamoto Y, Nomizu M, Yamada Y, Ito Y, Tanaka K, Sugioka Y (1996) Inhibition of angiogenesis, tumour growth and experimental metastasis of human fibrosarcoma cells HT1080 by a multimetric form of the laminin sequence Tyr-Ile-Gly-Ser-Arg (YIGSR). Br J Cancer 73:589–595
20. Kanemoto T, Reich R, Royce L, Greatorex D, Adler SH, Shiraishi N, Martin GR, Yamada Y, Kleinman HK (1990) Identification of an amino acid sequence from the laminin-A chain that stimulates metastasis and collagenase-IV production. Proc Natl Acad Sci U S A 87:2279–2283

21. Kosmehl H, Berndt A, Katenkamp D (1996) Molecular variants of fibronectin and laminin: structure, physiological occurrence and histopathological aspects. Virchows Arch 429: 311–322

22. LaFlamme SE, Auer KL (1996) Integrin signalling. Semin Cancer Biol 7:111–118

23. Levi E, Fridman R, Miao HQ, Ma YS, Yayon A, Vlodavsky I (1994) Matrix metalloproteinase 2 releases active soluble ectodomain of fibroblast growth factor receptor 1. Proc Natl Acad Sci U S A 93:7069–7074

24. Lochter A, Srebrow A, Sympson CJ, Terracio N, Werb Z, Bissell MJ (1997) Misregulation of stromelysin-1 expression in mouse mammary tumor cells accompanies acquisition of stromelysin-1-dependent invasive properties. J Biol Chem 272:5007–5015

25. Lopez-Conejo T, Olmo N, Turnay J, Navarro J, Lizarbe A (1996) Characterization of tumorigenic sub-lines from a poorly tumorigenic human colon-adenocarcinoma cell line. Int J Cancer 67:668–675

26. Low JA, Johnson MD, Bone EA, Dickson RB (1996) The matrix metalloproteinase inhibitor Batimastat (BB-94) retards human breast cancer solid tumor growth but not ascites formation in nude mice. Clin Cancer Res 2:1207–1214

27. MacDougall JR, Matrisian LM (1995) Contributions of tumor and stromal matrix metalloproteinases to tumor progression, invasion and metastasis. Cancer Metastasis Rev 14: 351–362

28. Merrilees MJ, Finlay GJ (1985) Human tumor cells in culture stimulate glycosaminoglycan synthesis by human skin fibroblasts. Lab Invest 53:30–36

29. Nabeshima K, Lane, W, Biswas, C (1996) Partial sequencing and characterization of the tumor-derived collagenase stimulatory factor. Arch Biochem Biophys 285:90–96

30. Noël A, Borcy V, Bracke M, Gilles C, Bernard J, Birembaut P, Mareel M, Foidart JM (1995) Heterotransplantation of primary and established human tumour cells in nude mice. Anticancer Res 15:1–8

31. Noël A, De Pauw-Gillet MC, Purnell G, Nusgens B, Lapière CM, Foidart JM (1993) Enhancement of tumorigenicity of human breast adenocarcinoma cells in nude mice by Matrigel and fibroblasts. Br J Cancer 68:909–915

32. Noël A, Emonard H, Polette M, Birembaut P, Foidart JM (1994) Role of matrix, fibroblasts and type IV collagenases in tumor progression and invasion. Pathol Res Pract 190:934–941

33. Noël A, Lefebvre O, Maquoi E, Vanhoorde L, Chenard MP, Mareel M, Foidart JM, Basset P, Rio MC (1996) Stromelysin-3 expression promote tumor take in nude mice. J Clin Invest 97:1924–1930

34. Noël A, Munaut C, Boulvain A, Calberg-Bacq CM, Lambert CA, Nusgens B, Lapière CM, Foidart JM (1992) Modulation of collagen and fibronectin synthesis in fibroblasts by normal and malignant cells. J Cell Biochem 48:150–161

35. Noël A, Simon N, Raus J, Foidart JM (1992) Basement membrane components (Matrigel) promote human breast adenocarcinoma MCF7 cells tumorigenicity and provide an in vivo model to assess cell responsiveness to estrogen. Biochem Pharmacol 43:1263–1267

36. Passaniti A, Isaacs JT, Haney JA, Adler SW, Cujdik TJ, Long PV, Kleinman HK (1992) Stimulation of human prostatic carcinoma tumor growth in athymic mice and control of migration in culture by extracellular matrix. Int J Cancer 51:318–324

37. Peyrol S, Raccurt M, Gerard F, Gleyzal C, Grimaud JA, Sommer P (1997) Lysyl oxidase gene expression in the stromal reaction to in situ and invasive ductal breast carcinoma. Am J Pathol 150:497–507

38. Polette M, Gilbert N, Stas I, Narowski B, Noël A, Remacle A, Stetler-Stevenson W, Birembaut P, Foidart JM (1994) Gelatinase A expression and localization in human breast cancers. An in situ hybridization study and immunohistochemical detection using confocal microscopy. Virchows Arch 424:641–645

39. Price JE (1996) Metastasis from human breast cancer cell lines. Breast Cancer Res Treat 39:93–102

40. Pulyaeva H, Bueno J, Polette M, Birembaut P, Sato H, Seiki M, Thompson EW (1997) MT1-MMP correlates with MMP-2 activation potential seen after epithelial to mesenchymal transition in human breast carcinoma cells. Clin Exp Metastasis 15:111–120

41. Rio MC, Lefebvre O, Santavicca M, Noël A, Chenard MP, Anglard P, Byrne JA, Okada A, Régnier CH, Masson R, Bellocq JP, Basset P (1996) Stromelysin-3 in the biology of the normal and neoplastic mammary gland. J Mammary Gland Neoplasia 1:231–240
42. Ronnov-Jenssen L, Petersen OW, Koteliansky VE, Bissell MJ (1995) The origin of the myofibroblasts in breast cancer: recapitulation of tumor environment in culture unravels diversity and implicates converted fibroblasts and recruited smooth muscle cells. J Clin Invest 95:859–873
43. Stack S, Gray RD, Pizzo SV (1991) Modulation of plasminogen activation and type IV collagenase activity by a synthetic peptide derived from the laminin A chain. Biochemistry 30:2073–2077
44. Streuli CH, Schmidhauser C, Bailey N, Yurchenco P, Skubitz APN, Roskelley C, Bissell MJ (1995) Laminin mediates tissue-specific gene expression in mammary epithelia. J Cell Biol 129:591–603
45. Taipale J Keski-Oja J (1997) Growth factors in the extracellular matrix. FASEB J 11:51–59
46. Talbot DC, Brown PD (1996) Experimental and clinical studies on the use of matrix metalloproteinase inhibitors for the treatment of cancer. Eur J Cancer 14:2528–2533
47. Taub M, Wang Y, Szcesny TM, Kleinman HK (1990) Epidermal growth factor or transforming growth factor a is required for kidney tubologenesis in Matrigel cultures in serum-free medium. Proc Natl Acad Sci U S A 87:4002–4006
48. Topley P, Jenkins DC, Jessup EA, Stables JN (1993) Effect of reconstituted basement membrane components on the growth of a panel human tumour cell lines in nude mice. Br J Cancer 67:953–958
49. Unden AB, Sandstedt B, Bruce K, Hedblad MA, Ståhle-Bäckdahl M (1996) Stromelysin-3 mRNA associated with myofibroblasts is overexpressed in aggressive basal cell carcinoma and in dermafibrosarcoma but not in dermatofibrosarcoma. J Invest Dermatol 107:147–153
50. van Roozendaal CEP, van Ooijen B, Klijn JGM, Claassen C, Eggermont AMM, Henzen-Logmans SC, Foekens JA (1992) Stromal influences on breast cancer cell growth. Br J Cancer 65:77–81
51. Verhoeven D, Bourgeois N, Noël A, Foidart JM, Buyssens N (1990) The presence of a type IV collagen skeleton associated with periductal elastosis in breast cancer. J Histochem Cytochem 38:245–255
52. Wang M, Liu YE, Greene J, Sheng S, Fuchs A, Rosen EM, Shi YE (1997) Inhibition of tumor growth and metastasis of human breast cancer cells transfected with tissue inhibitor of metalloproteinase 4. Oncogene 14:2767–2674
53. Weaver VM, Fisher AH, Peterson OW, Bissel MJ (1997) The importance of the microenvironment in breast cancer progression: recapitulation of mammary tumorigenesis using a unique human mammary epithelial cell model and a three-dimensional culture assay. Biochem Cell Biol 74:833–851
54. Wernert N (1997) The multiple roles of tumour stroma. Virchows Arch 430:433–443

# Hepatocyte Growth Factor Secreted by Human Liver Myofibroblasts Increases Invasiveness of Hepatocellular Carcinoma Cells

V. Neaud, S. Faouzi, J. Guirouilh, A. Monvoisin, J. Rosenbaum

## Abbreviations

| | |
|---|---|
| HCC | hepatocellular carcinoma |
| MF | myofibroblast |
| HGF | hepatocyte growth factor |
| DMEM | Dulbecco's modified Eagle medium |
| CM | conditioned medium |
| EGF | epidermal growth factor |
| SDS-PAGE | sodium dodecyl sulfate/polyacrylamide gel electrophoresis |
| cDNA | complementary deoxyribonucleic acid |
| ELISA | enzyme-linked immunosorbent assay |
| IgG | immunoglobulin G |

## 1 Introduction

Hepatocellular carcinoma (HCC) is one of the most frequent primary tumors in the world. It is a major complication of liver cirrhosis, although more rarely it will develop on a non-cirrhotic liver. Like many cancers, HCC is infiltrated by myofibroblast (MF)-like cells. They can be identified through their positive staining for

Current Topics in Pathology, Volume 93
A. Desmoulière, B. Tuchweber (Eds.)
© Springer-Verlag Berlin Heidelberg 1999

smooth muscle $\alpha$-actin. Their phenotype is very similar to that of MFs, which are the major source of fibrosis components in chronic liver diseases [6, 7, 27]. Interactions between tumor cells and mesenchymal cells have been demonstrated in several models of cancer. For example, the growth of several tumors in nude mice was markedly enhanced if fibroblasts were co-injected with tumor cells [8, 14]. Also, tumor-associated MFs have been shown to be involved in the in vivo and in vitro invasiveness of colon-cancer cell lines [5].

Hepatocyte growth factor (HGF) is a multifunctional cytokine, which has been implicated in the pathogenesis of several tumors. HGF is secreted as a latent, single-chain molecule. It is activated by proteolysis, yielding the active heterodimeric form. HGF acts on the cells via its specific receptor, c-met [2]. It has been shown, using in situ hybridization, that human liver MFs express HGF in patients with cirrhosis [10]. Although there are still some contradictory results, most studies indicate that HGF is expressed in human [4, 13, 18, 24] or murine [3, 9, 17] HCC.

The aim of our work was to study the effects of human hepatic MFs on the morphology, proliferation and invasiveness of two human HCC cell lines and to assess the role of HGF in these effects.

# 2 Material and Methods

## 2.1 Cells

HuH7 and HepG2 human HCC lines were cultured in Dulbecco's modified Eagle medium (DMEM) containing 10% fetal calf serum. Human hepatic MFs were obtained from explants of non-tumoral liver resected during partial hepatectomy, as previously described [29]. Isolated cells were characterized as previously described [1, 29]. Specifically, the procedure, which is based on the selective growth advantage of MFs in the culture conditions used, allowed for a 100% pure MF population, as shown by positive staining for smooth muscle $\alpha$-actin and vimentin, and negative staining for CD 68 (a Kupffer cell marker), von Willebrand factor (an endothelial cell marker), or cytokeratin (an epithelial cell marker). MFs were grown in DMEM containing 5% fetal calf serum, 5% human AB serum and 5 ng/ml recombinant human epidermal growth factor (EGF).

## 2.2 Collection of Myofibroblast Conditioned Medium

Confluent MF, were incubated for 24 h in serum-free DMEM. MF-conditioned medium (MF-CM) was then collected. MF-CM was prepared from six different isolates of MF and comparable results were obtained.

## 2.3 Western Blot for Hepatocyte Growth Factor

MF-CM was concentrated by adsorption on heparin-Sepharose, and resolved by sodium dodecyl sulfate-polyacrylamide gel electrophoresis (SDS-PAGE). The proteins were analyzed by means of Western blot with an anti-HGF antibody (R and D Systems), using enhanced chemiluminescence. In some experiments, HGF was also quantified with a commercial enzyme-linked immunosorbent assay (ELISA).

## 2.4 Northern Blot

Total RNA was prepared from cultured MFs and analyzed by Northern blot with a radiolabeled cDNA probe for human HGF.

## 2.5 Cell Proliferation Assay

Tumor cells were seeded in plastic 24-well plates. After 15 h, triplicates were counted to determine the number of cells that had adhered to the well. In other wells, tumor cells were incubated in triplicate in either serum-free DMEM (control medium) or MF-CM. For neutralization experiments, MF-CM was pre-incubated with anti-human HGF antibody, or non immune goat immunoglobulin G (IgG). Tumor cells were counted after 3 days of culture. Results were expressed as percentages of proliferation and compared with that in control medium. $P = (Ne - No/Nc - No) \times 100$, where $P$ = proliferation, $No$ = number of cells that had adhered to the plastic support at the time of seeding, $Nc$ = number of cells in the presence of control medium, and $Ne$ = number of cells in experimental samples.

## 2.6 Immunofluorescent Staining of Tumor Cells

Tumor cells were cultured for 3 days on glass coverslips in either control medium or MF-CM. They were stained with monoclonal antibodies anti desmosomal protein (clone ZK-31, Sigma), and anti-E-cadherin. After washing with phosphate-buffered saline, cells were incubated with fluorescein isothiocyanate (FITC)-conjugated anti-mouse IgG antibody.

## 2.7 Cell Invasion Assay

A Matrigel invasion assay was performed essentially as described [20]. For neutralization experiments, MFs were preincubated for 1 h at 37 °C with anti-HGF antibody. In some experiments, rHGF (100 ng/ml) was used instead of MF in the lower compartment. After a 48 h incubation, the cells on the upper surface of the filter were wiped with a cotton swab. Cells that invaded the lower surface of the filter were counted.

# 3 Results

## 3.1 Evidence that Myofibroblasts Synthesize and Secrete Hepatocyte Growth Factor

Northern-blot analysis of MF RNA with a cDNA probe to human HGF in early experiments showed a single band migrating at 6 kb. However, in some experiments, multiple bands were detected with sizes of 6, 4.5, 3, 1.9 and 1.3 kb (Fig. 1 A). Immunoblotting of serum-free MF-CM in non-reducing conditions showed a band migrating slightly higher than the recombinant human HGF used as a standard. In some experiments, an additional lower molecular weight band was also detected (Fig. 1 B). HGF levels were quantified by ELISA in MF-CM samples and ranged from 5 ng/ml to 40 ng/ml.

## 3.2 Effect of Human Hepatic Myofibroblasts on Tumor Cell Morphology

As shown in Fig. 2, HepG2 cells grew in control medium as dense clusters of tightly packed cells. Numerous desmosomes could be shown by immunofluorescence, and

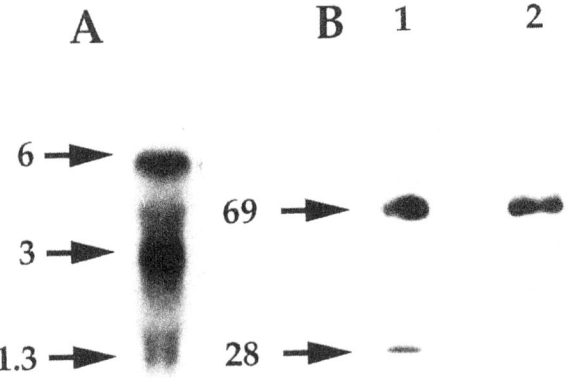

**Fig. 1.** Expression of hepatocyte growth factor (HGF) by cultured myofibroblasts (MFs). (A) Total RNA (13 µg) from cultured MFs was analyzed by means of Northern blot with a complementary DNA (cDNA) probe to human HGF. The size of the bands is indicated in kilobases. (B) Concentrated conditioned medium from MFs was analyzed by means of Western blot, in non-reducing conditions with a polyclonal antibody to human HGF. *Lane 1*: conditioned medium, *lane 2*: rHGF. Molecular weights are indicated on the left (kDa)

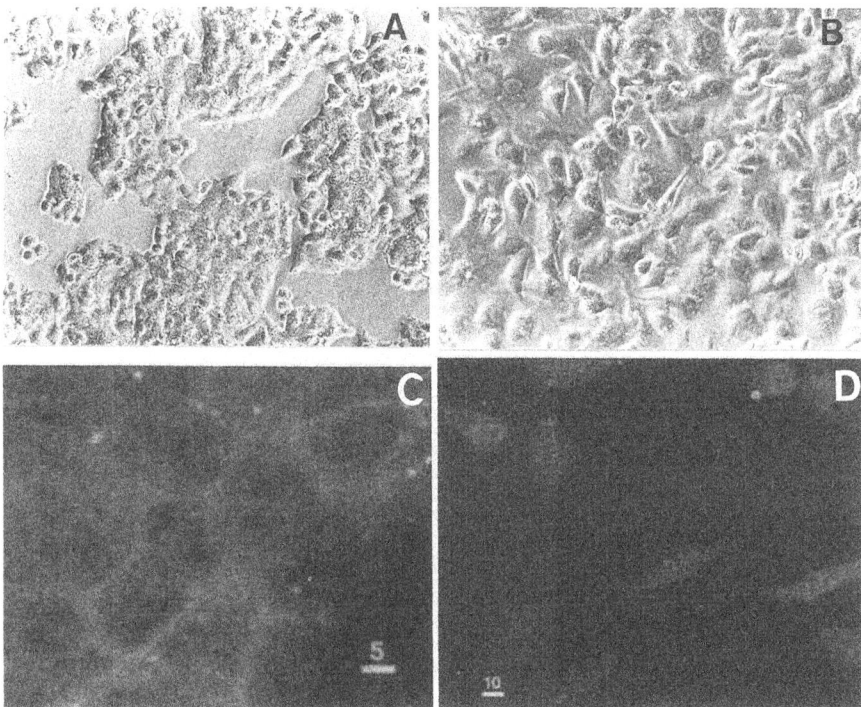

**Fig. 2 A – D.** Effect of human hepatic myofibroblast conditioned medium (MF-CM) on tumor cell morphology. HepG2 cells were cultured in control medium (**A, C**) or in MF-CM (**B, D**) for 24 h and photographed. **A, B** Phase-contrast microphotographs; note the scattering of HepG2 cells in MF-CM. **C, D** Staining with an anti-E-cadherin antibody. Bars indicate the size (µm)

the cells expressed E-cadherin. During incubation with MF-CM, HepG2 cells dissociated, their desmosomes disappeared and E-cadherin expression was lost. Many cells were elongated. This effect of MF-CM was reproduced by recombinant HGF. No morphological modifications of HepG2 cells could be observed when MF-CM had been neutralized with anti-HGF antibodies. The use of control IgG did not modify the effects of MF-CM. In contrast with HepG2 cells, MF-CM and rHGF did not induce morphological modifications of HuH7 cells, nor was labeling of desmosomes and E-cadherin affected (not shown).

## 3.3 Effect of Myofibroblast-Conditioned Medium on Tumor Cell Proliferation

As shown in Table 1, MF-CM induced a significant decrease of HepG2 cell growth, while it induced a significant increase of HuH7 cell proliferation ($p < 0.0001$ by means of analysis of variance). These effects were mimicked by HGF and were abolished after preincubation of MF-CM with anti-HGF antibodies.

**Table 1.** Effect of myofibroblast-conditioned medium (MF-CM) and hepatocyte growth factor (HGF) on tumor cell proliferation

|  |  | HepG2 | | HuH7 | |
| --- | --- | --- | --- | --- | --- |
|  |  | Percentage of control proliferation | SD | Percentage of control proliferation | SD |
| MF-CM | Alone | 32.5 | 8.3 | 160.3 | 18.7 |
|  | + Anti-HGF Ab | 109 | 11.5 | 76 | 5.2 |
|  | + Control Ab | 38.2 | 9 | 138.3 | 13.5 |
| rHGF |  | 27.9 | 4 | 127.7 | 14.5 |

*Ab*, antibody.

**Table 2.** Effect of myofibroblasts (MFs) and hepatocyte growth factor (HGF) on tumor cell invasiveness

|  |  | HepG2 | | HuH7 | |
| --- | --- | --- | --- | --- | --- |
|  |  | Number of invasive cells | SD | Number of invasive cells | SD |
| Tumor cells alone | | 10 | 4.3 | 44.7 | 11 |
| + MF | Alone | 1136 | 317 | 856.7 | 397.3 |
|  | + Anti-HGF Ab | 5.3 | 2.1 | 19.3 | 18.5 |
|  | + Control Ab | 1069.7 | 227.9 | 825.7 | 392.7 |
| rHGF |  | 982 | 217.1 | 800 | 333.4 |

*Ab*, antibody.

## 3.4 Effect of Human Hepatic Myofibroblasts on Tumor Cell Invasiveness

The invasive response of tumor cells is shown in Table 2. In control medium, only a few tumor cells could invade Matrigel. In contrast, MFs present in the lower compartment were able to greatly increase the invasiveness of HepG2 and HuH7 cells. This increase was lost after incubation with anti-HGF antibody. Increased invasiveness of both tumor cells types could be reproduced by adding HGF into the lower compartment.

## 4 Discussion

Our data show that human liver MFs modulate the phenotype of the two human HCC cell lines HepG2 and HuH7, with the most notable result being an increased invasiveness of these cell lines. Our results indicate that HGF is responsible for the effects of MF-CM on tumor cells. This is shown by: (1) expression of HGF mRNA and protein by MFs, (2) abolition of the effects of MF-CM in the presence of a specific anti-HGF antibody, and (3) reproduction of the effects of MF-CM by recombinant HGF.

MF-CM had divergent effects on HepG2 and HuH7 cells, with regard to cell proliferation. Growth of HepG2 was inhibited as previously described [25], while that of HuH7 was stimulated. This effect was due, in both cases, to HGF, since it could be inhibited by the anti-HGF antibody. Opposite effects of HGF on the growth of various cell types have already been reported [16].

As for cell growth, both tumor cell types behaved differently in their scattering responses. MF-CM readily induced the scattering of HepG2 cells, while HuH7 cells were unaffected. These effects were blocked by the anti-HGF antibody and mimicked by recombinant HGF. It has been suggested that the scatter response to HGF depends on the initial state of differentiation of the cells, the least differentiated having a stronger response [28].

MFs were able to greatly increase the invasiveness of both tumor cell lines in vitro across Matrigel. This effect was blocked by the anti-HGF antibody and could be reproduced by adding pure HGF instead of MFs in the lower compartment of the invasion chamber. Several reports have already shown that HGF can induce an invasive phenotype [11, 21]. The mechanism of the HGF-induced invasiveness has not been clearly demonstrated, but is likely to involve proteinases that can degrade the extracellular matrix [15, 19].

Our data suggest that HGF might be acting as a pro-tumorigenic mediator in liver cancer. Previous data in animal models of liver cancer have yielded contradictory results regarding the role of HGF [12, 22, 23, 26, 30]. Several explanations can be offered to explain the discrepancies. The context in which HGF is presented might be important; in these experimental models, HGF was either produced, unphysiologically, by transgenic hepatocytes or injected intravenously. Local production by MFs in a specific microenvironment could induce different effects. Also, MF-derived HGF might act synergistically with additional MF products, which are not present in these experimental models. Finally, our work deals with human HCC cells that might behave differently than murine cells.

**Acknowledgement.** This work was supported by grants from the Comité de la Gironde of the Ligue Nationale Française contre le Cancer, the Association pour la Recherche sur le Cancer, the Groupement des Entreprises Françaises pour la Lutte contre le Cancer, and the Conseil régional d'Aquitaine. SF was a recipient of a fellowship from the Comité de la Dordogne of the Ligue Nationale Française contre le Cancer.

## References

1. Blazejewski S, Préaux AM, Mallat A, Mavier P, Dhumeaux D, Schuppan D, Rosenbaum J (1995) Human myofibroblast-like cells obtained by outgrowth are representative of the fibrogenic cells in the liver. Hepatology 22:788–797
2. Bottaro DP, Rubin JS, Faletto DL, Chan AML, Kmiecik TE, Vande Woude GF, Aaronson SA (1991) Identification of the hepatocyte growth factor receptor as the c-met proto-oncogene product. Science 251:802–804
3. Burr AW, Hillan KJ, McLaughlin E, Ferrier R, Chapman C, Mathew J, Burt AD (1996) Hepatocyte growth factor levels in liver and serum increase during chemical hepatocarcinogenesis. Hepatology 24:1282–1287
4. D'Errico A, Fiorentino M, Ponzetto A, Daikuhara Y, Tsubouchi H, Brechot C, Scoazec JY, Grigioni W (1996) Liver hepatocyte growth factor does not always correlate with hepatocellular proliferation in human liver lesions: its specific receptor c-met does. Hepatology 24:60–64

5. Dimanche-Boitrel MT, Vakaet L, Pujuguet P, Chauffert B, Martin MS, Hamman A, Van Roy F, Mareel M, Martin F (1994) In vivo and in vitro invasiveness of a rat colon-cancer cell line maintaining E-cadherin expression: an enhancing role of tumor-associated myofibroblasts. Int J Cancer 56:512–521

6. Enzan H, Himeno H, Iwamura S, Onishi S, Saibara T, Yamamoto Y, Hara H (1994) α-smooth muscle actin-positive perisinusoidal stromal cells in human hepatocellular carcinoma. Hepatology 19:895–903

7. Friedman SL (1993) The cellular basis of hepatic fibrosis. Mechanisms and treatment strategies. N Engl J Med 328:1828–1835

8. Gleave ME, Hsieh JT, von Eschenbach AC, Chung LWK (1992) Prostate and bone fibroblasts induce human prostate cancer growth in vivo: implications for bidirectional stromal-epithelial interaction in prostate carcinoma growth and metastasis. J Urol 147:1151–1159

9. Herbst H, Cramet T, Bauer M, Schuppan D (1995) Cellular localization of hepatocyte growth factor in rat and human liver tissues (abstract). Hepatology 22:232A

10. Hu Z, Evarts RP, Fujio K, Omori N, Omori M, Marsden ER, Thorgeirsson SS (1996) Expression of transforming growth factor alpha/epidermal growth factor receptor, hepatocyte growth factor/c-met and acidic fibroblast growth factor/fibroblast growth factor receptors during hepatocarcinogenesis. Carcinogenesis 5:931–938

11. Jeffers M, Rong S, Vande Woude GF (1996) Enhanced tumorigenicity and invasion-metastasis by hepatocyte growth factor/scatter factor-met signalling in human cells concomitant with induction of the urokinase proteolysis network. Mol Cell Biol 16:1115–1125

12. Liu ML, Mars WM, Michalopoulos GK (1995) Hepatocyte growth factor inhibits cell proliferation in vivo of rat hepatocellular carcinomas induced by diethylnitrosamine. Carcinogenesis 16:841–843

13. Ljubimova JY, Petrovic LM, Wilson SE, Geller SA, Demetriou AA (1997) Expression of HGF, its receptor c-met, c-myc, and albumin in cirrhotic and neoplastic human liver tissue. J Histochem Cytochem 45:79–87

14. Loizidou MC, Carpenter R, Laurie H, Cooper AJ, Alexander P, Taylor I (1996) Growth enhancement of implanted human colorectal cancer cells by the addition of fibroblasts in vivo. Br J Surg 83:24–28

15. Moriyama T, Kataoka H, Seguchi K, Tsubouchi H, Koono M (1996) Effects of hepatocyte growth factor (HGF) on human glioma cells in vitro: HGF acts as a motility factor in glioma cells. Int J Cancer 66:678–685

16. Nagamine K, Shibamoto S, Takeuchi K, Miyazawa K, Kitamura N, Chatani Y, Kohno M, Ito F (1996) Dissociation of c-fos induction and mitogen-activated-protein kinase activation from the hepatocyte-growth-factor-induced motility response in human gastric carcinoma cells. Eur J Biochem 236:476–481

17. Nakayama N, Kashiwazaki H, Kobayashi N, Hamada JI, Ogiso Y, Itakura Y, Matsumoto K, Nakamura T, Koike T, Kuzumaki N, Takeichi N (1996) Hepatocyte growth factor and c-met expression in Long-Evans Cinnamon rats with spontaneous hepatitis and hepatoma. Hepatology 24:596–602

18. Noguchi O, Enomoto N, Ikeda T, Kobayashi F, Marumo F, Sato C (1996) Gene expressions of c-met and hepatocyte growth factor in chronic liver disease and hepatocellular carcinoma. J Hepatol 24:286–292

19. Pepper MS, Matsumoto K, Nakamura T, Montesano R (1992) Hepatocyte growth factor increases urokinase-type plasminogen activator (u-PA) and u-PA receptor expression in Madin-Darby canine kidney epithelial cells. J Biol Chem 267:20493–20496

20. Repesh LA (1989) A new in vitro assay for quantitating tumor-cell invasion. Invasion Metastasis 9:192–208

21. Rong S, Segal S, Anver M, Resau JH, Vande Woude GF (1994) Invasiveness and metastasis of NIH 3T3 cells induced by Met- hepatocyte growth factor/scatter factor autocrine stimulation. Proc Natl Acad Sci U S A 91:4731–4735

22. Sakata H, Takayama H, Sharp R, Rubin JS, Merlino G, LaRochelle WJ (1996) Hepatocyte growth factor/scatter factor overexpression induces growth, abnormal development, and tumor formation in transgenic mouse livers. Cell Growth Differ 7:1513–1523

23. Santoni-Rugiu E, Preisegger KH, Audolfsson T, Shiota G, Schmidt EV, Thorgeirsson SS (1996) Inhibition of neoplastic development in the liver by hepatocyte growth factor in a transgenic mouse model. Proc Natl Acad Sci U S A 93:9577–9582
24. Selden C, Farnaud S, Ding SF, Habib N, Foster C, Hodgson HJF (1995) Expression of hepatocyte growth factor mRNA, and c-met mRNA (hepatocyte growth factor) in human liver tumours. J Hepatol 21:227–234
25. Shiota G, Rhoads DB, Wang TC, Nakamura T, Schmidt EV (1992) Hepatocyte growth factor inhibits growth of hepatocellular carcinoma cells. Proc Natl Acad Sci U S A 89:373–377
26. Shiota G, Wang TC, Nakamura T, Schmidt EV (1994) Hepatocyte growth factor in transgenic mice: effects on hepatocyte growth, liver regeneration and gene expression. Hepatology 19:962–972
27. Terada T, Makimoto K, Terayama N, Suzuki Y, Nakanuma Y (1996) Alpha-smooth muscle actin-positive stromal cells in cholangiocarcinomas, hepatocellular carcinomas and metastatic liver carcinomas. J Hepatol 24:706–712
28. Weidner KM, Behrens J, Vandekerckhove J, Birchmeier W (1990) Scatter factor: molecular characteristics and effect on the invasiveness of epithelial cells. J Cell Biol 111:2097–2108
29. Win KM, Charlotte F, Cherqui D, Mavier P, Préaux AM, Dhumeaux D, Rosenbaum J (1993) Mitogenic effect of transforming growth factor-$\beta$1 on human Ito cells in culture: evidence for a mediation by endogenous platelet-derived growth factor. Hepatology 18:137–145
30. Yaono M, Hasegawa R, Mizoguchi Y, Futakuchi M, Nakamura T, Ito N, Shirai T (1995) Hepatocyte growth factor enhancement of preneoplastic hepatic foci development in rats treated with diethylnitrosamine and N-ethyl-hydroxyethylnitrosamine. Jpn J Cancer Res 86:718–723

# Interplay of Matrix and Myofibroblasts During Hepatic Fibrogenesis

D. Schuppan, J. J. Cho, J. D. Jia, E. G. Hahn

## 1 Myofibroblast-Like Cells in Hepatic Fibrogenesis

A variety of adverse stimuli, such as hepatotoxins, hepatotropic viruses, immune reactions to the liver, metabolic diseases, and biliary stasis can trigger liver fibrogenesis, i. e., the excess synthesis and deposition of extracellular matrix (ECM). Whereas in acute liver diseases, such as self-limited viral hepatitis, fibrogenesis is balanced by fibrolysis, i. e., the removal of excess ECM, repeated insults of sufficient severity, as occur in many chronic liver diseases, tilt the balance in favor of fibrogenesis, finally resulting in morphologically apparent fibrosis or cirrhosis. In fibrogenesis, damage to the hepatocyte or the bile duct epithelium leads to mononuclear cell activation, release of fibrogenic factors and activation of mesenchymal cells. It is the activated Kupffer cell, the macrophage and the proliferating bile duct epithelium that are thought to be the primary sources of the potentially fibrogenic cytokines and growth factors [1, 16–18, 26, 30, 33, 34, 37, 39] that finally target the hepatic stellate cell (HSC, the novel denomination for the perisinusoidal lipocyte or Ito cell) and the portal fibroblast (PF), those cell types that are responsible for excess ECM deposition in the liver [15, 17, 18, 22, 35, 36, 42, 46, 68].

Both HSC and PF have their correlates in other mesenchymal epithelial organs, such as the skin (the spectrum of dermal fibroblasts), the kidney (the mesangial cell and the interstitial fibroblast), the lung (the alveolar fibroblast and the interstitial fibroblast) and the intestine [13, 26, 35, 53] (Table 1). Upon activation by fibrogenic growth factors and disruption of their three-dimensional ECM environment, the usually quiescent HSCs and PFs undergo a transformation into a cellular phenotype that is characterized by a high proliferative potential and the capacity to produce an excess of ECM molecules. This transformation, which is accompanied by acquisition of the myofibroblast marker $\alpha$-smooth muscle actin [15, 17, 18, 21, 22, 35, 36, 42, 46, 48, 68], is central to a protective program aimed at rapid closure of a potentially lethal wound [13, 26, 34, 53]. This program is self limiting if the offending agent is present for a short period of time, but leads to fibrosis and cirrhosis when continuously activated. Some of the triggers, cells and

Current Topics in Pathology, Volume 93
A. Desmoulière, B. Tuchweber (Eds.)
© Springer-Verlag Berlin Heidelberg 1999

**Table 1.** Two classes of fibrogenic cell types. The phenotypes of fibrogenic cells of various organs show remarkable similarities

| Liver | Lung | Kidney | Intestine | Pancreas | Artery |
|-------|------|--------|-----------|----------|--------|
| Portal fibroblast | Interstitial fibroblast | Interstitial fibroblast | Interstitial fibroblast | Interstitial fibroblast | Intimal fibroblast |
| Stellate cell | Alveolar fibroblast | Mesangial cell | Subepithelial fibroblast | Stellate cell | Medial smooth muscle cell |

growth factors/cytokines that are involved in hepatic fibrogenesis are illustrated in Fig. 1.

In many chronic liver diseases, continued damage cannot be prevented and can only be mitigated at best. Furthermore, patients usually present with an already-advanced stage of structural and functional hepatic impairment. This necessitates the development of treatments that can either halt the progression of liver fibrosis or even reverse cirrhosis. Such strategies must target the fibrogenic factors, their cellular sources or the fibrogenic cell types. In addition, there is an urgent need for serum tests that allow a non-invasive assessment of fibrogenesis and fibrolysis in the liver, in order to monitor the efficiency of such treatment.

## 2 The Hepatic Extracellular Matrix

The ECM is not a metabolically inert material that merely serves as a framework for the functionally important parenchyma. The ECM can be defined as a complex assembly of macromolecules that rapidly undergoes remodeling after injury, to reestablish cellular functions and tissue homeostasis. Its macromolecules provide resident and immigrating (inflammatory) cells with signals that are necessary for

---

**Fig. 1.** Molecular and cellular mechanisms of liver fibrogenesis. This simplified scheme derives from numerous studies of liver fibrosis and fibrosis of other organs. A usually quiescent mesenchymal cell, such as the portal fibroblast and the hepatic stellate cell, is activated to transform into a myofibroblast-like cell that is characterized by actin stress fibers, a hypertrophied rough endoplasmic reticulum, a high rate of proliferation and an excessive extracellular-matrix (ECM) synthesis. A major source for fibrogenic growth factors and cytokines is the activated Kupffer cell/the activated macrophage (M$\Phi$). Other cell types, such as sinusoidal endothelial cells (which are central in angiogenesis and, once damaged, secrete fibrogenic factors), activated platelets (which release fibrogenic factors) and granulocytes (which produce reactive oxygen species and thus induce the release of cytokines in other cells) are also involved in the pathogenesis of liver fibrosis. Recently, proliferating bile-duct epithelial cells have been shown to secrete profibrogenic cytokines as well as basement-membrane proteins and collagenase (MMP-1). *bFGF*, basic fibroblast growth factor; *EGF*, epidermal growth factor; *HGF*, hepatocyte growth factor; *IF*, interferon; *IL*, interleukin; *TNF*, tumor necrosis factor; *TGF*, transforming growth factor; *PDGF*, platelet-derived growth factor; *MCP*, macrophage chemotactic peptide; *ET*, endothelin

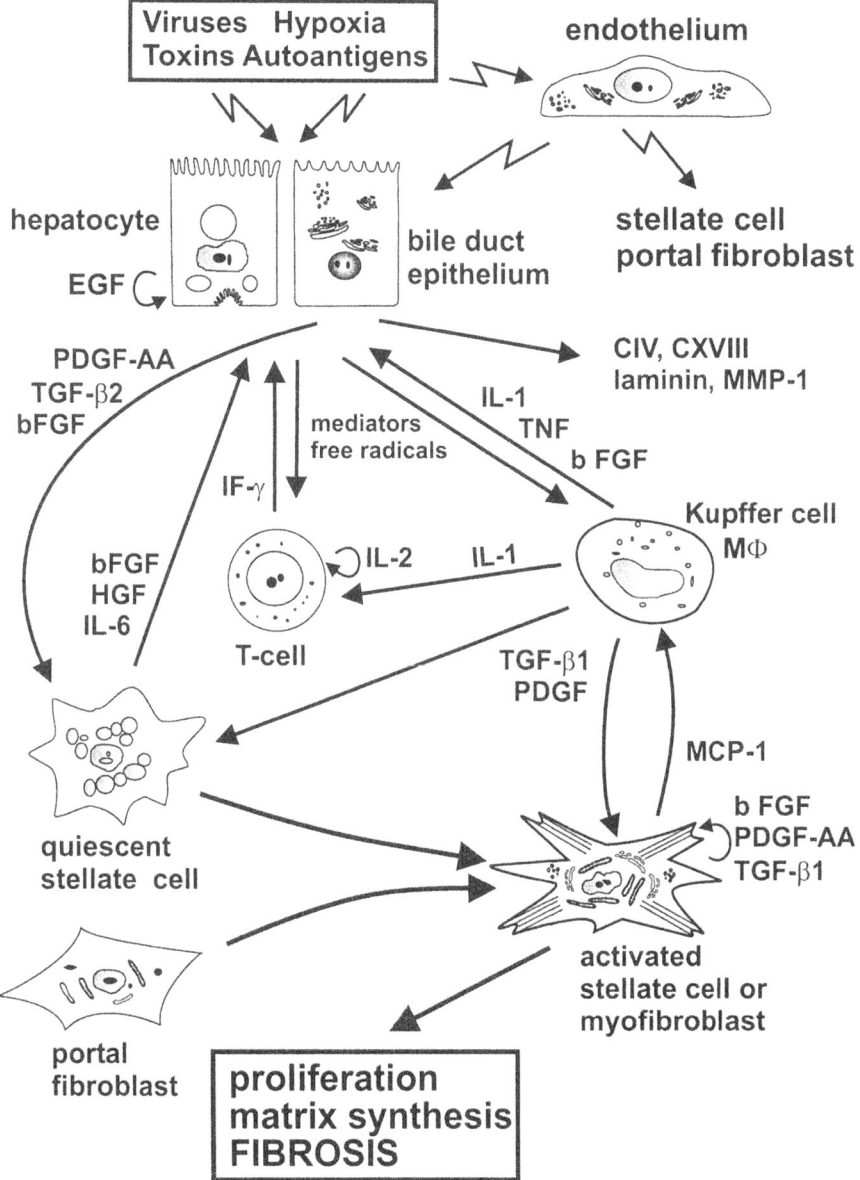

proliferation, differentiation, directed migration, or for the establishment of cell polarity [58, 59, 62, 64]. These signals are mediated by cellular receptors for ECM proteins such as the integrins.

The molecules of the ECM comprise collagens, noncollagenous glycoproteins, glycosaminoglycans, proteoglycans and elastin, and most of them are hybrids with structural and functional properties that are characteristic not only of a single class. In addition, other molecules that can specifically associate with the classical ECM components can be considered ECM constituents. Examples are ECM-degrading matrix metalloproteinases (MMPs) and their inhibitors (the tissue inhibitors of metalloproteinases, TIMPs) [2, 4, 64], certain crosslinking enzymes such as lysyl oxidase and tissue transglutaminase, and a variety of growth factors and cytokines. Binding of growth factors by certain matrix molecules leads to their storage in a matrix-dependent pattern and to modulation of their biological activities [38, 54, 58, 59, 63–65]. Once released by matrix-degrading enzymes, such as the MMPs, these factors can initiate cell proliferation, angiogenesis and ECM deposition – processes that are directed at the restitution of organ homeostasis.

## 3 Suitable In Vivo Models for Drug Testing

Animal models have proven indispensable for the study of the cell biology and pathobiochemistry of liver fibrosis, since studies in cell culture can never substitute for the far more complex events that occur in a multicellular organism in vivo (Fig. 2). However, in order to evaluate the antifibrotic potential of a given agent, selection of appropriate animal models that best reproduce human chronic liver diseases is central. Unfortunately, most of the past studies used models of injury that are caused by free radicals, severe necrosis, or inflammation, such as fibrosis due to carbon tetrachloride, dimethynitrosamine, choline deficiency and pig serum [40, 62, 67]. These models do not reflect the common human chronic liver diseases that are progressive yet characterized by moderate or even absent overt inflammation and necrosis. Along this line, many agents, such as radical scavengers, anti-oxidants, or anti-inflammatory drugs, prevent fibrosis in these animals but lack efficiency in man. Therefore, we favor a rat model of secondary biliary fibrosis induced by complete occlusion of the biliary system due to injection of the sclerosant sodium amidotrizoate (ethibloc). This model is characterized by the virtual absence of necrosis and inflammation but by a relentlessly progressing fibrosis, resulting in an eight- to tenfold increase of liver collagen within 6 weeks [6, 7, 16, 47, 62]. The following paragraph gives a subjective assessment of agents that appear to exert a more or less pronounced in vivo antifibrotic effect, either in suitable animal models or in man (as suggested by the non-invasive markers discussed below).

## 4 Potential Antifibrotic Agents

Apart from their antiviral activities, interferons suppress collagen synthesis in fibroblast cultures [50, 52]. In this regard, interferon-$\alpha$ is less potent than interferon-$\gamma$, and several studies have shown that parameters of fibrogenesis decrease in patients treated with interferon-$2\alpha$ for hepatitis B and C, in part irrespective of the antiviral response. Thus, liver procollagen mRNA [12], a histological score for liver fibrosis [32], $\alpha$-actin expression [21], and the aminoterminal propeptide of procollagen III (PIIINP), a presumed serum-marker of fibrogenesis [11, 12, 66], decreased in interferon-$2\alpha$-treated patients with hepatitis C. However, the anti-fibrotic effect of interferon-$\alpha$ in nonresponders could be due to better patient compliance with regard to alcohol consumption. Although even lower doses of interferon-$\gamma$ prevent the spontaneous activation of rat hepatic stellate cells in vitro, reducing the expression of procollagen and fibronectin mRNAs to levels between 3 % and 24 % of untreated controls, with total protein synthesis and cell survival remaining almost unaffected [50], required doses of this cytokine may be too toxic in man and may even trigger fibrogenesis in the more complex organism in vivo.

Prostaglandins E are antifibrotic in a rat models of liver fibrosis induced by bile duct ligation or nutrient deficiency [5, 55]. This effect is paralleled by a decreased serum-PIIINP (see below). However, in rat biliary fibrosis, much higher doses are needed, exceeding those tolerable by man [5].

Other hepatotropic drugs with negligible side effects that can be taken by oral route have reappeared in therapeutic trials. Polyunsaturated lecithin (PUL), with the active agent dilinoleyl-phosphatidyl-choline, prevented severe fibrosis and cirrhosis in baboons fed a diet containing 50 % ethanol, perhaps by upregulating HSC collagenase activity [28]. Silymarin, a phytopharmacon with the polyphenole silibinin as a major active ingredient can reduce collagen accumulation by 30 % in rat secondary biliary fibrosis (a preferred model for testing potential antifibrotic agents) even when given at a stage of advanced fibrosis [6]. This antifibrotic effect was also predicted by a reduction of serum PIIINP. Although previous experimental data suggested an antifibrotic effect of ursodeoxycholic acid in bile duct-ligated rats [44], we failed to reproduce these results despite having used large numbers of bile duct-occluded rats and despite an observed fall in serum cholestasis parameters [7]. Other drugs with antifibrotic potential include pentoxifylline [45, 47] and retinoids [57]. Since the actively collagen-producing cells of the liver have myofibroblastic and (in part) contractile properties, the endothelin system is involved in their activation. Thus, it has been shown that modulation of the endothelin receptors ETA-R and ETB-R by oral receptor antagonists may be useful for blocking fibrogenesis in vitro and in vivo [12a, 31, 51]. A personal summary of proven or disproven antifibrotic agents is given in Table 2.

Figure 2 shows the steps of collagen biosynthesis that have been established for the abundant fibril-forming collagens type I and type III that represent roughly 90 % of total collagen in fibrosis. All of these steps can be inhibited in vitro without causing major toxicity for the fibroblastic cells. A recent discovery is the identification of bone morphogenetic protein-1 (BMP-1) as the procollagen C-proteinase and the lysyl-oxidase-processing enzyme [25, 27]. Inhibition of BMP-1 should block extracellular collagen fibril assembly and crosslinking [14]. However, as mentioned above, multicellular organisms are far more complex, with interfering drugs either being inactive or too toxic – problems that mainly result from inefficient drug targeting of the key ECM-producing cells, the activated HSCs and PFs. As an example, the current inhibitors of prolyl hydroxylase, an enzyme that is

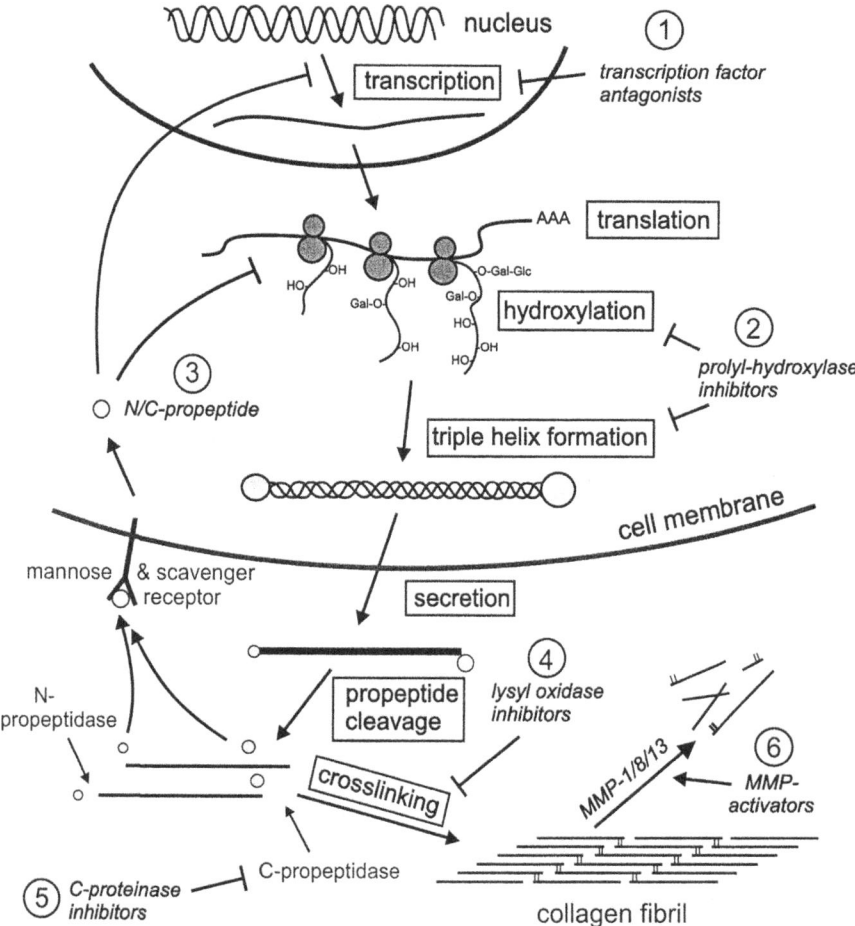

**Fig. 2.** Steps of collagen biosynthesis. The scheme applies to the well-studied fibril-forming collagens. Collagen mRNA is transcribed from the gene and translated into protein in the rough endoplasmic reticulum. During translation, the nascent polypeptide chains are hydroxylated on lysine and proline residues, glycosylated and assembled to the triple helix, starting from the C-terminal end. After secretion, N- and C-terminal propeptides are cleaved off by specific proteases and fibril growth occurs by quarter-staggered lateral assembly. Fibrils are then stabilized by formation of covalent crosslinks. Antifibrotic approaches could target either collagen biosynthesis by blocking: (**1**) collagen gene-specific transcription factors; (**2**) the production of thermodynamically stable triple helical collagen by inhibition of the enzyme prolyl hydroxylase; (**3**) collagen gene transcription and collagen mRNA translation by procollagen peptides (which are cleaved by extracellular propeptidases, and can be taken up by the cell to serve as feed-back inhibitors); (**4**) the matrix-bound enzyme lysyl oxidase which crosslinks and thus stabilizes the extracellular collagen fibrils; (**5**) the procollagen-processing enzyme procollagen C-proteinase (bone morphogenestic protein-1); or by (**6**) inducing the activation of collagenases

Table 2. Drugs for which an antifibrotic effect has been shown or disproven in vivo. This is a personal assessment based on studies in suitable animal models, such as rat secondary biliary fibrosis, or on clinical follow-up studies in man that used histological assessment and/or surrogate serum markers of liver fibrogenesis. 'Yes' or 'No' in parentheses indicates that, based on the data, an antifibrotic effect is probable or improbable, respectively. *ET-A-R*, endothelin A receptor

| Drug | Antifibrotic Effect | | Proposed Mechanism |
| --- | --- | --- | --- |
| | Animal | Man | |
| Colchicin | No | No | Secretion of collagenase and cytokines $\downarrow$ |
| D-Penicillamine | No | No | Collagen cross-links $\downarrow$ (lysyloxidase $\downarrow$) |
| Corticosteroids | No | (No) | Collagen synthesis $\downarrow$, immunsuppressant |
| Prolylhydroxylase-inhibitors | (No) | ? | Intracellular collagen degradation |
| HOE 077 | (Yes) | ? | HSC proliferation $\downarrow$ |
| Polyunsaturated lecithin | (Yes) | ? | Collagenase activity $\uparrow$ |
| Silymarin | Yes | (Yes) | Membrane modulation ?, antiinflammatory |
| Ursodeoxycholic acid | (No) | (?) | Anticholestatic, antiinflammatory |
| Pentoxifylline | Yes | ? | Intracellular collagen-degradation $\uparrow$, collagen $\downarrow$ |
| Prostaglandins E1/E2 | (Yes) | ? | Intracellular collagen-degradation $\uparrow$, collagen $\downarrow$ |
| Interferon $\gamma$ | Yes | ? | Collagenase $\uparrow$, collagen $\downarrow$, proliferation $\downarrow$ |
| Interferon $\alpha/\beta$ | (Yes) | (Yes) | Collagen $\downarrow$, proliferation $\downarrow$ |
| HGF | (Yes) | ? | Hepatocyte regeneration $\uparrow$ |
| anti-TGF-$\beta$ Mab | (Yes) | ? | Stellate cell collagen $\downarrow$ |
| ET-A-R-antagonists | ? | ? | Stellate cell matrix synthesis and proliferation $\downarrow$ (?) |
| Retinoic acid | ? | ? | Stellate cell matrix synthesis and proliferation $\downarrow$ (?) |

essential for the production of thermally stable collagen molecules, are ineffective, since they do not reach the fibroblastic cells in vivo.

Novel targeted approaches are based on the neutralization or localized removal of fibrogenic growth factors. This has been shown for transforming growth factor $\beta$1 (TGF-$\beta$1), a key fibrogenic mediator that can enhance ECM deposition and inhibit collagenase activity [8]. Intravenous injection of recombinant decorin, a small matrix proteoglycan that binds and sequesters TGF-$\beta$1 in the ECM, and intramuscular injection of the decorin gene, prevented renal granulation tissue formation in a model of antibody-mediated glomerular inflammation [9, 23]. A more specific approach may be based on neutralization of connective tissue growth factor (CTGF), the synthesis of which is upregulated in cells stimulated by TGF-$\beta$ and which increases cellular proliferation and collagen production in an autocrine manner [20, 27]. Since CTGF only appears to act on mesenchymal cells, it is devoid of the unwanted side effects of an anti-TGF-$\beta$ therapy, such as immuno-

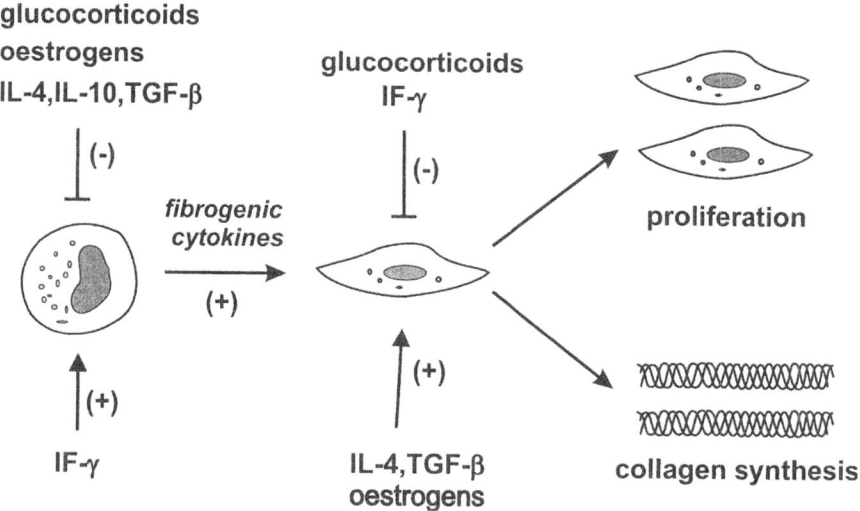

**Fig. 3.** Mediators display anti- or profibrogenic activities depending on the cellular context. By activating macrophages (monocytes, lymphocytes), interferon-γ (IF-γ) may be proinflammatory and potentially profibrogenic in early phases of wound healing, whereas it inhibits fibroblast collagen synthesis and proliferation in later (chronic) phases. The opposite is true for interleukin-4 (IL-4) and transforming growth factor-β (TGF-β), which can inhibit mononuclear cell activation, but are stimulators of fibroblast collagen synthesis. Although glucocorticoids block inflammation as well as fibroblast collagen synthesis, they may also suppress collagenase expression which is necessary to dissolve excess connective tissue

suppression and epithelial apoptosis [14]. Another example is the targeted modulation of the activities of platelet-derived growth factor (PDGF), a potent mitogen for hepatic stellate cells [41], and hepatocyte growth factor, a key mitogen for liver parenchymal cells, which bind to liver collagens at sites of excessive release [63, 65]. Since these interactions are mediated by a single acidic sequence present in the collagens, peptide analogues can be designed that remove or modify the deposition of these growth factors in the hepatic ECM.

Targeting of matrix receptors by ECM peptides and their biologically stable analogues (derived from signaling ECM molecules), is another approach for reversing the fibrogenic cellular phenotype. Thus, a stable analogue of the tripeptide Arg-Gly-Asp (RGD) that represents an integrin-binding motif in fibronectin and other ECM molecules, can inhibit fibrosis in a model of immune-mediated liver damage [10]. An interesting observation is that the extradomain-III (EIIIA), which is present in a splice-variant of fibronectin, can induce the myofibroblastic phenotype in cultured HSC and that a neutralizing antibody to this domain can reverse this step of activation [24]. A promising target is the induction of stress relaxation of fibrogenic cells, a process that is associated with a decrease in collagen synthesis and an increase in collagenase activity (Fig. 4). This stress relaxation also occurs once mesenchymal cells are placed from a stressed two-dimensional environment (mimicking a situation of wounding) into a relaxed three-dimensional environment (inducing quiescence) [19]. Stress relaxation mitigates or even abrogates signals transferred via the receptors for PDGF and other mitogenic growth factors [29], which can be explain-

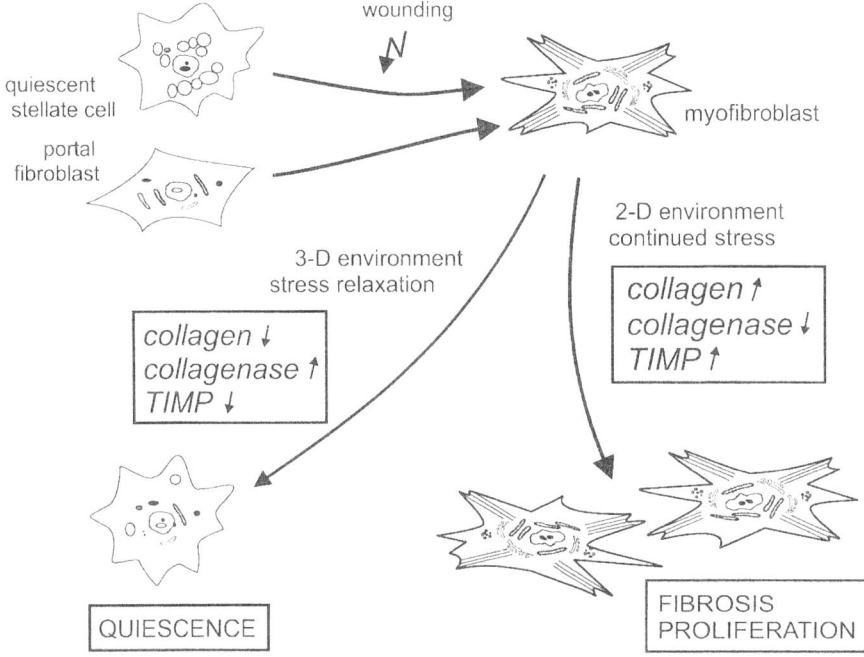

**Fig. 4.** Stress relaxation and induction of cellular quiescence. Continued mechanical stress triggers and maintains the fibrogenic phenotype. This phenotype is characterized by a responsive (stressed) conformation of certain extracellular-matrix (ECM) receptors, such as the integrins $\alpha 1 \beta 1$, $\alpha 2 \beta 1$ and $\alpha 5 \beta 1$, that serve as ECM-directed environmental sensors. Furthermore, it may be accompanied by an enhanced expression of the cellular receptors for fibrogenic growth factors such as transforming growth factor $\beta$ (TGF-$\beta$), basic fibroblast growth factor (bFGF) and platelet-derived growth factor (PDGF). Independently of growth factors, stressed integrins can enhance the expression of collagens and the tissue inhibitor of metalloproteinases (TIMP-1), and downregulate collagenase (MMP-1). This program is aimed at rapid wound closure, is usually self limited and subsides once the wound is filled with an appropriate ECM. However, it remains continuously operative in active liver fibrosis. Novel therapies can be designed that utilize adhesive recognition sequences from ECM molecules to compete with the ECM receptors, inducing a relaxed mesenchymal phenotype, with subsequent upregulation of collagenases and downregulation of collagens and TIMPs

ed by the necessity of integrin-mediated ECM-signals for growth factor-induced signal transduction [59, 64]. Thus, the recent finding that multimeric soluble collagen-VI in nanomolar amounts serves as a potent growth factor for various mesenchymal cells, including stellate cells, merits attention [3]. Since the collagen-VI-induced stress and growth response depends on receptor clustering, collagen-VI-derived peptides can be used to induce stress relaxation and thus a nonfibrogenic cellular phenotype.

## 5 Serum Markers for Liver Fibrosis

Suitable serum assays for liver fibrosis should fulfill the following requirements. They ought to (1) be specific to the liver, with no major contribution by other organs; (2) be sensitive to detect minor changes of fibrogenesis and fibrolysis; (3) reflect either fibrogenesis, fibrolysis or the amount of connective tissue deposited in the liver; (4) have a known biological half-life and known major routes of disposal and excretion, thus allowing a better interpretation of changing serum levels in patients with reduced kidney or liver function; (5) derive from a defined cellular source in the diseased liver (mainly the activated mesenchymal cells), in order to exclude interference by a functionally and synthetically compromised parenchyma; (6) be measurable by sensitive, rapid and easy-to-perform assay formats, such as the enzyme-linked immunosorbent assay (ELISA)-technique, thus obviating expensive equipment or a nuclear medicine department; and (7) be standardized and validated by reference laboratories, to ensure comparability of results.

Presently, the available serum markers for liver fibrosis do not meet the requirements of ideal parameters [reviewed in 18, 43, 49, 60–62], although biochemical, animal experimental and clinical studies have provided information that permits a preliminary judgment of the extent to which certain markers might mirror fibrogenesis and/or fibrolysis in the liver. Most of the measurable connective tissue antigens show the highest levels in active liver diseases, with only minor contributions from other systemic inflammatory or fibrotic conditions, such as pulmonary fibrosis, rheumatoid arthritis and the collagen diseases. When selecting assays for liver fibrosis, one has to consider the source and distribution of the measured antigen. Thus, collagen-/procollagen-I, the major ECM protein of liver, is also the main structural protein of bone, making its various assays unsuitable for the monitoring of fibrogenic liver diseases. A problem is the heterogeneity of circulating antigens usually encountered, which requires a characterization of the proteins or fragments which are detected by a given assay. An example is PIIINP. PIIINP immunoreactivity in serum elutes as four major fractions: the intact aminopropeptide of $Mr$ 50 kDa, a prominent fraction of its degradation product, fragment Col 1 of $Mr$ 10 kDa; and, two fractions of higher $Mr$, probably the dimeric propeptide and propeptide linked to the collagen helix.

In acute liver disease, the proportion of the intact propeptide of $Mr$ 50 kDa may increase relative to the other fractions. Only intact PIIINP that is released in stoichiometric amounts when newly secreted procollagen III is incorporated into the growing collagen fibril can be attributed to fibrogenesis. Reports of the predictive value of PIIINP as an independent parameter predicting prognosis or fibrogenesis in chronic liver diseases range from enthusiastic to disappointing. This may relate, in part, to the low sensitivity of PIIINP and many other serum fibrosis markers to detect early stages of the disease and subtle differences in collagen turnover, or to variant assays that were marketed in recent years.

Table 3 lists some of the serum fibrosis markers that may be useful in future studies of antifibrotic drug effects in the liver. It must be kept in mind that these markers still await validation in large prospective follow-up studies of patients with liver diseases and of controls. A study that will involve 500 patients, with biopsies taken at the beginning and after 18–24 months, incorporating an improved

**Table 3.** Serum assays for liver fibrosis

|  | Fibrogenesis | Fibrolysis | Liver specificity |
|---|---|---|---|
| PIIINP | + | (+) (acute) | + |
| PIIICP | + | – | + |
| PIVCP | – (?) | + | + |
| PIVNP | – (?) | + | + |
| Collagen VI | + | + (mesench. stress) | (+) |
| Undulin | – | + (portal) | + |
| Tenascin | + (lobular) | – | (+) |
| Laminin | + (?) | + (?) | (+) |
| Hyaluronan | + (?) | + (?) | (+) |
| TIMP-1 | + | – | + (?) |
| MMP-1 | – | + | + (?) |

*Liver specificity* denotes that the highest levels are observed in liver diseases. PIIINP may reflect fibrolysis in acute bouts of hepatitis. For further details refer to the text.
*PIIINP*, N-terminal propeptide of procollagen III; *PIVCP*, C-terminal propeptide of procollagen-IV (NC1-fragment); *PIVNP*, N-terminal propeptide of procollagen-IV (7-S collagen); *TIMP-1*, tissue inhibitor of metalloproteinases-1; *MMP-1*, matrix metalloproteinase-1 (interstitial collagenase).

histological method to quantify fibrosis, as well as a broad spectrum of fibrosis markers at a 3-month interval, is currently underway in Europe. In addition, by quantitative reverse-transcription polymerase chain reaction (RT-PCR), quantitative protein extraction and Western blotting [56], collagen synthesis and expression of various MMPs can now be quantified based on fractions of diagnostic biopsies, thereby allowing a direct correlation with concurrently measured serum fibrosis markers.

Therefore, the stage is set to attack fibrogenesis in chronic liver diseases. Trials should include well-defined methods to assess histological progression of fibrosis and a selected spectrum of serum fibrosis markers. Some of these markers may soon be validated and prove useful in predicting fibrogenesis or fibrolysis, thus enabling us to predict an antifibrotic effect in individual patients within a few weeks.

# References

1. Adachi Y, Bradford BA, Bojes HK, Thurman RG (1994) Inactivation of Kupffer cells prevents early alcohol-induced liver injury. Hepatology 20:453–460
2. Arthur MJP (1995) Collagenases and liver fibrosis. J Hepatol 22:43–48
3. Atkinson J, Ruehl M, Becker J, Ackermann R, Schuppan D (1996) Collagen VI regulates normal and transformed mesenchymal cell proliferation in vitro. Exp Cell Res 228:283–291
4. Birkedahl-Hansen H (1995) Proteolytic remodeling of the extracellular matrix. Curr Opin Cell Biol 7:728–735
5. Beno DWA, Espinal R, Edelstein BM, Davis BH (1993) Administration of prostaglandin E1 analog reduces rat hepatic and Ito cell collagen gene expression and accumulation after bile duct ligation injury. Hepatology 17:707–714
6. Boigk G, Stroedter L, Herbst H, Waldschmidt, Riecken EO, Schuppan D (1997a) Silymarin retards hepatic collagen accumulation in early and advanced biliary fibrosis secondary to bile duct obliteration in the rat. Hepatology 26:643–649

7. Boigk G, Stroedter L, Herbst H, Waldschmidt J, Riecken EO, Schuppan D (1997b) Ursodeoxy-cholic acid ameliorates parameters of cholestasis, but does not prevent collagen accumulation in rat secondary biliary fibrosis (abstract). Gastroenterology 112:A372

8. Border WA, Ruoslahti E (1992a) Transforming growth factor-$\beta$ in disease: the dark side of tissue repair. J Clin Invest 90:1-7

9. Border WA, Noble NA, Yamamoto T, Harper JR, Yamaguchi Y, Pierschbacher MD, Ruoslahti E (1992b) Natural inhibitor of transforming growth factor-$\beta$ protects against scarring in experimental kidney disease. Nature 360:361-365

10. Bruck R, Hershkoviz R, Lider O, Aeed H, Zaidel L, Matas Z, Barg J, Halpern Z (1996) Inhibition of experimentally-induced liver cirrhosis in rats by a nonpeptidic mimetic of the extracellular matrix-associated Arg-Gly-Asp epitope. J Hepatol 24:731-738

11. Camps J, Castilla A, Ruiz J, Civeira MP, Prieto J (1993) Randomised trial of lymphoblastoid $\alpha$-interferon in chronic hepatitis C. Effects on inflammation, fibrogenesis and viremia. J Hepatol 17:390-396

12. Castilla A, Prieto J, Fausto N (1991) Transforming growth factors beta-1 and alpha in chronic liver disease: effects of interferon-alpha therapy. N Engl J Med 324:933-940

12a. Cho JJ, Jia JD, Hocher B, Ruehl M, Somasundaram R, Riecken EO, Schuppan D. The specific endothelium A receptor antagonist LU 135252 reduces collagen accumulation but increases mortality in rats with secondary binary cirrhosis (abstract). Hepatology 28:547A

13. Floege J, Eng E, Young BA, Johnson RJ (1993) Factors involved in the regulation of mesangial cell proliferation in vitro and in vivo. Kidney Int Suppl 39:S47-S54

14. Franklin TJ (1997) Therapeutic approaches to organ fibrosis. Int J Biochem Cell Biol 29: 79-89

15. Friedman SL (1993) The cellular basis of hepatic fibrosis. N Engl J Med 328:1826-35

16. Gerling B, Becker M, Waldschmidt J, Schuppan D (1996) Elevated serum aminoternal pro-collagen-III-peptide parallels collagen accumulation in rats with secondary biliary fibrosis. J Hepatol 25:79-84

17. Gressner AM (1996) Transdifferentiation of hepatic stellate cells (Ito cells) to myofibroblasts: a key event in hepatic fibrogenesis. Kidney Int Suppl 54:S39-45

18. Gressner AM, Schuppan D (1998) Cellular and molecular pathobiology, pharmacological intervention, and biochemical assessment of liver fibrosis. In: Bircher J, Benhamon JP, McIntyre N, Rizetto M, Rodes J (eds) Oxford textbook of clinical hepatology. Oxford University Press (in press)

19. Grinnell F (1994) Fibroblasts, myofibroblasts and wound contraction. J Cell Biol 124:401-404

20. Grotendorst GR, Okochi H, Hayashi N (1995) A novel transforming growth factor beta response element controls the expression of the connective tissue growth factor gene. Cell Growth Differ 7:469-480

21. Guido M, Rugge M, Chemello L, Leandro G, Fattovich G, Giustina G, Cassaro M, Alberti A (1996) Liver stellate cells in chronic viral hepatitis: the effect of interferon therapy. J Hepatol 24:301-307

22. Hautekeete ML, Geerts A (1997) The hepatic stellate (Ito) cell: its role in human liver disease. Virchows Arch 430:195-207

23. Isaka Y, Brees DK, Ikegaya K, Kaneda Y, Imai E, Noble NA, Border WA (1996) Gene therapy by skeletal muscle expression of decorin prevents fibrotic disease in rat kidney. Nat Med 2:418-423

24. Jarnagin WR, Rockey DC, Koteliansky VE, Wang SS, Bissell DM (1994) Expression of variant fibronectins in wound healing: cellular source and biological activity of the EIIIA segment in rat hepatic fibrogenesis. J Cell Biol 127:2037-2048

25. Kessler E, Takahara K, Biniaminov L, Brusel M, Greenspan DS (1996) Bone morphogenetic protein-1: the type I procollagen C-proteinase. Science 271:360-362

26. Kovacs EJ, DiPietro LA (1994) Fibrogenic cytokines and connective tissue production. FASEB J 8:854-861

27. Lee S, Solo-Cordero DE, Kessler E, Takahara K, Greenspan DS (1997) Transforming growth factor beta regulation of bone morphogenetic protein-1/procollagen C-proteinase and related proteins in fibrogenic cells and hkeratinocytes. J Biol Chem 272:19059-19066

28. Lieber CS, Robins SJ, Li J, deCarli LM, Mak KM, Fasuolo LJM, Leo MA (1994) Phosphatidyl-choline protects against fibrosis and cirrhosis in the baboon. Gastroenterology 106:152-159

29. Lin YC, Grinnell F (1993) Decreased level of PDGF-stimulated receptor autophosphorylation by fibroblasts in mechanically relaxed collagen matrices. J Cell Biol 122:663–672
30. McClain C, Hill D, Schmidt J, Diehl AM (1993) Cytokines and alcoholic liver disease. Semin Liver Dis 13:170–181
31. Mallat A, Preaux AM, Serradeil-Le Gal C, Raufaste D, Gallois C, Brenner DA, Bradham C, Maclouf J, Iourgenko V, Fouassier L, Dhumeaux D, Mavier P, Lotersztajn S (1996) Growth inhibitory properties of endothelin-1 in activated human hepatic stellate cells: a cyclic adenosine monophosphate-mediated pathway. Inhibition of both extracellular signal-regulated kinase and c-Jun kinase and upregulation of endothelin B receptors. J Clin Invest 98:2771–2778
32. Manabe N, Chevallier M, Chossegros P, Causse X, Guerret S, Trepo C, Grimaud JA (1993) Interferon-α2b therapy reduces liver fibrosis in chronic non-A non-B hepatitis: a quantitative histologic evaluation. J Hepatol 18:1344–1349
33. Matsumoto K, Fuji H, Michalopoulos G, Fung JJ, Demetris AJ (1994) Human biliary epithelial cells secrete and respond to cytokines and hepatocyte growth factor in vitro: interleukin-6, hepatocyte growth factor, and epidermal growth factor promote DNA synthesis in vitro. Hepatology 20:376–382
34. Matthes H, Herbst H, Schuppan D, Stallmach A, Milani S, Stein H, Riecken EO (1992) Cellular localization of procollagen gene transcripts in inflammatory bowel dieseases. Gastroenterology 102:431–442
35. Milani S, Herbst H, Schuppan D, Riecken EO, Stein H (1990) Procollagen expression by nonparenchymal rat liver cells in experimental biliary fibrosis. Gastroenterology 98:175–184
36. Milani S, Herbst H, Schuppan D, Surrenti C, Riecken EO, Stein H (1990) Cellular localization of type I, III and IV procollagen gene transcripts in normal and fibrotic human liver. Am J Pathol 137:59–70
37. Milani S, Herbst H, Schuppan D, Stein H, Surrenti C (1991) Transforming growth factors $\beta$1 and $\beta$2 are differentially expressed in fibrotic liver disease. Am J Pathol 139:1221–1229
38. Nathan C, Sporn M (1991) Cytokines in context. J Cell Biol 113:981–946
39. Perez Napoli J, Prentice D, Niinami C, Bishop GA, Desmond P, McCaughan GW (1997) Sequential increases in the intrahepatic expression of epidermal growth factor, basic fibroblast growth factor, and transforming growth factor $\beta$ in a bile duct ligated rat model of cirrhosis. Hepatology 26:624–633
40. Perez Tamayo R (1984) Is cirrhosis of the liver experimentally produced by CCl$_4$ an adequate model of human cirrhosis? Hepatology 3:112–120
41. Pinzani M, Gesualdo L, Sabbah GM, Abboud HE (1989) Effects of platelet-derived growth factor and other mitogens on DNA synthesis and growth of cultured rat liver fat storing cells. J Clin Invest 84:1786–1794
42. Pinzani M (1995) Hepatic stellate (Ito) cells: expanding roles for a liver-specific pericyte. J Hepatol 22:700–706
43. Plebani M, Burlina A (1991) Biochemical markers of hepatic fibrosis. Clin Biochem 24:219–239
44. Poo JI, Feldmann J, Erlinger S et al. (1992) Ursodeoxycholic acid limits liver histologic alterations and portal hypertension induced by bile duct ligation in the rat. Gastroenterology 102:1752–1759
45. Preaux AM, Mallat A, Rosenbaum J, Zafrani ES, Mavier P (1997) Pentoxifylline inhibits growth and collagen synthesis of cultured human hepatic myofibroblast-like cells. Hepatology 26:315–322
46. Ramadori G (1991) The stellate cell (Ito-cell, fat-storing cell, lipocyte, perisinusoidal cell) of the liver. New insights into pathophysiology of an intriguing cell. Virchows Arch B Cell Pathol 61:147–158
47. Raetsch C, Boigk G, Stroeter L, Waldschmidt J, Herbst H, Riecken EO, Schuppan D (1996) Pentoxifyllin inhibits hepatic collagen deposition in early but not advanced rat biliary fibrosis (abstract). Gastroenterology 110:A1301
48. Reeves HL, Burt AD, Wood S, Day CP (1996) Hepatic stellate cell activation occurs in the absence of hepatitis in alcoholic liver disease and correlates with the severity of steatosis. J Hepatol 25:677–683

49. Risteli L, Risteli J (1990) Noninvasive methods for detection of organ fibrosis. In: Rojkind M (ed) Focus on connective tissue in health and disease. CRC Press, Boca Raton, pp 61–98
50. Rockey DC, Maher JJ, Jarnagin WR, Gabbiani G, Friedman SL (1992) Inhibition of rat lipocyte activation in culture by interferon-γ. Hepatology 16:776–784
51. Rockey DC, Chung JJ (1996) Endothelin antagonism in experimental hepatic fibrosis. Implications for endothelin in the pathogenesis of wound healing. J Clin Invest 98:1381–1388
52. Rosenbloom J, Feldman G, Freundlich G, Jimenez SA (1984) Transcriptional control of human diploid fibroblast collagen synthesis by interferon. Biochem Biophys Res Commun 123:365–372
53. Ross R (1993) The pathogenesis of atherosclerosis: a perspective for the 1990's. Nature 362:801–809
54. Ruoslahti E, Yamaguchi Y (1991) Proteoglycans as modulators of growth factor activities. Cell 64:867–869
55. Ruwart MJ, Wilkinson KF, Rush BD, Vidmar TJ, Peters KM, Henley KS, Appelman HD, Kim KY, Schuppan D, Hahn EG (1989) The integrated value of serum procollagen III peptide over time predicts hepatic hydroxyproline content and stainable collagen in a model of dietary cirrhosis in the rat. Hepatology 10:801–806
56. Schöpper H, Bechstein WO, Neuhaus P, Riecken EO, Schuppan D (1997) Quantification of collagenase (MMP-1) from Menghini biopsies of human liver (abstract). J Hepatol 26 [Suppl]:273
57. Schuppan D (1992) Vitamin A and liver fibrosis: cure or villain. J Lab Clin Med 119:590–591
58. Schuppan D, Herbst H, Milani S (1993) Matrix, matrix synthesis and molecular networks. In: Zern MA, Reid LM (eds) Extracellular matrix: chemistry, biology and pathobiology with emphasis on the liver. Marcel Dekker, New York, pp 201–254
59. Schuppan D, Somasundaram R, Dieterich W, Bauer M (1994) The extracellular matrix in cellular differentiation and proliferation. In: Molecular and cell biological aspects of gastroenteropancreatic neuroendocrine tumour disease. Ann NY Acad Sci 733:87–102
60. Schuppan D, Stölzel U, Oesterling C, Somasundaram R (1995) Serum assays for liver fibrosis. J Hepatol 22 [Suppl 2]:82–88
61. Schuppan D, Aksü T, Libuda P, Koszka C, Herbst H (1996) Serum markers for liver fibrosis – current and future developments. In: Reichen J, Poupon R (eds) Surrogate markers to assess efficacy of treatment in chronic liver diseases. Kluwer, Dordrecht, pp 105–122
62. Schuppan D, Jia JD, Boigk G, Oesterling C (1997) Liver fibrogenesis – therapy and non-invasive assessment. In: Galmiche JP, Gournay J (eds) Recent advances in the pathophysiology of gastrointestinal and liver diseases. John Libbey, Paris, pp 243–257
63. Schuppan D, Schmid M, Somasundaram R, Ackermann R, Nakamura T, Rühl M, Riecken EO (1998) Collagens retain hepatocyte growth factor (HGF) in the liver extracellular matrix. Gastroenterology 114:139–152
64. Schuppan D, Gressner AM (1999) Function and metabolism of collagens and other extracellular matrix proteins. In: Bircher J, Benhamou JP, McIntyre N, Rizetto M, Rodes J (eds) Oxford textbook of clinical hepatology, 2nd edn, Oxford University Press (in press)
65. Somasundaram R, Schuppan D (1996) Platelet derived growth factor (PDGF AA, AB and BB) binds to collagens type I-VI: evidence for common collagenous epitopes. J Biol Chem 271:26884–26891
66. Suou T, Hosho K, Kishimoto Y, Horie Y, Kawasaki H (1995) Long-term decrease in serum N-terminal propeptide of type III procollagen in patients with chronic hepatitis C treated with interferon alpha. Hepatology 22:426–431
67. Tsukamoto H, Matsuoka M, French SW (1990) Experimental models of hepatic fibrosis: an overview. Semin Liver Dis 10:56–65
68. Tuchweber B, Desmouliere A, Bochaton-Piallat LL, Rubbia-Brandt L, Gabbiani G (1997) Proliferation and phenotypic modulation of portal fibroblasts in the early stages of cholestatic fibrosis in the rat. Lab Invest 74:265–278

# Subject Index

# Index of Volumes 90–92 Current Topics in Pathology

The manufacturer's authorised representative in the EU is Springer
Nature Customer Service Centre GmbH, Europaplatz 3, 69115 Heidelberg,
Germany. If you have any concerns regarding our products, please
contact ProductSafety@springernature.com

Printed and bound by CPI Group (UK) Ltd, Croydon, CR0 4YY

24/04/2026

02096316-0005